# Homelessness Among U.S. Veterans

# Homelessness Among U.S. Veterans

## CRITICAL PERSPECTIVES

EDITED BY JACK TSAI, Ph.D.

OXFORD
UNIVERSITY PRESS

Oxford University Press is a department of the University of Oxford. It furthers
the University's objective of excellence in research, scholarship, and education
by publishing worldwide. Oxford is a registered trade mark of Oxford University
Press in the UK and certain other countries.

Published in the United States of America by Oxford University Press
198 Madison Avenue, New York, NY 10016, United States of America.

Library of Congress Cataloging-in-Publication Data
Names: Tsai, Jack, editor.
Title: Homelessness among U.S. Veterans : Critical Perspectives / [edited by] Jack Tsai.
Other titles: Homelessness among United States veterans
Description: Oxford ; New York : Oxford University Press, [2019] |
Includes bibliographical references and index.
Identifiers: LCCN 2018022566 | ISBN 9780190695132 (hardcover : alk. paper)
Subjects: | MESH: Veterans Health | Homeless Persons—psychology |
Veterans—psychology | United States
Classification: LCC RC455.2.P85 | NLM WA 360 | DDC 305.9/08408697—dc23
LC record available at https://lccn.loc.gov/2018022566

9 8 7 6 5 4 3 2 1

Printed by Sheridan Books, Inc., United States of America

# Contents

# Foreword

PHILIP F. MANGANO

Not long ago in San Bernardino County, about an hour's drive east of Los Angeles, a group of County government agencies, providers, faith leaders, law enforcement, developers, and other stakeholders were convened by the County CEO. Just as with other social problems, a concerted effort was about to be focused on what seemed an intractable element in the social landscape.

Living in washes, on the streets, in encampments, and in a few government-sponsored transitional programs, homeless Veterans were living out the long misery of homelessness right before our eyes. The worsening physical and psychological conditions were chronicled by pedestrians, police, and the Sheriff's HOPE Team that engaged these lives on the periphery of communities and out in the high desert.

While there were, indeed, efforts being made on their behalf, at best they were bailing the leaking boat of homelessness—some were moved out, more fell in.

Back in mid-2016 we were told by the local VA medical center that their research showed that 401 Veterans were homeless in San Bernardino County. The community responded. The CEO-led Advisory Board was convened with the intent of remedying the homelessness of 401 Veterans in the next year.

By Thanksgiving Eve that same year, 401 homeless Veterans had been identified and housed. How did what seemed so intractable, so beyond resolving, yield so readily? How were those lives so desperate, so hopeless, engaged and finally offered what they most wanted, a place to live, a lock on the door to insulate their vulnerable and often disabled minds and bodies from the vagaries of the world?

# A Conspiracy Informed by Research

The elements that brought resolution to the cohort of homeless Veterans in San Bernardino—a resolution that has now engaged and housed more than 1,000 homeless Veterans there—are well known in political and business circles:

- *Political will,* local and national
- *Strategic thinking,* what Malcolm Gladwell tells us informs *intelligent action*
- *Innovation adoption,* avoiding what Einstein defined as "insanity"

These elements informed by data and research made the difference for San Bernardino Veterans as well as Veterans all across the country. Without the research, none of these elements would have worked individually, nor would they have worked collectively. We would have imposed on homeless Veterans what had been commonly mistaken to inform policy—conjecture and anecdote. Whatever in the past looked good on paper would be pursued. "Evidence-based" and "field-tested" were academic verbiage that had little to do with the responses that were funded to keep the "bailing" going.

In my advocacy efforts in Massachusetts before I became the so-called Homeless Czar under President Bush and for a time under President Obama, we learned early on that our best friend to move and shape policy for homeless people was a good snowstorm. Our job was to touch hearts, and we did. We received resources and promptly spent them on programs that shaped a status quo that was immune to outcomes and results.

Only when a new administration came in and our snow advocacy was met with little effect, and we were asked for numbers, did we learn that our halcyon days of anecdote and guesswork were probably over. So we began to collect the numbers at the front and back doors of homeless programs to create a far more sophisticated advocacy informed by research that talked about discharge planning, housing placements, and outcomes.

When I was appointed by President Bush I was heartened to discover that our new approach was part of the President's Management Agenda. I read and re-read the document while I awaited the completion of my background check. I boiled that document down to three key components:

1. That all investments should be data and research driven. Again, the days of conjecture and anecdote were history. All federal resources were to be considered an investment that required a "return."
2. That all investments should be performance oriented and mission informed.
3. That all investments should be results oriented.

These were certainly not the elements of federal policy back then shaping the response to homelessness! We set out to make that difference—to ensure that investment, research, performance, and results were the new nomenclature not only of federal policy but also of our 10-Year Plans in partnership with cities, counties, and states.

## Innovation

To put into practice these new themes of investment, research, performance, and results, we understood that spending money in a system that was only seeing constant increases in homelessness made no sense. We began to look for initiatives that had proven results in ending people's homelessness.

Given the fact that consecutive VA Secretaries—Principi, Nicholson, Peake—had prioritized homeless Veterans, a focus of ours was on this subpopulation. We discovered that a Veteran-specific initiative that has been conceived by HUD Secretary Jack Kemp in the early 1990s had good results in ending homelessness for Veterans. The pilot had been implemented for two years and then studied for three.

We dusted off the shelved research and determined in those documents that the outcomes were significant. The HUD-VASH program had worked but had been mothballed for more than a dozen years. In dusting off the research we uncovered an innovative program that met a policy objective—reducing homelessness among Veterans.

At the same time, based on data and research emanating from New York City, we embraced another innovative initiative that was achieving policy ends—reducing homelessness among those experiencing chronic homelessness. The researchers had informed policy by identifying a cohort of street and sheltered homeless people who had been homeless for a year or more and had a disabling condition. The focus was amended to include those who had multiple episodes of homelessness over four years and a disabling condition. Policy was shaped around this research, and as an Administration we committed to reducing the homelessness of this population—those experiencing what the researchers called "chronic homelessness."

The idea was old-fashioned. Rather than relying on conjecture and anecdote, what was untested and looked good on paper, we began with the research and allowed the data to shape policy and investment of resources to implement evidence-based practices.

The two innovative initiatives—HUD-VASH and Housing First—were eventually united in a reinvigorated HUD-VASH initiative that has substantially reduced Veteran homelessness in our country in the past decade and a half.

Truthfully, the VA was a reluctant adopter of Housing First. Despite the data and research and despite HHS deeming Housing First an evidence-based practice, the VA bureaucracy would be identified in the diffusion study for the dissemination of Housing First as the laggard.

Fortunately, through the resolute political will and research respect from Secretaries Shinseki and McDonald, the VA eventually acceded to the innovation, and the number of housed Veterans increased dramatically. The VA Center on Homelessness Among Veterans in Philadelphia, under the leadership of Vince Kane and the research credibility of UPenn's Dr. Dennis Culhane, was an essential partner in ensuring that data and research came to inform VA's policy regarding HUD-VASH and Housing First. The status quo of Veterans in a perpetual state of "transitioning" was replaced by a trajectory that ended in housing and stability.

## Political Will and Strategic Planning

There is no question that without the concerted political will of successive VA Secretaries, the progress achieved in reducing the numbers of homeless Veterans by 45% in 8 years would have been undoable. All the Secretaries that I have mentioned—Principi, Nicholson, Peake, Shinseki, and McDonald—prioritized homelessness in budget matters.

The resuscitation of HUD-VASH and adoption of Housing First in the Bush Administration and the heightened focus and investment in the Obama Administration once again confirm that this issue is beyond partisanship. One Administration built on the practice of the other to create and invest in the innovative ideas that made policy palpable on the ground and in the field.

In each case the adoption of these innovations was informed and incented by the research that had been done, the data that had been gathered. Superseding the old "what looks good on paper" with data on the paper upgraded homelessness policy and implementation and contributed to the creation of what homeless people want—a place to live.

The evolution of policy through research and data has become the sine qua non for elected officials at every level of government. Continued research to evaluate initiatives, to refine objectives and goals, and to identify new populations is a necessary part of any governmental response. So, for example, the evolving attention to the needs of female Veterans and unaccompanied homeless women in the general population has been led by research and data gathering. Without these "scanners," we would not be cognizant that one in every four homeless adults is a woman.

The efficacy of strategic planning to implement policy directives relies on a certain degree of business acumen. In my time in Washington, the development of local 10-Year Plans shaped around business principles and practices required a strategic planning emphasis beyond creating "wish lists" and lighting candles. Too frequently communities either weren't involved or were content with a status quo that did not produce results.

The upgrade in planning that incented jurisdictional elected and appointed leaders to engage in planning was the reliance on certifiable data and research. "Does Housing First, so counterintuitive, actually work?" "Well, here are the data from seven cities your size in which the research carried out from day one, client one, demonstrates an 87% retention rate over 2 years." Sold! "Do Veterans actually stay in HUD-VASH housing?" "Well, here are the data from across the country that demonstrate that 90% of all Veterans placed in HUD-VASH units are still there." Sold!

We who are on the front lines of policy, advocacy, and implementation are beholden to our research partners for the tools to initiate and sustain political and civic will on an issue that has been "soft on data" in the past—the data that tell us what works and, equally important, what doesn't work; the data that tell us how many are housed and how many aren't; the data that tell us how expensive homeless people can be in the mainstream health and law enforcement systems; the research that identifies which programs are delivering the desired outcomes; the research that quantifies the magnitude of the problem, establishes baselines, indicates best practices, and quantifies budget implications.

All of these are vital to evolving our response and upgrading our initiatives. In many regards researchers should lead and the rest of us follow. To accomplish the mission for homeless Veterans, researchers are our partners in the vanguard.

# Contributors

**Jessica Blue-Howells, LCSW**
National Coordinator, Health
  Care for Reentry Veterans and
  CHALENG
U.S. Department of Veterans Affairs

**Emily Brignone, PhD**
Postdoctoral Fellow
Center for Health Equity Research
  and Promotion
VA Pittsburgh Healthcare System

**Thomas H. Byrne, PhD**
Assistant Professor, Boston
  University School of Social Work
Investigator, Center for Healthcare
  Organization and Implementation
  Research (CHOIR), Edith Nourse
  Rogers Memorial Veterans
  Hospital
Investigator, VA National Center on
  Homelessness Among Veterans

**Sean Clark, JD**
National Coordinator, Veterans
  Justice Outreach
U.S. Department of Veterans Affairs

**Dennis Culhane, PhD**
The Dana and Andrew Stone
  Professor of Social Policy
University of Pennsylvania
Director of Research
National Center on Homelessness
  Among Veterans
U.S. Department of Veteran Affairs

**Sarah L. Cutrona, MD, MPH**
Co-Director, Medication
  Optimization Program
Center for Healthcare Organization
  Implementation Research
Edith Nourse Rogers Memorial VA
  Hospital
Associate Professor of Medicine and
  Quantitative Health Sciences
Division of Health Informatics and
  Implementation Science
University of Massachusetts
  Medical School

**Melissa E. Dichter, PhD, MSW**
Core Investigator, VA Center for
Health Equity Research and
Promotion, Crescenz VA Medical
Center (Philadelphia, PA)
Assistant Professor, Department of
Family Medicine and Community
Health, University of Pennsylvania
Perelman School of Medicine

**Eric B. Elbogen, PhD**
Local Recovery Coordinator, Durham
VA Health Care System
Professor of Psychiatry and
Behavioral Sciences
Duke University School of Medicine

**Jamison Fargo, PhD**
Professor, Department of Psychology
Utah State University
Research Scientist
National Center on Homelessness
Among Veterans
U.S. Department of Veteran Affairs

**Andrea K. Finlay, PhD**
Researcher-in-Residence, Veterans
Justice Programs–Homeless
Programs Office
VA Health Services Research and
Development (HSR&D) Service
Research Health Scientist, HSR&D
Center for Innovation to
Implementation, VA Palo Alto
Health Care System
Affiliated Researcher, National
Center on Homelessness Among
Veterans, U.S. Department of
Veterans Affairs

**Sonya Gabrielian, MD, MPH**
Psychiatrist, VA Greater Los Angeles
Core Investigator, VA Desert
Pacific Mental Illness Research,
Education, and Clinical Center
Assistant Professor of Psychiatry and
Biobehavioral Sciences
University of California–Los Angeles
Geffen School of Medicine

**Lillian Gelberg, MD, MSPH**
Professor, Department of Family
Medicine
University of California–Los Angeles
Geffen School of Medicine
Department of Health Policy and
Management
University of California–Los Angeles
Fielding School of Public Health
Office of Healthcare Transformation
and Innovation
VA Greater Los Angeles
Healthcare System

**Ashton M. Gores, MPH**
Graduate Research Assistant
Yale School of Public Health

**Philip F. Mangano**
Former Executive Director, White
House United States Interagency
Council on Homelessness
(2002–2009)
President, American Round Table to
Abolish Homelessness

**D. Keith McInnes, ScD, MSc**
Investigator, Center for Healthcare
    Organization and Implementation
    Research
Edith Nourse Rogers Memorial VA
    Hospital
Research Associate Professor,
    Department of Health Law, Policy
    and Management
Boston University School of
    Public Health

**Stephen Metraux, PhD**
Health Sciences Researcher, National
    Center for Homelessness Among
    Veterans
Department of Veterans Affairs
Associate Professor, School of Public
    Policy & Administration
University of Delaware

**Ann Elizabeth Montgomery, PhD**
Investigator, VA National Center on
    Homelessness Among Veterans
Investigator, Birmingham VA
    Medical Center Health Services
    Research & Development
Assistant Professor, University of
    Alabama at Birmingham, School of
    Public Health

**Maria J. O'Connell, PhD**
Director of Research and Evaluation,
    Yale Program for Recovery and
    Community Health
Associate Professor of Psychiatry,
    Yale University School of
    Medicine

**Thomas P. O'Toole, MD**
Senior Medical Advisor, Office of
    Assistant Deputy Undersecretary
    for Health for Clinical Operations,
    Veterans Health Administration
Professor of Medicine, Alpert
    Medical School at Brown
    University

**Robert A. Rosenheck, MD**
Senior Investigator, VA New
    England Mental Illness Research,
    Education, and Clinical Center
Professor of Psychiatry and of Public
    Health, Yale University School of
    Medicine

**John A. Schinka, PhD**
Investigator, VA National Center on
    Homelessness Among Veterans
James A. Haley VA Medical Center
Professor of the School of Aging
    Studies, University of South
    Florida

**R. Tyson Smith, PhD**
Senior Program Manager, Research
    and Evaluation, Camden Coalition
    of Healthcare Providers

**Christine Timko, PhD**
Senior Research Career Scientist,
    VA Health Services Research and
    Development (HSR&D) Service
Senior Investigator, HSR&D Center
    for Innovation to Implementation,
    VA Palo Alto Health Care System
Clinical Professor, Department
    of Psychiatry and Behavioral
    Sciences, Stanford University
    School of Medicine

# 1

# Introduction and History of Veteran Homelessness

JACK TSAI

> Let us strive on to finish the work we are in, to bind up the
> nation's wounds, to care for him who shall have borne the
> battle and for his widow and his orphan, to do all which may
> achieve and cherish a just and lasting peace among ourselves
> and with all nations.
> —Abraham Lincoln, *Second Inaugural Address, March 4, 1865*

Homelessness is a long-standing, complex, and interdisciplinary problem that affects individuals, their loved ones, and their communities. I begin this book and this introductory chapter with an illustrative example. The example is not meant to form a caricature of a homeless Veteran in the reader's mind. Certainly, homeless Veterans come from diverse walks of life with different backgrounds and pathways to homelessness; they are a very heterogeneous group. Instead, I think it is important to put a face to homeless Veterans before delving into the history, research, and clinical practice concerning homeless Veterans. Several other chapters in this book also provide case examples and quotes from homeless Veterans for this purpose. In this introductory chapter, after I describe an example of a homeless Veteran, I briefly define homelessness, discuss the importance of homeless Veterans as a population, and describe the history of homelessness among Veterans up to contemporary time. I conclude this chapter with a discussion about the purpose of this book and provide a brief overview of the diverse chapters of the book, which together provide a comprehensive text on the topic.

# Illustrative Example

Ray Marks was only 19 years old when he left his hometown of Indianapolis, Indiana, to enlist in the Army to join the Vietnam War. He served in the Infantry for several years and achieved the rank of Lieutenant. Lieutenant Marks was involved in firefights and watched some of his comrades die as well as participated in killing soldiers of the Viet Cong. He was involved in alcohol and drug use while in the military. He sustained several leg injuries during the war that did not heal properly, but he was eventually honorably discharged. After he left the military, Lieutenant Marks returned to his hometown in Indianapolis. He received a harsh homecoming because there were nationwide protests against the Vietnam War at the time. Ray was still a young man when he left the military, but he returned to live with his parents for several years before finding his own apartment. He had trouble finding employment and worked odd jobs for many years. He was not interested in going to the local U.S. Department of Veterans Affairs (VA) hospital for his health care needs because the hospital had a poor local reputation.

With his free time, the memories of war, the lack of support for Vietnam Veterans at the time, and a difficult job market, Ray began using drugs with his friends. He started with marijuana and cocaine, but eventually began using heroin. The heroin use began taking up his money and time until he eventually became homeless. He would borrow money from friends and family, but he eventually "burned bridges" with them as he tried to maintain his drug habits.

Ray was homeless for many years, at times living on the streets and other times staying with friends or in shelters or temporary housing. A VA social outreach worker found him at a homeless shelter and referred him to the VA's homeless services. He was admitted to a VA transitional housing program and provided a place to stay. He also began receiving medical and mental health services through the VA. He received assistance applying for VA disability compensation and was granted a monthly amount. Several months after being in VA transitional housing, he was referred and admitted to the VA's supported housing program. Through the VA's supported housing program, Ray was able to get a housing voucher and found an apartment that would take his voucher, which paid for most of his rent.

Ray maintained his apartment through the VA's supported housing program for many years. He had girlfriends and worked occasional construction jobs when his physical health allowed him to, although he developed chronic back pain. Unfortunately, Ray eventually relapsed with his drug use. He was arrested for a drug-related offense and served some time before being paroled. He lost his apartment and was readmitted to the VA's transitional housing program and began his recovery process again. He began regularly seeing his VA mental health and primary care providers. Currently, he reports that he is working on his recovery and dreams of getting married and owning his own home someday.

## Definition of Homelessness

Homelessness is a persistent problem in the United State and one that has been a public health concern among Veterans for more than three decades (Lewin, 1987; U.S. Department of Housing and Urban Development, 2013). Homelessness can be defined as not having a "fixed, regular, and adequate nighttime residence" or residing "in a shelter or place not meant for human habitation" (The McKinney-Vento Homeless Assistance Act, as amended by S. 896 Homeless Emergency Assistance and Rapid Transition to Housing [HEARTH] Act of 2009) and includes moving frequently between different types of accommodations and staying in homeless shelters and places not meant for human habitation (e.g., vehicles, abandoned buildings). Some consider homelessness a violation of a basic human right—the right to have access to safe and secure housing (United Nations, 1948, 1976). Homelessness is also a concern because it is associated with a host of other negative outcomes, including a wide range of serious medical problems (Hwang, 2001; Schanzer, Dominguez, Shrout, & Caton, 2007), mental health and substance abuse problems (Fazel, Kholsa, Doll, & Geddes, 2008; Folsom et al., 2005), premature mortality (Hibbs et al., 1994; O'Connell, 2005), frequent hospitalizations and excessive costs per hospital stay (Gladwell, 2006; Rosenheck & Seibyl, 1998; Salit, Kuhn, Hartz, Vu, & Mosso, 1998), and incarceration (McGuire, 2007; Tsai, Rosenheck, Kasprow, & McGuire, 2014).

## Why Focus on Homeless Veterans?

The United States has the most comprehensive system of health care and social services for Veterans of any nation in the world. The VA is the second largest federal department in the country after the Department of Defense and includes the Veterans Health Administration, which operates the largest integrated health care system in the country with at least one VA medical center in each state and hundreds of medical facilities, clinics, and affiliated centers nationally.

Veterans constitute a unique segment of the U.S. population because of their honored service to the country as reflected in their access to special federal and state government benefits such as VA health care, disability and education benefits, and home-loan guarantees. The presence of Veterans within the general U.S. homeless population is regarded as a point of shame by many, and there has been great public concern for the health and well-being of homeless Veterans for many years (Donovan & Shinseki, 2013). In 2009, Secretary Shinseki of the VA pledged to end homelessness among Veterans by the end of 2015 and has since poured billions of dollars into creating new VA homeless services and expanding existing ones (U.S. Department of Veterans Affairs, 2009). The efforts to address Veteran homelessness have continued to the present day.

During the past two decades, there has also been increased widespread concern for homelessness in the general U.S. population and large public support for spending federal funds to address the problem (Tsai, Lee, Byrne, Pietrzak, & Southwick, 2017). The economic recessions in 2001 and 2007–2009 also were times when there were high rates of unemployment and housing instability, which personally affected many individuals and exposed them to the risks of homelessness themselves. But homelessness among Veterans holds a special place in the American psyche and deserves special concern because of Veterans' service to the country and the promise that is made to them after their service, as exemplified in the quote at the beginning of the chapter. In the next section, we detail how Veteran homelessness has evolved and the key events that shaped the current zeitgeist about Veteran homelessness.

## History of Veteran Homelessness

Box 1.1 provides a detailed historical timeline of major events and wars that occurred in U.S. history that affected homelessness among Veterans. Some of these milestone events are briefly described here.

Homelessness among Veterans spans the history of the United States and has been documented as early as the Reconstruction Era in the 1860s and 1870s. After the American Civil War, hundreds of thousands of soldiers were displaced and many were homeless as the country strived to recover from the death and devastation of war during Reconstruction (Robertson, 1987). Many of the nomads riding the railroads and congregating in cities were Civil War Veterans with physical injuries and trauma.

After World War I, Veterans became a major political force for change when they marked on Washington in 1932 as the "Bonus Marchers," which homeless Veterans were part of. President Herbert Hoover ordered the Veterans to be removed from all government property and their campsites cleared out. This became a debacle as Army Chief of Staff Douglas MacArthur commanded the infantry and cavalry supported by six tanks to drive the Bonus Marchers and their wives and children out. The scene brought the struggle of World War I Veterans into the awareness of the public and was seared into the nation's memory. Many World War I Veterans were also affected by the Great Depression, during which

*Box 1.1*

- 1861–1865 American Civil War

  The American Civil War involved more than 3 million soldiers and more than 600,000 deaths. The war displaced many Veterans and left many homeless. After the war, the country entered an economic recession for several years, and there were thousands of new homeless, including Veterans.

- 1912 Sherwood Act

  The Sherwood Act extends military pensions to all Veterans. Union, Mexican, and Civil War Veterans now automatically receive pensions until the age of 62 years, regardless of injury or disability. Before this act, military pensions were only available to soldiers discharged due to illness or disability inflicted during service.

- 1914–1918 World War I

  World War I involved nearly 5 million U.S. soldiers, with more than 100,000 dead and 200,000 wounded.

- 1929–1939 The Great Depression

  The Great Depression was the longest, deepest, and most widespread depression of the 20th century. It has been estimated that nearly 25% of America's work force were homeless or living in "shantytowns" during this time period.

- 1930 Veterans Administration Established

  President Herbert Hoover signs an Executive Order elevating the Veterans Bureau to a federal administration—the Veterans Administration—to "consolidate and coordinate government activities affecting war Veterans."

- 1939–1945 World War II

  More than 16 million U.S. soldiers served during World War II, which led to more than 400,000 deaths during service and 600,000 wounded.

- 1944 GI Bill passed

  The Servicemen's Readjustment Act, known as the GI Bill, provided returning Veterans with unemployment compensation and financial resources for education to help them reintegrate after military service.

- 1950–1953 Korean War

  Over 1.5 million U.S. soldiers served during the Korean War, with over 30,000 deaths and 100,000 wounded.

*(continued)*

*Box 1.1 (Continued)*

- 1955–1975 Vietnam War

  More than 3 million U.S. solders served during the Vietnam War, with more than 50,000 deaths and 100,000 wounded. During the war and its aftermath, it is estimated there were more than 50,000 homeless Veterans in a given night.
- 1990–1991 Persian Gulf War

  More than half a million U.S. soldiers served during the Gulf War, with more than 300 deaths and 400 wounded.
- 2001–Present War on Terror

  To date, more than 2.5 million U.S. soldiers have served during the conflicts in Iraq and Afghanistan with more than 6,000 deaths and 900,000 wounded. More than 100,000 Veterans have used homeless services offered through the Veterans Health Administration during this time period. This period has included various operations, including Operations Enduring Freedom/Iraqi Freedom/New Dawn and Operation Inherent Resolve begun in 2014.
- 2009–2015 Federal Initiative to End Veteran Homelessness

  The U.S. Department of Veterans Affairs announces goal to end Veteran homelessness. The first federal strategic plan to end Veteran homelessness is created, and billions of federal dollars have been spent on homeless programs and services for Veterans.
- 2014–Present Mayors Challenge to End Veteran Homelessness

  As part of the Joining Forces Initiative, First Lady Michelle Obama developed a growing coalition of mayors, governors, and county official committed to ending Veteran homelessness in their communities. As of 2018, the Mayors Challenge consists of a network of 530 elected officials.

there was tremendous poverty and mass numbers of people who were homeless (Dickson & Allen, 2006).

The homelessness crisis of the Great Depression began to dramatically abate by the early 1940s with the enlistment of tens of thousands of Americans in the military and the wartime economic upswing of World War II (Kusmer, 2002). Homelessness re-emerged as a major problem in many cities after World War II, but efforts were to made to help World War II Veterans with the passing of the Servicemen's Readjustment Act, which is more commonly known as the GI Bill. The bill offered Veterans the opportunity to be financially supported while they enter schools instead of the labor market so that they could be better prepared to be employed afterward.

While not specific to Veterans, in the 1960s, deinstitutionalization of patients in mental institutions resulted in thousands of people being moved out of hospitals into communities, and many of them became homeless (Lamb, 1984). As the problem grew over time, homelessness entered the public consciousness and began to be recognized as a major public health problem—one that could be addressed with mental health and social services (Bassuk, 1984; Rossi, 1990). The advent of the Vietnam War in the early 1980s really began to bring the problem of homeless Veterans to the attention of the general public (Kusmer, 2002). Many Vietnam Veterans returned with mental health, substance abuse, and social adjustment issues. The VA began to create health care programs to serve homeless Veterans with severe mental illness, and there were several large evaluation efforts at this time to understand the needs of these Veterans (Rosenheck, Gallup, & Leda, 1991).

After the Vietnam War, a period characterized by high inflation and two economic recessions, homelessness specifically among Veterans began to be viewed as an important social and public health problem that needed further government intervention (Lewin, 1987; Rosenheck et al., 1989; Wright, 1988). A new wave of homeless individuals in their 20s and 30s began to appear on the streets. This "new" homeless could be seen sleeping in doorways, in cardboard boxes, in abandoned cars, in bus stations, or in other public places, and hardly anybody could remain oblivious (Rossi, 1990). This is contrasted to the "old homeless" of previous decades, during which homelessness blighted some sections of major cities but could be largely ignored because it was concentrated in skid row or fringe neighborhoods. Many of these "new" homeless individuals were Veterans who suffered from posttraumatic stress disorder, substance use disorders, and physical disabilities and they were highly visible (Kusmer, 2002; Rossi, 1990).

The following next decades saw many major efforts by the federal government to address homelessness in general, and specifically among Veterans. In 1992, a major response to Veteran homelessness was the creation of the VA's supported housing program through the joint effort of the U.S. Department of Housing and Urban Development (HUD) and the VA to create the HUD-VA Supportive Housing (HUD-VASH) program (Rosenheck et al., 1998; Tsai, O'Connell, Kasprow, & Rosenheck, 2011). In 2000, the National Alliance to End Homelessness released a 10-year strategy to end homelessness in the United States. The Bush Administration then began an initiative to end chronic homelessness in 10 years, and more than 200 cities nationwide created local plans to end homelessness in their communities (National Alliance to End Homelessness, 2014). In 2010, *Opening Doors* was released, which was the nation's first federal strategic plan to end homelessness and represents a joint action by the 19 member agencies of the U.S. Interagency Council on Homelessness and local and state partners in the public and private sectors (U.S. Interagency Council on Homelessness, 2010).

In 2009, the Obama Administration and VA Secretary Eric Shinseki announced a five-year federal initiative to end homelessness specifically among Veterans by 2015. This commitment to end Veteran homelessness included increased capital funding for supported housing units and housing vouchers; supportive services for low-income Veterans and their families; increased employment opportunities for Veterans; a national referral center to link Veterans to local service providers; and various preventive measures like providing outreach to Veterans involved in the criminal justice system and developing a homeless screener for Veterans. The National Center on Homelessness Among Veterans was also created to address policy, research, and practice issues related to homeless Veterans.

After September 11, 2001, the United States became involved in military conflicts in Afghanistan (2001–present) and in Iraq (2003–2011). A new generation of Veterans returned from war zones with medical and behavioral health problems (Hoge, Auchterlonie, & Milliken, 2006; Seal, Bertenthal, Miner, Sen, & Marmar, 2007). Unlike the Vietnam War, the nation rallied behind its troops returning from Afghanistan and Iraq, and there was increased scrutiny on the health care and social services available to returning Veterans. When Robert McDonald succeeded Eric Shinseki as VA Secretary in 2014, VA Secretary McDonald continued the commitment to prevent and end Veteran homelessness, and programs like the HUD-VASH program have continued to be funded to the present day. In 2017, VA Secretary David Shulkin under the Trump Administration proposed and then retracted plans to reallocate funding for VA homeless programs to other VA programs (U.S. Department of Veterans Affairs, 2017). National backlash from various Veteran service organizations and community providers caused the retraction and demonstrated the tremendous sustained national support that exists for homeless Veterans (Allen & Woellert, 2017). There may also be overlap between addressing Veteran homelessness and other clinical priorities that have arisen under Secretary Shulkin, such as reducing Veteran suicides (Tsai, Trevisan, Huang, & Pietrzak, in press).

## Overview of the Book

This book provides a contemporary, comprehensive overview of major topics related to Veteran homelessness featuring well-known homeless researchers in the field. The book is intended for a wide audience of people who are interested in research and services for homeless populations, including academics, policymakers, program administrators, clinicians, and students. While the book is focused on homeless Veterans, much of the content may extend to other homeless populations in the United States and abroad.

Beginning with Chapter 2, Emily Brignone, Jamison Fargo, and Dennis Culhane describe more than two decades of work on the definition and epidemiology of Veteran homeless, including the prevalence and incidence of homelessness in the U.S. Veteran population. They also summarize recent numbers on sheltered and unsheltered homeless Veterans. In Chapter 3, Sonya Gabrielian, Ashton Gores, Lillian Gelberg, and myself delve into the literature on the two largest risk factors for Veteran homelessness: mental illness and substance abuse. We specifically examine conditions like posttraumatic stress disorder and military sexual trauma that are highly prevalent among Veterans and describe how mental illness and substance use disorders may lead to pathways to homelessness.

In Chapter 4, Thomas O'Toole reviews current knowledge on the health care needs of homeless Veterans, including common medical conditions. In addition, he discusses in depth the role of primary care in homeless health care and VA service models developed to deliver quality primary care services to homeless Veterans. In Chapter 5, Maria O'Connell and Robert Rosenheck describe the development, operations, and outcomes of the VA's supported housing program, which serves tens of thousands of Veterans annually. They also discuss the Housing First model, which has become the predominant approach to supported housing. In Chapter 6, Jessica Blue-Howells, Christine Timko, Sean Clark, and Andrea Finlay focus on criminal justice issues among homeless Veterans and the intersection between homelessness and incarceration. They present data on these topics and describe major interventions in the VA to address criminal justice issues.

In Chapter 7, Eric Elbogen discusses the important, oft-ignored problem of money mismanagement among homeless Veterans, how it can be addressed, and what money management programs exist. In Chapter 8, Ann Elizabeth Montgomery, Thomas Byrne, and Melissa Dichter focus on the growing subgroup of homeless female Veterans and discuss the numbers, characteristics, and unique health care and social needs of homeless female Veterans, including those with dependent children. In Chapter 9, Steve Metraux and Tyson Smith focus on homelessness among the youngest generation of Veterans who served after September 11, 2001. They identify multiple protective and risk factors for homelessness in this important subgroup of homeless Veterans. In Chapter 10, John Schinka and Thomas Byrne shift to focusing on the other age spectrum of homeless Veterans, including aging, mortality, and the needs of older homeless Veterans. And finally, in Chapter 11, Keith McInnes and Sarah Cutrona conclude the book with a future-facing chapter about the role of information technology and its potential in addressing the needs of homeless Veterans.

Together, this book highlights the great advancements and development of services for homeless Veterans in recent decades. The VA has spent tens of billions of dollars to address Veteran homelessness, and this book describes the programs created, knowledge gained, and thousands of Veterans served through the public's support and concern on the topic. As the nation continues to strive to prevent and end Veteran homelessness, we must build on the knowledge and progress that have already been attained.

# References

Allen, A., & Woellert, L. (2017, December 7). VA kills plan to cut homeless-vet program after outcry. *Politico.* Retrieved from https://www.politico.com/story/2017/12/06/homeless-veterans-benefits-trump-207781?cid=apn

Bassuk, E. L. (1984). The homelessness problem. *Scientific American, 251*(1), 40–45.

Dickson, P., & Allen, T. B. (2006). *The bonus Army: An American epic.* New York: Walker & Company.

Donovan, S., & Shinseki, E. K. (2013). Homelessness is a public health issue. *American Journal of Public Health, 103*(S2), S180–S180.

Fazel, S., Kholsa, V., Doll, H., & Geddes, J. (2008). The prevalence of mental disorders among the homeless in Western countries: Systematic review and meta-regression analysis. *PLoS Medicine, 5*(12), e225.

Folsom, D. P., Hawthorne, W., Lindamer, L. A., Gilmer, T., Bailey, A., Golshan, S., . . . Jeste, D. (2005). Prevalence and risk factors for homelessness and utilization of mental health services among 10,340 patients with serious mental illness in a large public mental health system. *American Journal of Psychiatry, 162*(2), 370–376.

Gladwell, M. (2006, February 13). Million-dollar Murray. *The New Yorker,* 96.

Hibbs, J. R., Benner, L., Klugman, L., Spencer, R., Macchia, I., Mellinger, A., & Fife, D. K. (1994). Mortality in a cohort of homeless adults in Philadelphia. *New England Journal of Medicine, 331*(5), 304–309.

Hoge, C. W., Auchterlonie, J. L., & Milliken, C. S. (2006). Mental health problems, use of mental health services, and attrition from military service after returning from deployment to Iraq or Afghanistan. *Journal of the American Medical Association, 295*(9), 1023–1032.

Hwang, S. W. (2001). Homelessness and health. *Canadian Medical Association Journal, 164*(2), 229–233.

International Covenant on Economic, Social and Cultural Rights, Article 11 (1976).

Kusmer, K. (2002). *Down and out, on the road: The homeless in American history.* New York: Oxford University Press.

Lamb, H. R. (1984). Deinstitutionalization and the homeless mentally ill. *Hospital and Community Psychiatry, 35,* 899–907.

Lewin, T. (1987, December 30). Nation's homeless veterans battle a new foe: Defeatism. *The New York Times,* A10.

McGuire, J. (2007). Closing a front door to homelessness among veterans. *Journal of Primary Prevention, 28*(3–4), 389–400.

The McKinney-Vento Homeless Assistance Act. (2009, May 20). As amended by S. 896 Homeless Emergency Assistance and Rapid Transition to Housing (HEARTH) Act of 2009, Pub. L. No. 111-022.

National Alliance to End Homelessness. (2014). Ten year plan. Retrieved from http://www.endhomelessness.org/pages/ten-year-plan

O'Connell, J. J. (2005). *Premature mortality in homeless population: A review of the literature.* Nashville, TN: National Health Care for the Homeless Council.

Robertson, M. J. (1987). Homeless veterans: An emerging problem? In R. D. Bingham, R. E. Green, & S. B. White (Eds.), *The homeless in contemporary society* (pp. 64–81). Newbury Park, CA: Sage Publications.

Rosenheck, R. A., Gallup, P., & Leda, C. (1991). Vietnam era and Vietnam combat veterans among the homeless. *American Journal of Public Health, 81*(5), 643–646.

Rosenheck, R. A., Harkness, L., Johnson, B., Sweeney, C., Buck, N., Deegan, D., & Kosten, T. (1998). Intensive community-focused treatment of veterans with dual diagnoses. *American Journal of Psychiatry, 155*(1429–1433).

Rosenheck, R. A., Leda, C., Gallup, P., Astrachan, B., Milstein, R., Leaf, P., . . . Errera, P. (1989). Initial assessment data from a 43-site program for homeless chronic mentally ill veterans. *Hospital and Community Psychiatry, 40*(9), 937–942.

Rosenheck, R. A., & Seibyl, C. L. (1998). Homelessness: Health service use and related costs. *Medical Care, 36*(8), 1256–1264.

Rossi, P. H. (1990). The old homeless and the new homelessness in historical perspective. *American Psychologist, 45*(8), 954–959.

Salit, S. A., Kuhn, E. M., Hartz, A. J., Vu, J. M., & Mosso, A. L. (1998). Hospitalization costs associated with homelessness in New York City. *New England Journal of Medicine, 338*(24), 1734–1740.

Schanzer, B., Dominguez, B., Shrout, P. E., & Caton, C. L. (2007). Homelessness, health status, and health care use. *American Journal of Public Health, 97*(3), 464–469.

Seal, K. H., Bertenthal, D., Miner, C. R., Sen, S., & Marmar, C. (2007). Bringing the war back home: Mental health disorders among 103,788 US veterans returning from Iraq and Afghanistan seen at Department of Veterans Affairs Facilities. *Archives of Internal Medicine, 167*(5), 476–482.

Tsai, J., Lee, C. Y. S., Byrne, T., Pietrzak, R. H., & Southwick, S. M. (2017). Changes in public attitudes and perceptions about homelessness between 1990 and 2016. *American Journal of Community Psychology, 60*(3–4), 599–606.

Tsai, J., O'Connell, M., Kasprow, W. J., & Rosenheck, R. A. (2011). Factors related to rapidity of housing placement in Housing and Urban Development—Department of Veterans Affairs Supportive Housing program of 1990s. *Journal of Rehabilitation Research and Development, 48*(7), 755–762.

Tsai, J., Rosenheck, R. A., Kasprow, W. J., & McGuire, J. F. (2014). Homelessness in a national sample of incarcerated veterans in state and federal prisons. *Administration and Policy in Mental Health and Mental Health Services Research, 41*(3), 360–367.

Tsai, J., Trevisan, L., Huang, M., & Pietrzak, R. H. (2018). Addressing veteran homelessness to prevent veteran suicides. *Psychiatric Services*, April 2 [Epub ahead of print]. https://doi.org/10.1176/appi.ps.201700482

Universal Declaration of Human Rights, Article 25 (1), (1948).

US Department of Housing and Urban Development. (2013). *The 2013 Annual Homeless Assessment Report (AHAR) to Congress: Part 1, point-in-time estimates of homelessness.* Retrieved from https://www.hudexchange.info/resources/documents/ahar-2013-part1.pdf

US Department of Veterans Affairs. (2009). Secretary Shinseki details plans to end homelessness for veterans. Retrieved from http://www1.va.gov/opa/pressrel/pressrelease.cfm?id=1807

US Department of Veterans Affairs. (2017, December 6). Statement by Secretary Shulkin—Homeless funding. Retrieved from https://va.gov/opa/pressrel/pressrelease.cfm?id=3985

US Interagency Council on Homelessness. (2010). *Opening doors: Federal strategic plan to prevent and end homelessness.* Washington, DC: United States Interagency Council on Homelessness.

Wright, J. D. (1988). The worthy and unworthy homeless. *Society, 25*(5), 64–69.

# 2

# Epidemiology of Homelessness Among Veterans

EMILY BRIGNONE, JAMISON FARGO, AND DENNIS CULHANE

> Now is not the time to let up or get complacent. With our
> goals in sight in many communities across the country, we all
> need to work harder and smarter towards achieving them.
> —Secretary Erik Shinseki, *May 30, 2014*

## Introduction

In this chapter, we address the epidemiology of Homelessness Among U.S. Veterans, including a discussion of the methodological challenges relevant to the enumeration and description of homelessness as well as a presentation of current estimates and trends in homelessness among Veterans. The chapter begins with a brief overview of homelessness among Veterans historically, with the remainder of the chapter focusing on the prevalence and incidence of homelessness among Veterans over the past decade. The methodological considerations discussed in this chapter include issues surrounding conceptual definitions of homelessness, implications related to the time frame used for estimates, a comparison between point prevalence, period prevalence, and incidence, and a description of various approaches for using primary and administrative data to estimate the magnitude and composition of homelessness among Veterans. Finally, we present recent national estimates of the prevalence and incidence of homelessness among Veterans, along with a summary of trends over time, and segmentation of estimates by demographic, geographic, and housing status characteristics.

# Historical Overview

Homelessness Among U.S. Veterans has been documented as early as the post–Civil War period, when a considerable number of former soldiers became "vagrants."[1 (p. 67)] Later, many World War I Veterans were affected by the homelessness crisis of the Great Depression.[1 (p. 319)] With the expansion of Veterans' benefits through the G.I. Bill and the economic upswing of the 1940s, homelessness among Veterans declined substantially, and it remained relatively low throughout the 1950s and 1960s.[2] In the years following the Vietnam War, however, the presence of Vietnam Veterans among the homeless became more highly visible, and the link between military service and homelessness began to enter public awareness.[1 (p. 382)]

Rates of homelessness continued to rise through the 1970s and 1980s due to economic recessions, decreases in affordable housing, the war on drugs, and the deinstitutionalization of patients with serious mental illness.[3,4] By this time, the modern concept of homelessness was established, and homelessness among Veterans became a major concern often regarded by the public and media as a national failure and source of shame. Community surveys conducted in the 1980s indicated that Veterans were overrepresented among the homeless population compared with the general population.[5] Subsequent national surveys following the Gulf War corroborated this finding.[5,6]

With the return of a new era of service members from post-9/11 conflicts in Iraq and Afghanistan (Operations Iraqi Freedom, Enduring Freedom, and New Dawn [OEF/OIF/OND]), patterns of homelessness among Veterans began to change. In contrast to Vietnam-era Veterans, who generally did not become homeless until 5 to 10 years after their discharge from service, significant numbers of OEF/OIF/OND Veterans are becoming homeless soon after discharge.[7] For example, results from one population-based study indicate that during the present era, half of new homelessness episodes occur within 3 years of discharge.[8] Many experts point to the hallmark injuries of these conflicts, posttraumatic stress disorder (PTSD) and traumatic brain injury (TBI), as potential contributors to the shift toward more rapid development of homelessness.[9,10]

In late 2009, a five-year plan to end homelessness among Veterans was enacted by the U.S. Department of Veterans Affairs (VA) under the direction of Secretary Eric Shinseki and President Barack Obama.[11] Billions of dollars have since been invested in the expansion of services for homeless Veterans.[8,12] The overall framework for ending Veteran homelessness was developed by the VA and National Center for Homelessness Among Veterans,[13] and adopted by the U.S. Interagency Council on Homelessness in the Federal Strategic Plan to Prevent and End Homelessness, *Opening Doors*.[14] This plan, originally presented to Congress in 2010 and most recently updated in 2015, focuses on several key areas, including providing affordable housing and permanent supportive housing, increasing meaningful and sustainable employment opportunities, reducing the financial vulnerability of Veterans, and transforming the homeless crisis response system with a focus on prevention and rapid rehousing.

## Why Study the Epidemiology of Homelessness Among Veterans?

Establishing reliable estimates of the incidence, prevalence, and composition of homelessness among Veterans is important for several reasons. First, these estimates are necessary for evaluating how the rates of homelessness among Veterans are changing in response to policies, programming, and other contextual factors. Such estimates are also important for service provision planning because the size and composition of the homeless Veteran population directly affects the budgetary and staffing needs of prevention and intervention programs. Relatedly, like the changing characteristics of the overall Veteran population, the characteristics of Veterans who experience homelessness are also in transition. There is considerable variability in the demographic and health characteristics of Veterans who experience homelessness, in the frequency and chronicity of their homelessness experiences, and in their relative state of deprivation. Understanding the composition of this population, including anticipated changes over time, can improve the tailoring of services to meet the needs of this diverse and evolving population.

## Conceptual Definitions Relating to Homelessness Among Veterans

To begin to examine the epidemiology of homelessness among Veterans, definitional issues relating to the terms "homelessness" and "Veteran" must be addressed. For the purposes of eligibility for VA services, these terms are defined in Title 38 of U.S. Code.[15] In Title 38, "Veteran" refers to "a person who served in the active military, naval, or air service, and who was discharged or released from service under conditions other than dishonorable." This definition of Veteran status is often not completely aligned with definitions used in other studies that attempt to quantify and describe homelessness among Veterans. For example, studies that use data from outside the VA often consider the term "Veteran" to include anyone who self-reports as having served in the military, regardless of active-duty or discharge status. There are both practical and theoretical reasons for this. It may not be feasible for researchers to validate the official Veteran status of each individual who self-reports having served in the military. Alternatively, researchers may be interested in the housing experiences of individuals who served in the military but are not eligible for VA services. Notably, even self-reported measures of Veteran status likely result in the underestimation of Veterans among the homeless population. Recent studies indicate that approximately one-third of Veterans experiencing homelessness did not identify as Veterans to community homeless service providers.[16,17]

One example of the difference between VA-defined Veteran status and Veteran status as operationalized in research literature is the Annual Homeless Assessment Report (AHAR),[18] which is the most complete source for the prevalence and incidence of homelessness among Veterans. For the purposes of this report, Veteran status is self-reported, and the population of Veterans includes Veterans with every active-duty or discharge status, regardless of VA eligibility. Given that several hundreds of thousands of Veterans are ineligible for VA benefits as a result of their discharge status, along with research suggesting that these Veterans may be overrepresented among the homeless,[19,20] this definitional difference could potentially result in nontrivial discrepancies in estimates across studies from these sources.

Veterans are considered by the VA to be homeless if they meet the definition of "homeless" that is codified in section 103(a) of the McKinney-Vento Act.[21] The different ways in which an individual or family may be defined as homeless under this section of McKinney-Vento are described here:

*Literal Homelessness:* Homelessness that occurs when an individual or family lacks a fixed, regular, and adequate nighttime residence. This can include:

- Having a primary nighttime residence that is a public or private place not designed for or ordinarily used as a regular sleeping accommodation for human beings, including a car, park, abandoned building, bus or train station, airport, or camping ground;
- Living in a supervised publicly or privately operated shelter designated to provide temporary living arrangements (including hotels and motels paid for by charitable organizations or federal, state, or local government programs);
- Exiting an institution where one temporarily resided (such as a jail or hospital) and having resided in a shelter or place not meant for human habitation.

*Imminent Homelessness:* Homelessness that occurs when individuals will imminently lose their housing, including housing they own, rent, or live in without paying rent or housing they are sharing with others, and rooms in hotels or motels not paid for by charitable organizations or federal, state, or local government. This can include:

- Receiving a court order resulting from an eviction action that notifies the individual or family that they must leave within 14 days;
- Having a primary nighttime residence that is a room in a hotel or motel and lacking the resources necessary to reside there for more than 14 days;
- Having credible evidence indicating that the owner or renter of the housing will not allow the individual or family to stay for more than 14 days;
- Having no subsequent residence identified and lacking the resources or support networks needed to obtain other permanent housing.

Homelessness may also be defined among Veterans in families with children and youth under other federal statutes under the following circumstances:

- Having experienced a long-term period without living independently in permanent housing or having experienced persistent instability as measured by frequent moves over such a period, and expecting to continue as such for an extended period of time because of chronic disabilities, chronic physical health or mental health conditions, substance addiction, histories of domestic violence or childhood abuse, the presence of a child or youth with a disability, or multiple barriers to employment.

Definitions of homelessness may also vary slightly between studies and may also change over time. Notably, under Title 38, the conditions specified under section 103(b) of the McKinney-Vento statute do not constitute homelessness. This section, which was added to McKinney-Vento under the 2009 Homeless Emergency Assistance and Rapid Transition to Housing (HEARTH) Act,[21] designates individuals fleeing domestic violence or other life-threatening conditions as homeless. Several bills containing provisions that would update the VA definition to include section 103(b) have been introduced, but none had passed at the time that this chapter was written.

## Challenges to Identifying and Enumerating Homelessness Among Veterans

In addition to variation in the conceptual definitions of homelessness across studies, other issues exist that can complicate the epidemiological examination of homelessness. These include methodological considerations relating to the time frame specified for estimates, data sources and the associated operationalization of conceptual definitions, and practical challenges inherent in finding an often hidden and transitory population.

## TIME FRAME FOR ESTIMATES

Depending on the time frame selected for the enumeration of homelessness, estimates can represent counts of individuals experiencing homelessness at a particular point in time (point prevalence), counts of individuals who experienced homelessness at any point during a certain time frame (period prevalence), or counts of individuals who became newly homeless during a certain time frame (incidence). Although each type of estimate provides unique and valuable information, the time frame selected has considerable implications for the overall magnitude of counts and the types of homelessness identified in counts.

Point prevalence counts generally take place on a single night and provide an unduplicated estimate of the magnitude of homelessness at a particular point in time. These counts help to inform short-term service provision planning, such as determining shelter capacity needs. However, because of the dynamic nature of homelessness, counting only those experiencing homelessness on a single night underestimates the true magnitude of homelessness. Homelessness is frequently characterized on the basis of frequency and chronicity of episodes. A single, brief episode of homelessness followed by a return to permanent housing is referred to as temporary or transitional. Homelessness characterized by multiple brief episodes of homelessness is referred to as episodic. Finally, as currently defined by the U.S. Department of Housing and Urban Development (HUD), chronic homelessness refers to homelessness occurring among individuals with disabling conditions that lasts at least one year, or four or more separate episodes of homelessness occurring within three years with a combined time spent homeless of at least 12 months.[22,23] Point prevalence estimates tend to capture individuals experiencing chronic homelessness while underrepresenting those who are experiencing temporary or episodic homelessness.[24,25] Because different types of homelessness are associated with different individual characteristics and service needs, descriptions of the homeless population that are based on individuals identified in point prevalence counts are likely skewed toward the characteristics of the chronically homeless.

Period prevalence counts, on the other hand, tend to provide more comprehensive estimates of the magnitude of homelessness than point prevalence estimates. They are also more likely to reflect the true diversity of homelessness experiences and of the individuals who experience homelessness. This is important for informing policy and programming that appropriately balances remedial services for the chronically homeless with preventive efforts that target the distinct needs of individuals who experience or are at-risk for temporary or episodic homelessness.[26]

## SELECTION OF DATA SOURCES

Both administrative and primary data sources can provide important insights regarding the epidemiology of homelessness among Veterans, with certain benefits and limitations inherent in each. Data from administrative sources are generally inexpensive and nonintrusive, can be collected relatively quickly, and can often provide individual-level data for samples covering vast geographic areas. They often include longitudinal data, which can provide insights into the dynamic patterns of homelessness, and their retrospective nature allows for flexibility in the selection of time frames for estimates.

Because of the integrated nature of the VA Health Care System and the broad range of homeless services it provides, researchers have the unique opportunity to estimate homelessness among Veterans through the use of VA administrative health care data. Diagnoses related to homelessness and use of homelessness-related services can be administratively monitored to identify Veterans experiencing homelessness. To this end, the VA maintains a centralized database of Veterans who receive services in VA-funded homeless programs called Homeless Operations Management and Evaluation System (HOMES). Records pertaining to homelessness may also be linked at the individual level to demographic and health care data within the VA system, allowing for high-level analysis of the relationships between homelessness and demographic and military service characteristics, health care utilization patterns, and medical and mental health status. When linked, such data can be used to evaluate conceptual and statistical models that advance our understanding of homelessness among Veterans. Outside of the VA, other administrative systems are used to track homelessness among Veterans. One example is the Homeless Management Information System (HMIS) that is employed by state and local governments to record information, including Veteran status, about individuals who receive homeless services in their communities.

Despite the many benefits of administrative data, there are certain limitations to their use in estimating the prevalence and composition of homelessness among Veterans. Most important, this approach operationally defines homelessness based on the presence of homelessness-related clinical care or social service use, thus excluding individuals who do not or cannot use these services. This issue is particularly relevant for VA-based services because VA eligibility depends on military service and character of discharge criteria.[27] Veterans who experience homelessness but are ineligible for VA services are not represented in these data, despite potentially being at higher risk for homelessness for reasons related to their eligibility. Unlike administrative data from VA, representation in HMIS is not dependent on VA eligibility factors. However, for Veterans experiencing homelessness to be entered into HMIS, they must initiate homelessness-related services, which may not occur for a variety of reasons.

Thus, dependence on service engagement for the identification of homelessness among Veterans may result in incomplete counts as well as samples containing bias because of systematic differences between those who do and those do not engage in homeless services. However, estimates based on HMIS data are highly useful for service provision planning because these data are likely to be largely representative of those who will seek similar services in the future.

Primary data collection can allow researchers to examine homelessness among Veterans independently of eligibility factors or use of homeless services. However, the collection of primary homelessness data presents several practical challenges. First, in addition to potentially substantial underreporting of Veteran status,[16,17] homelessness, particularly temporary and episodic homelessness, is often not easily identifiable. For example, individuals lacking permanent housing may sleep in motels, cars, or vacant buildings. Many stay with family members or friends on a short-term basis, often moving in and out of homelessness from one unstable housing situation to the next.[28] Thus, enumeration efforts that rely on the visibility of homelessness will inevitably miss a considerable portion of this population. This is especially true for in-person counts because these estimates usually represent point prevalence because of the labor-intensive nature of data collection. Another method for examining homelessness among Veterans is through primary data collection methods such as surveys that assess self-reported experiences of homelessness. Using this approach, researchers can specify one or more time frames of interest for homelessness, such as currently homeless, homeless at any point in the past year, or homeless at any point in the past. This allows for both point and period prevalence counts. However, representative sampling that allows for broader inference with respect to homelessness is particularly difficult. Given the relatively rare nature of homelessness, large samples are required. In addition, multiple sampling frames may be needed to ensure sufficient coverage of hard-to-reach populations that are more likely to experience homelessness.

## ESTIMATES OF VETERAN HOMELESSNESS

While determining the exact prevalence and incidence of homelessness among Veterans is not possible because of the practical and methodological issues discussed in the preceding sections, a careful comparison of estimates gathered using a variety of methods can provide insights that, in aggregate, provide a meaningful and holistic view of the epidemiology of homelessness among Veterans. This strategy is often referred to as the "family of studies" approach and is frequently discussed and endorsed in the general homelessness literature.[28,29] In the summaries that follow, we present several recent estimates of homelessness among Veterans, including point prevalence, annual prevalence, and incidence, as well as changes over time. These estimates are based on the highest quality national data sources available, including AHAR,[18] HMIS,[30] American Community Survey,[31] administrative databases maintained by the VA and the VA Office of Inspector General (OIG),[8] and the National Health and Resilience in Veterans Study.[32] These studies are summarized and synthesized in the remaining sections of the chapter.

## ANNUAL HOMELESS ASSESSMENT REPORTS TO CONGRESS

The most comprehensive and current source of estimates of homelessness among Veterans is the AHAR,[18] a report that has been produced by HUD and submitted to the U.S. Congress annually since 2007. The AHAR includes both point prevalence and period prevalence estimates of homelessness as well as estimates of the extent of sheltered homelessness (living in transitional housing, emergency shelters, or safe havens) and unsheltered homelessness (living in locations not suitable for human habitation) on a national level. The data provided in the AHAR are used to track progress of the goals set forth in the Federal Strategic Plan to Prevent and End Homelessness and to inform federal, state, and local strategies to prevent and intervene in homelessness.

The AHAR is presented as a two-part report. Part 1 of the AHAR includes point prevalence estimates based on a point-in-time count of homeless individuals. These counts are conducted by local jurisdictions called Continuums of Care (CoCs). CoCs are responsible for coordinating homeless services within a particular geographic area. In the AHAR, CoCs are classified into three categories according to the size and type of area they cover. "Major City CoCs" cover the 50 largest cities in the United States, and "Balance of State (BoS) or Statewide CoCs" are composed of multiple rural counties or an entire state. The remaining CoCs fall somewhere in between these categories and are classified as "Smaller city, county, and regional CoCs." Point-in-time counts are conducted on a single night in January and provide unduplicated, one-night estimates of homelessness, including separate counts for individuals experiencing sheltered and unsheltered homelessness. Veteran status is recorded for all individuals counted, and since 2009, AHAR has included separate point-in-time counts of homeless Veterans.

Part 2 of each annual AHAR is released the following year and includes period prevalence estimates based on HMIS data. Each CoC maintains its own HMIS and records individual-level information on sheltered homelessness as evidenced by receipt of homeless services. These one-year estimates include individuals who experienced sheltered homelessness at any point during the given year. Certain client characteristics, including Veteran status, are also captured. Each HMIS may be tailored to meet local needs, but all must conform to federal standards to allow for aggregation and comparisons at the national level.

Each CoC submits point-in-time and one-year estimates to HUD. These reports may then be aggregated to form statewide and nationwide estimates. Since the origination of the AHAR nearly 10 years ago, estimates of homelessness among Veterans have improved considerably, and they continue to improve as a result of high CoC participation, refinement, and clarification of procedures, as well as the integration of VA-funded community-based Veterans housing services into HMIS. With more than 400 CoCs providing data, recent estimates effectively cover the entire United States. The most recent AHAR reports available at the time this chapter was written were Part 1 of the 2016 AHAR[33] and Part 2 of the 2015 AHAR.[34]

On the night of the 2016 point-in-time count, 39,471 Veterans were identified as homeless. These estimates indicate that the representation of Veterans among the homeless on a given night is roughly proportional to their representation in the overall adult population (9.2%). However, Veterans remain overrepresented among the sheltered homeless population on a given night, making up approximately 10% of that group.

Demographic characteristics for these Veterans are presented overall and separately by sheltered and unsheltered status in Table 2.1. Approximately 91% of Veterans experiencing homelessness on a given night are men, 8% are women, and less than 1% are transgender. Hispanic ethnicity is reported by 9%. Roughly 60% are White and 30% are Black or African American; the remaining 10% are Veterans who identify as multiracial, Native American, Pacific Islander, or Asian. The vast majority of Veterans (97%) experiencing homelessness on a given night are not part of households that include children. Approximately two-thirds are sheltered and one-third are unsheltered.

There is substantial variability between states and CoCs regarding the proportion of Veterans experiencing homelessness in that area who are unsheltered. In terms of states, on the high end, between 58% and 61% of Veterans experiencing homelessness on a given night in Hawaii, Mississippi, and California are unsheltered. On the low end, between 0% and 4% of Veterans experiencing homelessness on a given night in Rhode Island, New Hampshire, and Massachusetts are unsheltered.

Since the AHAR began tracking Veteran status since 2009, point-in-time counts of homelessness among Veterans have decreased by 46% (33,896 fewer Veterans in 2016 than in 2009). These declines have been steeper among unsheltered relative to sheltered homeless Veterans, reflecting a decrease of 56% versus 39%, respectively. Figure 2.1 illustrates the annual point-in-time counts overall as well as separately for sheltered and unsheltered homelessness among Veterans from 2009 through 2016.

Between 2009 and 2016, declines were seen across all categories of CoC (major city CoCs; smaller city, county, and regional CoCs; and balance of state or statewide CoCs), as well as in 43 states and the District of Columbia. California,

*Table 2.1* **Demographic Characteristics of Veterans Included in the 2016 Point-In-Time Count of Homelessness**

| Characteristic | Overall 39,471 (100%) N (%) | Sheltered 26,404 (%) | Unsheltered 13,037 (%) |
|---|---|---|---|
| **Gender** | | | |
| Female | 3,328 (8.4%) | 2,208 (8.4%) | 1,120 (8.6%) |
| Male | 35,955 (91.1%) | 24,104 (91.3%) | 11,851 (90.7%) |
| Transgender | 188 (0.5%) | 92 (0.4%) | 96 (0.7%) |
| **Ethnicity** | | | |
| Non-Hispanic | 35,913 (91%) | 24,513 (92.8%) | 11,400 (87.2%) |
| Hispanic | 3.558 (9%) | 1,891 (7.2%) | 1,667 (12.8%) |
| **Race** | | | |
| White | 22,965 (58.2%) | 14,974 (56.7%) | 7,991 (61.2%) |
| Black or African American | 12,987 (32.9%) | 9,869 (37.4%) | 3,118 (23.9%) |
| Asian | 253 (0.6%) | 153 (0.6%) | 100 (0.8%) |
| Native American | 1,087 (2.8%) | 501 (1.9%) | 586 (4.5%) |
| Pacific Islander | 331 (0.8%) | 125 (0.5%) | 206 (1.6%) |
| Multiple races | 1,848 (4.7%) | 782 (3%) | 1,066 (8.2%) |

Adapted from Part 1 of the 2016 AHAR Report

New York, and Florida saw the largest absolute decreases in terms of numbers of homeless Veterans (4,233–8,361 fewer Veterans); Louisiana, New York, and Kansas saw the largest percentage decreases (74%–80% lower). Hawaii, Utah, and South Carolina saw the largest increases in terms of absolute numbers (109–171 more Veterans), while Utah, Vermont, and Hawaii saw the largest percentage increases (34%–102% higher).

One-year estimates of Veteran homelessness as reported in the AHAR are still considerably higher than point-in-time estimates, despite only reflecting sheltered homelessness. By expanding the time frame of the measurement from one night to one year, many more experiences of temporary and episodic homelessness are captured. In 2015, sheltered homelessness was recorded for 132,847 Veterans. This equates to approximately one in 170 Veterans. Veterans are overrepresented among the one-year estimates, making up 11.5% of adults who experience sheltered homelessness during the year but only 9.2% of the

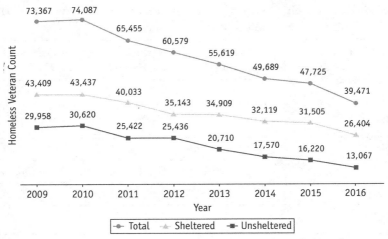

*Figure 2.1*  Point-in-time estimates of Veterans experiencing sheltered and unsheltered homelessness, 2009–2016.  Data sources: US Department of Housing and Urban Development. (2016). *The 2016 Annual Homeless Assessment Report (AHAR) to Congress: Part 1 Point-in-Time Estimates of Homelessness.* Retrieved from Washington, DC: https://www.hudexchange.info/resource/5178/2016-ahar-part-1-pit-estimates-of-homelessness/

general adult population. This contrasts with the point prevalence estimates in the point-in-time portion of the AHAR, in which Veterans' share of homeless and general populations are similar. This is likely a reflection of their higher propensity for sheltered relative to unsheltered homelessness, as is reflected in the point-in-time count.

Men make up approximately 91% of Veterans who experience homelessness during the year, which is similar to their representation among the general Veteran population. For several other demographic characteristics, however, there are major differences between the general Veteran population and the sheltered homeless Veteran population. More than 50% of Veterans who experience sheltered homelessness during the year identify as a race other than White, whereas only 21% of the general Veteran population identifies as such. Veterans aged 62 years and older are vastly underrepresented among Veterans who experience sheltered homelessness. While Veterans in this age group make up more than half of the general Veteran population, they make up less than 15% of the sheltered homeless Veteran population. Conversely, Veterans between the ages of 41 and 51 years are overrepresented, making up less than 20% of the general Veteran population but 40% of the population of sheltered homeless Veterans. Finally, 53% of Veterans who experience sheltered homelessness have a disability compared with 28% among the general Veteran population.

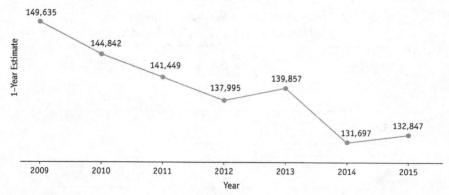

*Figure 2.2* One-year estimates of Veterans experiencing sheltered homelessness, 2009–2015. Data sources: US Department of Housing and Urban Development. (2016). *The 2016 Annual Homeless Assessment Report (AHAR) to Congress: Part 2 Point-in-Time Estimates of Homelessness.* Retrieved from Washington, DC: https://www.hudexchange. info/resources/documents/2016-AHAR-Part-2.pdf

Between 2009 and 2015, one-year estimates of sheltered homelessness declined by 11.2% (16,788 fewer Veterans), despite slight increases recorded in 2013 and 2015. Annual one-year estimates for this period are illustrated in Figure 2.2.

There have been several shifts in the demographic composition of Veterans who experience sheltered homelessness since these data were first collected in 2009. First, while the number of Veterans experiencing sheltered homelessness is decreasing among men, it is increasing among women. The proportion of Veterans experiencing sheltered homelessness during the year who are Black or African American is also increasing, as is the proportion of those who are aged 51 years older. Table 2.2 includes a comparison of the demographic characteristics of Veterans experiencing sheltered homelessness in 2009 and 2015.

The AHAR is a valuable resource for understanding current and historical trends in the epidemiology of homelessness because it constitutes a nearly nationwide effort that uses complex methodologies to describe both sheltered and unsheltered homelessness over the long term. However, the AHAR is subject to certain limitations. First, the AHAR gives little information regarding the incidence of homelessness. Reports do not distinguish between individuals who are homeless for the first time and those who have episodic or chronic patterns of homelessness. This makes it more difficult to use these findings to develop strategies specifically geared toward primary prevention. There is also considerable variability between CoCs in terms of geography, population density, and the balance of unsheltered versus sheltered homelessness, which may lead to some degree of nonuniformity in the practical implications of the results.

*Table 2.2* **Characteristics of Veterans Experiencing Sheltered Homelessness, 2009 and 2015**

|  | 2009<br>N = 149,633 | 2015<br>N = 132,847 |
|---|---|---|
|  | % |  |
| **Gender** | | |
| Male | 92.6% | 91.1% |
| Female | 7.4% | 8.9% |
| **Ethnicity** | | |
| Hispanic | 10.9% | 7.6% |
| Non-Hispanic | 89.1% | 92.4% |
| **Race** | | |
| White, Non-Hispanic | 49.3% | 49.8% |
| White, Hispanic | 8% | 5.1% |
| Black or African American | 34.2% | 38.6% |
| Other One Race | 4.1% | 3.5% |
| Multiple Races | 4.4% | 3.2% |
| **Age (years)** | | |
| 18–30 | 8.2% | 9.1% |
| 31–50 | 44.7% | 33.2% |
| 51–61 | 38.5% | 43.3% |
| 62 and older | 8.8% | 14.5% |
| **Household size** | | |
| One person | 99.7% | 99.9% |
| Two or more people | 0.3% | 0.1% |
| **Disability status** | | |
| Disabled | 52.7% | 53.1% |
| Not disabled | 47.3% | 46.9% |

Data are drawn from Exhibit 5.16 in the 2015 Annual Homeless Assessment Report (AHAR) to Congress, Part 2: Estimates of Homelessness in the United States.[34]

## VA OFFICE OF INSPECTOR GENERAL STUDY

In 2012, the VA OIG released *Homeless Incidence and Risk Factors for Becoming Homeless in Veterans,*[8] a study that estimated the rate of homelessness in the five years following discharge from active-duty military service. This study offers the unique benefit of establishing the incidence of homelessness in sample of Veterans with no history of homelessness. This allows for a specific focus on the epidemiology of first-time homelessness during the potentially vulnerable re-integration period, which may be considerably different than the epidemiology of repeat episodes of homelessness, or homelessness occurring as part of a pro-tracted episode. These insights may help to inform the development of primary prevention strategies.

The population for this study included Veterans who were discharged from active-duty service between July 2005 and September 2006. The final cohort in-cluded 310,685 Veterans who were aged 17 to 64 years, used U.S. Department of Defense (DoD) or VA care following discharge, and had not experienced home-lessness before their service discharge.

This cohort was administratively followed for evidence of homelessness from the time of their discharge from service through September 2010. As discussed earlier in the chapter, because of the broad range of homelessness-related services provided by the VA, homelessness may be ascertained based on the presence of homelessness-related services and diagnoses recorded in the VA electronic medical records of Veterans. For the purposes of this study, Veterans were considered homeless if their electronic medical records reflected use of VA specialized homeless programs, completion of a VA health care for homeless Veterans intake assessment, or receipt of a diagnostic code indicating lack of housing.

Over the course of study follow-up, 5,574 Veterans became homeless (1.8%), with an overall median time of approximately 3 years to the first evidence of homelessness. Using the Kaplan-Meier method to account for variability in the length of administrative follow-up, the estimated homeless incidence (newly homeless) rate for the 5-year period immediately following discharge from active-duty service was 3.7%.

Service in OEF/OIF conflicts was associated with a shorter median time to first homelessness and a higher homeless incidence rate. There were also demo-graphic differences between those who became homeless during study follow-up (homeless cohort) and those who did not (domiciled cohort). While the median time to first homelessness was shorter among men, homeless incidence rates were higher among women. On average, those in the homeless cohort were younger at their time of separation from service than those in the domiciled (never homeless) cohort and were more likely than those in the domiciled cohort to have a pay grade in the lower enlisted range of E1 through E4.

Although this study offers several useful insights regarding the incidence of homelessness among newly returning Veterans, it is also subject to certain limitations. The population of Veterans who separated from the military during the specified period was 491,800, yet the analytic sample only included 310,685 Veterans (63%). The reason for nearly all of these exclusions was lack of VA or DoD care following separation from military service. Some portion of the sample excluded may not have met the official VA definition for "Veteran." Others were likely eligible for VA or DoD care but chose not to use it. It is unknown how results from the analytic sample might generalize to Veterans who choose non-VA services or no services at all. Further, as discussed earlier in this chapter, factors related to eligibility may relate to risk for homelessness. Thus, results from this study may underestimate the incidence of homelessness among a more broadly defined Veteran population.

## ONE-YEAR INCIDENCE AND PREDICTORS OF HOMELESSNESS STUDY

More recently, Tsai and colleagues used administrative data from the VA to estimate the incidence of homelessness among a particular population: Veterans who were referred to VA specialty mental health clinics.[35] In this 2017 study, a retrospective cohort design was used to estimate the one-year incidence of homeless among 306,351 Veterans who were referred to anxiety and PTSD clinics over a four-year period. Similarly to the previously described study, homeless incidence was defined as use of VA homeless services or a diagnostic code indicating lack of housing.

Of the total sample, 5.6% experienced homelessness within 1 year after referral to VA specialty mental health care. Risk for homelessness varied along sociodemographic and diagnostic lines. Women had higher risk for homelessness than men (7.6% vs. 5.4%). Veterans aged 55 years and younger were at highest risk by age, with particularly high risk among those aged 46 to 55 years (9.3%). Risk was also higher among Veterans who were Black relative to White (9.5% vs. 4.9%) and divorced or never married relative to married (8.2% vs. 3%). Veterans who were diagnosed with alcohol use disorders (12.1% vs. 4.6%) or drug use disorders (17.2% vs. 4.5%) had higher risk than those without these diagnoses. Finally, those who did not have a VA service–connected disability rating had higher risk than those who did (7.2% vs. 3.6%). Additional sociodemographic and clinical correlates of homelessness among Veterans are discussed in detail in subsequent chapters.

While this study is subject to similar limitations as the previously described study, these estimates are particularly useful in that they represent a population of Veterans that is both high risk and accessible to VA providers. Thus, they may help to inform efforts to prevent homelessness through early monitoring of known vulnerable populations.

## PREVALENCE AND RISK OF HOMELESSNESS AMONG U.S. VETERANS STUDY

In a 2012 study by Fargo and colleagues,[36] the prevalence of Veterans among the homeless population, poverty population, and general populations was estimated. HMIS data were obtained for 130,554 individuals experiencing homelessness across seven CoCs in 2008. The American Community Survey (ACS), a survey administered by the U.S. Census Bureau annually that collects demographic, social, and economic characteristics from a sample of households in all U.S. counties,[31] was used to estimate the total Veteran and non-Veteran populations for each of the seven CoCs.

Of the 130,554 adults who received homeless services in the seven selected CoCs, 8.2% were Veterans. In comparison, Veterans made up a smaller portion of both the ACS poverty and the ACS general population (3.3% and 7%, respectively). Results of this study indicated that both male and female Veterans were overrepresented in the population experiencing homelessness compared with Veterans living in the general population (1.3 and 2.1 times higher for males and females, respectively) or the population living in poverty (2.1 and 3 times higher for males and females, respectively). Homelessness was also experienced to a greater degree among both male and female Veterans compared with non-Veterans for both the general population (1.4 and 2.3 times higher for males and females, respectively) and the population living in poverty (2.2 and 3 times higher for males and females, respectively).

This study offered unique insights into the prevalence of Veterans experiencing homelessness, the overrepresentation of homelessness among Veterans relative to both the general and the poverty populations, and homeless non-Veterans. Limitations of this study include self-reported Veteran status as available in HMIS and use of a convenience sample of seven CoCs, which although representing 10% of the U.S. homeless population in terms of absolute numbers, may not have been representative of the entire U.S. homeless Veteran population.

## NATIONAL HEALTH AND RESILIENCE IN VETERANS STUDY

In a 2016 study, Tsai and colleagues estimated the lifetime prevalence of homelessness among Veterans using data from the National Health and Resilience in Veterans Survey.[32] The National Health and Resilience in Veterans Survey is nationally representative survey of Veterans that is ascertained from a larger, probability-based, nonvolunteer sample of U.S. households. The study sample included 1,533 Veterans with a broad range of sociodemographic and military service characteristics.

Overall, 8.5% of surveyed Veterans reported experiencing homelessness during their adult life. Among these, the average cumulative duration of homelessness was nearly two years, and only 17.2% reported using VA homeless or social services during the time that they were homeless. Those who were White or lived in rural areas were less likely to have used VA homeless services. As noted by the study authors, it was unclear how ineligibility for VA services may have contributed to nonuse. In any case, this study provides additional evidence that VA-based homelessness estimates likely miss a significant portion of Veterans who experience homelessness.

The study also identified several correlates of lifetime homelessness. Veterans with a history of homelessness had lower incomes and reported more physical and mental health symptoms. Interestingly, although older respondents were expected to be at greater risk for lifetime homelessness due to more years at risk, the likelihood of lifetime homelessness was greatest among Veterans aged 35 to 44 years. As suggested by the authors, higher rates of premature mortality among older Veterans who experienced homelessness may have contributed to this effect.

Because this survey assessed history of homelessness over the long term, responses may have been subject to some recall bias. The survey also did distinguish between different types of homelessness (e.g., episodic vs. chronic) and did not ascertain how long ago homelessness occurred. For this reason, changes to homelessness over time are difficult to infer. Regardless of these limitations, this study provides novel insights into the lifetime prevalence of homelessness among Veterans and provides important context for other estimates, including sociodemographic, clinical, and service use characteristics of Veterans who experience homelessness.

## Summary and Conclusions

Reliable estimates of the size and composition of the population of Veterans that experience homelessness are needed to inform appropriate prevention and intervention efforts. Because of the practical and methodological complexities involved in understanding the epidemiology of homelessness, no single study provides complete details. However, the collective evaluation of estimates yielded by diverse methodologies provides a nuanced view of these epidemiological issues, including point prevalence, period prevalence, and incidence rates; sheltered and unsheltered status; and the demographic, military service, and geographic characteristics of the Veterans who experience homelessness.

In the past decade, homelessness among Veterans has declined substantially. When Veteran status was first recorded in the HUD point-in-time count in 2009, 73,367 Veterans experiencing homelessness were identified. In the 2016 point-in-time count, 39,471 were identified—a decline of nearly 50%. There have also been significant declines in one-year estimates of sheltered homelessness among Veterans over this period. Between 2009 and 2015, the number of Veterans experiencing sheltered homelessness declined 11%, from 149,635 to 132,847 individuals.

The differentially larger decline in point-in-time estimates relative to one-year estimates suggest that the average length of time spent homeless by Veterans who do experience homelessness has decreased. This is reflective of progress toward achieving what is referred to as "functional zero" in homelessness among Veterans. Functional zero refers to a system in which episodes of homelessness are rare, brief, and nonrecurring; in which shelter is provided in the event of homelessness; and in which individuals who experience homelessness are moved quickly to permanent housing.[37] While these recent declines are encouraging, Veterans continue to be overrepresented among the homeless, particularly among those who experience sheltered homelessness over the course of a year. Despite making up approximately 9.2% of the overall adult population, Veterans made up 11.5% of adults who experienced sheltered homelessness in 2015.

The epidemiology of homelessness among Veterans will continue to evolve in response to a variety of factors. Broader economic conditions, including employment opportunities, availability of affordable housing, and access to health care, may also contribute to the growth or mitigation of homelessness among Veterans. Continued funding and availability of homeless and related supportive services that are responsive to these conditions is needed to sustain the declines that have occurred in recent years.

The future of homelessness among Veterans also relates closely to the changing composition of the Veteran population. As the proportion of women Veterans increases, the proportion of women among the population of homeless Veterans can also be expected to increase. In addition, the housing-related needs of Veterans will change as the Veteran population ages. Finally, changes to the military workforce, including the overall size of the force, the background and characteristics of service members and new recruits, and the members' service-related experiences and exposures, may also eventually manifest in changes to the prevalence or incidence of homelessness. Several of these issues are discussed in detail in the later chapters of this book.

While recent years have brought significant improvements in the estimation of homelessness among Veterans, future research may provide more refined and actionable estimates through the integration of higher quality data and analytic techniques. This may include technological advancements in data collection efforts. For example, in 2015, a mobile app was made available to assist communities with point-in-time counts.[38] The app captures GPS location coordinates for each survey. This detailed information can improve service deployment by helping CoCs to understand the specific locations where outreach and services are needed. This and other similar tools have the potential to improve quality, consistency, and precision of large-scale data collection efforts. Longitudinal data may also become more highly integrated into research, including details related to the initial entry into homelessness, the length of homelessness episodes, and returns to homelessness following rehousing. These high-level epidemiological details can be used to develop sophisticated profiles of homelessness that facilitate more precise targeting and tailoring of strategies to prevent homelessness, reduce the length of homelessness episodes, and prevent the reoccurrence of homelessness following rehousing.

# References

1. Kusmer K. *Down and Out, on the Road: The Homeless in American History*. New York, NY: Oxford University Press; 2002.
2. Rossi PH. The old homeless and the new homelessness in historical perspective. *Am Psychol*. 1990;45(8):954–959.
3. O'Flaherty B. *Making Room: The Economics of Homelessness*. Cambridge, MA: Harvard University Press; 1998.
4. Burt MR. *Over the Edge: The Growth of Homelessness in the 1980s*. New York, NY: Russell Sage Foundation; 1992.
5. Rosenheck R, Frisman L, Chung A. The proportion of Veterans among homeless men. *Am J Public Health*. 1994;84(3):466–469.
6. Gamache G, Rosenheck R, Tessler R. The proportion of Veterans among homeless men: A decade later. *Soc Psychiatry Psychiatr Epidemiol*. 2001;36(10):481–485. doi:10.1007/s001270170012.
7. Badkhen A. Shelters take many vets of Iraq, Afghan wars. *Boston Globe*. August 7, 2007. http://archive.boston.com/news/local/articles/2007/08/07/shelters_take_many_ vets_of_ iraq_afghan_wars/. Accessed June 5, 2017.
8. US Department of Veterans Affairs Office of Inspector General. Homeless incidence and risk factors for becoming homeless in Veterans. http://www.va.gov/oig/pubs/VAOIG-11-03428-173.pdf. Accessed June 1, 2017.
9. Tanielian T. Invisible wounds of war. 2008. http://www.rand.org/pubs/monographs/MG720.html. Accessed June 1, 2017.
10. Institute of Medicine Committee on the Initial Assessment of Readjustment Needs of Military Personnel, Veterans, and Their Families. Returning home from Iraq and Afghanistan: Preliminary assessment of readjustment needs of Veterans, service members, and their families. 2010. https://www.nap.edu/download/12812. Accessed June 10, 2017.
11. US Department of Veterans Affairs. Secretary Shinseki details plan to end homelessness for Veterans. Office of Public and Intergovernmental Affairs. November 3, 2009. https://www.va.gov/opa/pressrel/pressrelease.cfm?id=1807. Accessed June 26, 2017.
12. VA Programs for Homeless Veterans. US Department of Veterans Affairs website. https://www.va.gov/HOMELESS/for_homeless_Veterans.asp. Accessed June 26, 2017.

13. National Center for Homelessness Among Veterans. US Department of Veterans Affairs website. https://www.va.gov/HOMELESS/nchav/index.asp. Accessed July 25, 2017.

14. United States Interagency Council on Homelessness. Opening Doors: Federal Strategic Plan to Prevent and End Homelessness. https://www.usich.gov/resources/uploads/asset_library/ USICH_OpeningDoors_Amendment2015_FINAL.pdf. Accessed June 16, 2017.

15. Title 38 U.S.C. § 101.

16. Tregalia D. National Center on Homelessness Among Veterans. Identifying and serving Veterans accessing community-based homeless services: A study of three U.S. cities. https:// www.va.gov/HOMELESS/docs/Treglia_brief.pdf. 2016. Accessed July 25, 2017.

17. Metraux S, Stino M, Culhane DP. Validation of self-reported veteran status among two sheltered homeless populations. *Public Health Rep.* 2014;129(1):73–77.

18. AHAR Reports, Guides, Tools, and Webinars. US Department of Housing and Urban Development website. https://www.hudexchange.info/programs/hdx/guides/ahar/#report. Accessed October 22, 2017.

19. Gundlapalli AV, Fargo JD, Metraux S, et al. Military misconduct and Homelessness Among US Veterans separated from active duty, 2001–2012. *JAMA.* 2015;314(8), 832–834.

20. Metraux S. Homelessness and risk factors for homelessness among Veterans from the era of the Afghanistan (OEF) and Iraq (OIF/OND) conflicts. National Center on Homelessness Among Veterans. 2013. http://www.endVeteranhomelessness.org/sites /default/files/research/Metraux OEF-OIF research brief.pdf. Accessed June 2, 2017.

21. Title 42 U.S.C. § 11302.

22. Kuhn R, Culhane, D. Applying cluster analysis to test a typology of homelessness by pattern of shelter utilization: Results from the analysis of administrative data. *Am J Commun Psychol.* 1998;26(2):210–212.

23. Government Publishing Office. Federal Register Volume 80, Number 233. December 4, 2015. https://www.gpo.gov/fdsys/pkg/FR-2015-12-04/pdf/2015-30473.pdf Accessed June 28, 2017.

24. Balshem H, Christensen V, Tuepker A, Kansagara D. VA Health Services Research and Development Service Evidence-based Synthesis Program. A critical review of the literature regarding homelessness among Veterans. 2011. https://www.hsrd. research.va.gov/ publications/esp/homelessness.cfm. Accessed June 1, 2017.

25. Culhane D, Dejowski EF, Ibanez J, et al. Public shelter admission rates in Philadelphia and New York City: the implications of turnover for shelter population counts. *Housing Policy Debate.* 1994;5(2):107–140.

26. Wong YI. Patterns of homelessness: A review of longitudinal studies. In: Culhane DP, Hornburg, SP, eds. *Understanding Homelessness: New Policy and Research Perspectives.* Washington, DC: Fannie Mae Foundation; 1997.

27. Szymendera, SD. *Who Is a "Veteran"? Basic Eligibility for Veterans' Benefits.* (CRS Report No. R42234). Washington, DC: Congressional Research Service. 2016.

28. Cordray DS, Pion GM. What's behind the numbers? Definitional issues in counting the homeless. *Housing Policy Debate. 1991;* 2(3):585–616.

29. Burt MR, Cohen BE. The Urban Institute. 1989. America's homeless: Numbers, characteristics, and programs that serve them. http://webarchive.urban.org/publications/ 203042. html. Accessed June 1, 2017.

30. Homeless Management Information System. HUD Exchange website. https://www.hud exchange.info/programs/hmis/. Accessed June 25, 2017.

31. American Community Survey (ACS). US Census Bureau website. https://www.census.gov/ programs-surveys/acs/. Accessed June 7, 2017.

32. Tsai J, Link B, Rosenheck RA, Pietrzak RH. Homelessness among a nationally representative sample of US veterans: Prevalence, service utilization, and correlates. *Soc Psychiatry Psychiatr Epidemiol.* 2016;51(6):907–916.

33. US Department of Housing and Urban Development. The 2016 Annual Homeless Assessment Report (AHAR) to Congress. Washington, DC. 2016. https://www.hudexchange.info/resources/documents/2016-AHAR-Part-1.pdf. Accessed June 1, 2017.

34. US Department of Housing and Urban Development. The 2015 Annual Homeless Assessment Report (AHAR) to Congress. Washington, DC. 2015. https://www.hudexchange.info/onecpd/assets/File/2015-AHAR-Part-2.pdf. Accessed June 1, 2017.

35. Tsai J, Hoff RA, Harpaz-Rotem I. One-year incidence and predictors of homelessness among 300,000 U.S. Veterans seen in specialty mental health care. *Psychol Serv.* 2017;14(2):203–207.

36. Fargo J, Metraux S, Byrne T, Munley E, Montgomery A, Jones H. Prevalence and risk of Homelessness Among US Veterans. *Prev Chronic Dis.* 2012;9(15):1–9.

37. Ending Homelessness Among Veterans Overview. US Department of Veterans Affairs website.    https://www.va.gov/HOMELESS/ssvf/docs/Ending_Veterans_Homelessness_Overview.pdf. Accessed June 26, 2017.

38. HUD Releases Point-in-Time Mobile Application. HUD Exchange website. https://www.hudexchange.info/news/hud-releases-point-in-time-mobile-application/. Accessed October 22, 2017.

# 3

# Mental Illness and Substance Use Disorders Among Homeless Veterans

SONYA GABRIELIAN, ASHTON M. GORES, LILLIAN GELBERG,
AND JACK TSAI

> When we do come across someone who is struggling . . . we
> have to develop a culture of open arms and acceptance so that
> they feel comfortable saying, "I'm a Veteran. And by the way,
> I need a little help." . . . [T]his is something we need to do in
> this country around mental health as a whole: de-stigmatizing
> mental health.
> —Michelle Obama, 2015

There is a complex and mutually reinforcing interplay between mental illness, substance use disorders (SUDs), and homelessness. Psychiatric symptoms (e.g., depression, hearing voices, or feeling paranoid) and SUDs can make it difficult to obtain and sustain independent housing.[1] Serious psychiatric symptoms or SUDs often pose barriers to many household tasks and social relationships. Attachments to family and friends often become strained, leading to social disconnectedness that increases risk for homelessness.[2] In addition, persons with serious mental illness (SMI, defined as a schizophrenia spectrum or other psychotic disorder, bipolar disorder, major depressive disorder, or post-traumatic stress disorder [PTSD])[3] often have difficulty managing even routine tenant-landlord conflicts,[4] increasing their risk for eviction. Yet, when on the streets, homeless persons with mental health problems suffer from high rates of victimization, which can worsen quality of life, psychiatric symptoms, and SUDs.[5]

This chapter examines the nuanced interplay of mental illness, SUDs, and homelessness among Veterans. First, we describe risks for experiencing homelessness conferred by mental illness, SUDs, or co-occurrence of these disorders (CoD). Second, we present prevalence data on mental illness and SUDs among Veterans who have experienced homelessness, as well as comparative studies between homeless Veterans and other non-Veteran adults. Third, we explore the diverse pathways to homelessness among Veterans with mental illness, SUDs, and/or CoD. Last, we review supported housing outcomes for this vulnerable Veteran subgroup.

## Mental Illness and Substance Use Disorders as Risk Factors for Veteran Homelessness

Regardless of Veteran status, the presence of a mental health problem (encompassing psychiatric symptoms and SUDs) is hailed as one of the strongest risk factors for experiencing homelessness.[6] The overrepresentation of mental health problems in homeless persons is in part due to deinstitutionalization (the transfer of care for persons with SMI from long-stay hospitals to community-based settings) and a dearth of affordable housing.[1,4,7] Persons with mental health problems who experience homelessness are often difficult to engage in psychiatric care, SUD treatment, and/or social services, including supported housing or other evidence-based practices to address homelessness.[8] Moreover, much of the community mental health system is poorly equipped to prevent and treat homelessness.[4]

A systematic review of risk factors for homelessness among Veterans, across 31 studies from 1987 to 2014,[9] revealed that SUDs and mental illness conferred the strongest and most consistent risk for Veteran homelessness. In particular, SUDs and schizophrenia spectrum and other psychotic disorders[10] posed particularly high risk.[9,11-13] Individual studies included in this review quantified different estimates of specific risks conferred by these diagnoses; one of the most rigorous studies,[9] a secondary database analysis of 1.1 million U.S. Department of Veterans Affairs (VA) mental health service users, found that the presence of any illicit drug use disorder increased a Veteran's odds of experiencing homelessness by nearly eight times.[14] This study also described that Veterans with an alcohol use disorder were almost five times more likely to have experienced recent homelessness than their peers who did not have this disorder[14]; a diagnosis of schizophrenia increased a Veterans' odds of homelessness by approximately three times.[14] Of note, Veterans with CoD are more likely to have experienced homelessness than Veterans without both mental illness and SUD diagnoses.[15]

In contrast, the literature is mixed with regard to risks conferred by a diagnosis of PTSD (which is more prevalent among Veterans than the general population) compared with other mental health disorders.[9,13,16] While one study found that a positive PTSD screening increased homeless women Veterans' odds of experiencing homelessness by five times,[17] a contrasting study of male Veterans suggested that the effects of PTSD on homelessness were likely accounted for by symptoms (e.g. depression or anxiety) that overlap with related psychiatric disorders.[18] Overall, data linking PTSD to homelessness are hindered by the small number of studies in this area and by nongeneralizable sampling methods employed in existing research.[2]

Though the linkages between mental illness, SUDs, and homelessness among Veterans parallel patterns observed in the general adult population, more homeless Veterans have mental health problems than their non-Veteran counterparts.[19] Some speculate that risks for homelessness conferred by mental illness, SUDs, and CoD among Veterans are enhanced by specific military experiences, such as the psychological implications of combat exposure or military sexual trauma (MST).[2] Figure 3.1 presents a conceptual model of risk factors for Veteran homelessness. Military-related trauma (physical, emotional, or sexual) is a known risk factor for the development of mental illness and/or SUDs,[20] which in turn may convey risks for experiencing homelessness.[2] Similarly, prolonged combat exposure is associated with psychiatric symptoms, employment problems, and decreased social support, all of which are risk factors for experiencing homelessness.[2] Military culture, including disruptive service tours that often include

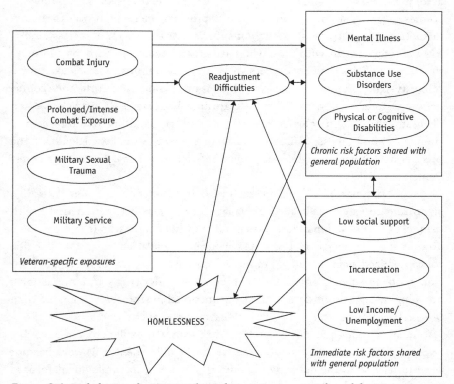

*Figure 3.1* Risk factors for Veteran homelessness: conceptual model. Adapted from Balshem H, Christensen V, Tuepker A, Kansagara D. A critical review of the literature regarding homelessness among Veterans. *VA-ESP Project #05-225*. April 2011:1–64.

geographic relocation and/or combat exposure, may increase the likelihood of negative psychosocial outcomes (including homelessness) from SUDs.[2] Risks for incarceration and unemployment increase for Veterans with SUDs, which increases the risk for homelessness. Though Veterans benefit from the VA's comprehensive services and health care access (presumed resources for homelessness prevention that are more robust than many community resources for non-Veterans), adjustment challenges subsequent to military discharge may outweigh the protective benefits of available VA services.[2] Moreover, this vulnerable population faces notable barriers to care. Homeless Veterans underuse VA primary care (a key gateway to homeless services at VA) relative to their housed peers.[21] Though homeless Veterans with SMI use more VA outpatient and emergency department services than their nonhomeless Veteran counterparts, the homeless group fills fewer psychotropic medication prescriptions (controlling for demographic factors, diagnoses, and health services use),[22] which increases risks for psychiatric hospitalization and poor psychosocial functioning.

An inherent challenge in discussing risk factors for Veteran homelessness (including but not limited to mental illness, SUDs, and CoD) is the absence of a comprehensive explanatory model for Veteran homelessness.[2,9] Numerous studies suggest that, though mental health problems increase the risk for homelessness, these problems alone are not sufficient as a cause for homelessness.[7,23] Even among persons with SMI, who have greater symptom burdens and more functional deficits than their peers with other mental health problems, only a minority experience homelessness.[7] There is little known about the time course between stated risk factors and Veteran homelessness (e.g., the relative and likely interdependent roles of pre-military, military, and post-military mental trauma, mental illness, SUDs, and CoD). Moreover, we know little about the precise mechanisms by which any given risk factor conveys increased risk for homelessness.[9]

In contrast, particularly for persons with SMI (Veterans and non-Veterans), significant research[24-27] has led to explanatory models between mental health diagnoses and functional outcomes outside of housing status (e.g., vocational attainment and social relationships). For this population, cognitive deficits, conceptualized as impairments in memory, speed of mental processing, attention, problem-solving, and the mental processes underlying social interactions, are a highly significant determinant of functional outcomes,[28,29] more so than psychiatric symptoms, e.g., hallucinations, or mood disturbances.

Similarly, though some research[30-33] has explored explanatory models between SUDs and functional outcomes, such as employment, this work has not been translated to the outcome of housing. Though such employment-focused research is limited by loosely defined vocational outcome criteria (e.g., a specific amount of dollars earned per year) and the use of descriptive, nonexperimental designs,[30] it begins to elucidate the multidimensional relationships between

SUDs and employment status. Specifically, person-level characteristics (e.g., educational attainment, motivation, criminal justice involvement) interplay with the social network consequences of SUDs (decreased social support) and environmental factors (high-risk environments) to influence the attainment and retention of employment.[30-33] Additional research is needed to translate these findings to the functional outcome of housing. There is a pressing need to better conceptualize the potential explanatory roles of cognitive deficits, symptoms, or other factors associated with mental illness in conveying homelessness risk among Veterans, as well as to elucidate the specific linkages between aspects of SUDs and the experience of Veteran homelessness.

# Epidemiology of Mental Illness and Substance Use Disorders Among Homeless Veterans

Chapter 2 of this book presented data on the prevalence and incidence of homelessness among Veterans; here, we dive deeper into these figures, presenting data relevant to specific psychiatric diagnoses and SUDs among Veterans who have experienced homelessness. Of note, overall, homeless Veterans are more likely than other homeless adults to have health and social conditions linked to an increased risk for death[34]; relevant to this discussion, tri-morbidity (CoD and at least one physical illness) confers profound risks for morbidity and mortality, is higher in Veteran than non-Veteran homeless populations (27.34% vs. 21.94%, respectively),[34] and highlights the importance of understanding rates of mental illness, SUDs, and CoD in this vulnerable population.

The prevalence rates of affective disorders (depressive and bipolar disorders), anxiety disorders (including PTSD), and schizophrenia spectrum and other psychotic disorders are substantially higher in homeless than housed populations, regardless of Veteran status.[35-37] Similarly, SUDs and CoD are essentially pandemic among homeless persons.[36] A systematic review of literature assessing the prevalence of psychiatric illness and SUDs in homeless Veterans found that most studies relied on populations of Veterans seeking services (as opposed to prevalence in the entire population of homeless Veterans).[2] Moreover, between studies, there was significant variance in methodologies used to capture the presence versus absence of various disorders, ranging from self-report, to diagnoses associated with receipt of VA services, to standardized screening instruments (most of which are not validated in homeless Veteran populations).[2] Despite these limitations, the review concluded that there is adequate and consistent evidence, across studies, to assert that the prevalence of mental illness and SUDs is very high in homeless Veterans, despite access to comprehensive VA mental health services and addiction treatment.[2]

One study published in 2008 employed cluster analysis on interview data collected from 3,333 Veterans who used VA homeless services (in VA hospitals, outpatient clinics, prisons, and community-based Veterans' centers) in one geographic VA region (primarily from Pennsylvania, but spanning West Virginia, Delaware, New Jersey, New York, and Ohio)[36]; this analysis classified Veterans into homogenous groups with shared clinical characteristics, derived from interview ratings of the presence or absence of alcohol use disorder, drug use disorder, psychosis, depression, bipolar disorder, personality disorders, PTSD, and adjustment disorders.[36] Clustering was favored over simple prevalence estimates for its ability to identify core patterns of clinically meaningful subtypes of psychopathology, which in turn could aid with planning for VA and community-based mental health services for Veterans with a history of homelessness.[36] The average linkage method was employed for cluster analyses, computing the average of the similarity of variables collected for any given Veteran's case with all other Veterans' cases in a cluster; any given Veteran's case joined a cluster if a specific level of similarity was achieved.[36]

Three distinct clusters were deemed statistically and clinically significant: "addiction" (92%), a heterogeneous group with SUDs, depression, bipolar disorders, and adjustment disorders; "psychosis" (6.5%), encompassing persons with schizophrenia spectrum and other psychotic disorders, sometimes with comorbid affective disorders or SUDs; and "personality disorders" (1.6%), including persons with personality disorders, sometimes with accompanying adjustment disorders, without comorbid SUDs.[36] Though each cluster was associated with its own constellation of symptoms, demographic characteristic and housing status were similar across clusters.[36] Overall, this analysis highlighted the predominance of CoD among homeless Veterans, primarily consisting of affective disorders and comorbid SUDs, and suggested the value of tailoring the VA's CoD services for Veterans experiencing homelessness.

Other studies report more traditional prevalence estimates of psychiatric diagnoses and SUDs. Table 3.1 presents data from a cross-sectional, community-based survey of 425 homeless men in Pittsburgh and Philadelphia that compared the prevalence of various diagnoses among homeless Veterans ($n = 127$, 29.9% of the sample) with other homeless adults ($n = 298$, 70.1% of the sample).[38] Surveys were administered in unsheltered sites (e.g., abandoned buildings, on the streets), congregate eating facilities, emergency shelters, transitional housing facilities, and single-room occupancy (SRO) settings.[38] More homeless Veterans reported having any psychiatric condition than homeless non-Veterans (61.4% vs. 54.2%, respectively); of note, this between-group difference was not statistically significant ($P = 0.2$).[38] Rates of PTSD (18.1%/8.1%) and the presence of two or more psychiatric conditions (33.1%/22.2%) were significantly ($P < 0.05$) higher in homeless Veterans than non-Veteran homeless adults; rates of depression (37.8%/34.3%), anxiety disorder (16.5%/12.8%), and

*Table 3.1* **Prevalence of Mental Health Diagnoses in Homeless Veterans vs. Homeless Non-Veterans in Pittsburgh and Philadelphia**

| Diagnoses | Homeless Veterans (n = 127, 29.9%) | Homeless Non-Veterans (n = 298, 54.2%) | P Value |
|---|---|---|---|
| At least one psychiatric condition | 61.4% | 54.2% | 0.20 |
| Depression | 37.8% | 34.3% | 0.51 |
| Bipolar disorder | 10.2% | 6.4% | 0.23 |
| Post-traumatic stress disorder* | 18.1% | 8.1% | <0.01 |
| At least one substance use disorder | 79.5% | 82.6% | 0.49 |

*$P < 0.05$.
Adapted from O'Toole et al., 2003[38]

bipolar disorder (10.2%/6.4%) did not have any significant differences between the two groups (all $P > 0.05$).[38] Though current SUDs rates were similar between homeless Veterans and non-Veteran homeless adults, rates in both groups were strikingly high (79.5% and 82.6%, respectively).[38]

These rates contrast those reported in a study of 29,143 formerly homeless Veterans engaged in the U.S. Department of Housing and Urban Development–VA Supported Housing (HUD-VASH) program from 2008 to 2011.[39] In this study, 40.33% of participants did not have an SUD, 32.08% had both alcohol and drug use disorders, 16.64% had only an alcohol use disorder, and 10.96% had only drug use disorders.[39] Of note, by nature of this sample having derived from Veterans engaged in VA housing services, these prevalence rates may underrepresent the prevalence of SUDs in the general homeless Veteran population. There are several potential reasons for this discrepancy. First, supported housing (e.g., HUD-VASH) improves SUD outcomes for some homeless adults.[40] Second, though HUD-VASH is a Housing First program,[41,42] without treatment or sobriety mandates, participants may be reluctant to disclose SUDs to VA providers for fear of losing their housing. Third, the literature is mixed as to the effectiveness of supported housing for persons with severe and active addiction to drugs or alcohol[43,44]; as such, homeless Veterans with severe and recalcitrant SUDs may simply struggle to engage in this program. However, despite these limitations, Veterans with SUDs in HUD-VASH had longer histories of homelessness; Veterans with both alcohol and drug use disorders had demographic characteristics that predispose them to vulnerability: they were more likely to be older, never married, male, and to have had combat exposure.[39]

Though the methodologies employed for these studies (and others estimating prevalence) make it difficult to assess the severity of these mental illness and SUD diagnoses, a secondary analysis of national inpatient VA administrative data showed that homeless Veterans represented 12.1% of all hospitalized patients but made up 42.3% of patients with primary SUDs diagnoses and 20.2% of patients with primary psychiatric diagnoses at discharge.[45] Because acute care use (including inpatient stays) is a proxy for disease severity, this study suggests significant morbidity of these conditions among homeless Veterans. To better conceptualize the prevalence and severity of mental illness and SUDs among homeless Veterans, further research is needed to assess for the presence versus absence of mental illness and SUDs, as well as the severity of these problems, across diverse groups of homeless Veterans (regardless of VA eligibility, current housing status, or engagement in VA or community mental health care).

## MILITARY SEXUAL TRAUMA AND PREVALENCE OF MENTAL ILLNESS AND SUBSTANCE USE DISORDERS AMONG HOMELESS VETERANS

With an increasing number of women serving in the military,[2] the impacts of MST on Veteran homelessness have gained more attention. MST is conceptualized as sexual assault and/or severe and threatening sexual harassment during military service and is associated with a breadth of mental health disorders (including SUDs, PTSD, other anxiety disorders, and adjustment disorders).[46,47] The experience of homelessness in and of itself is coined a "traumatic lifestyle"; that is, trauma, including MST, compounds the core traumatic conditions that accompany substandard housing, such as the struggle to meet basic needs for food, clothing, and shelter.[48]

Rates of MST are high among homeless Veterans; of 126,598 homeless Veterans who used VA outpatient services in fiscal year 2010, 39.7% of women and 3.3% of men screened positive for MST[46] (compared with 16.7% of women and 3% of men who report a history of sexual violence in the general population).[49] Among homeless Veterans in this outpatient sample, this study presented the prevalence of mental health conditions by MST status and gender. Across both genders, adjusting for demographic characteristics (age, race, ethnicity, and marital status), homeless Veterans who screened positive for MST had more mental health conditions than their peers without MST (2.9 vs. 2 for men and women, $P < 0.001$).[46] Table 3.2 presents the prevalence of mental health conditions by MST status and by gender. For both genders, rates of depression, PTSD, other anxiety disorders, bipolar disorders, personality disorders, and SUDs were higher ($P < 0.05$) among Veterans with MST than those without MST. Among homeless Veteran men only, the prevalence of schizophrenia spectrum and other psychotic disorders was significantly ($P < 0.05$)

Table 3.2 **Prevalence of Mental Health Diagnoses by MST Status and by Gender**

| Diagnoses | Female Homeless Veterans | | | Male Homeless Veterans | | |
| --- | --- | --- | --- | --- | --- | --- |
| | Positive MST Screen (n = 3,538) | Negative MST Screen (n = 5,377) | Adjusted Odds Ratio[†] | Positive MST Screen (n = 3,915) | Negative MST Screen (n = 113,768) | Adjusted Odds Ratio[†] |
| Depression | 73% | 59.7% | 1.78* | 66.9% | 50.1% | 1.95* |
| Bipolar disorder | 22.5% | 15.5% | 1.53* | 17.9% | 10.3% | 1.82* |
| PTSD) | 64.8% | 23% | 6.24* | 51.3% | 21.9% | 3.80* |
| Other anxiety disorder (excluding PTSD) | 35.2% | 27% | 1.42* | 28.9% | 19.8% | 1.57* |
| Schizophrenia spectrum and other psychotic disorders | 10.6% | 9.7% | 1.12 | 18.0% | 11.8% | 1.67* |
| Personality disorders | 16.5% | 9% | 1.9* | 12.8% | 6.1% | 2.15* |
| Adjustment disorders | 16.8% | 19.7% | 0.84 | 16.1% | 16.1% | 0.98 |
| Substance use disorders | 45.3% | 33.4% | 1.62* | 68.6% | 61.9% | 1.32* |

MST, military sexual trauma; PTSD, post-traumatic stress disorder.

*P < 0.05.

†Adjusted for age, race, ethnicity, and marital status.

Adapted from Pavao et al., 2013.[46]

higher among those with MST than those without MST.[46] Differential rates of PTSD were particularly salient in this study: among female homeless Veterans, PTSD was present in 64.8% compared with 23% who screened positive versus negative for MST, respectively; among male homeless Veterans, PTSD was present in 51.3% compared with 21.9% who screened positive versus negative for MST, respectively.[46]

Interestingly, though rates of MST are higher among female than male Veterans, a cohort study of 601,892 Veterans who separated from the military between fiscal years 2001 and 2011 found that positive screens for MST are a stronger risk factor for homelessness among men than women.[47] Overall, Veterans who screen positive for MST receive more frequent and intensive VA mental health services.[46] However, men with MST may be more reluctant to seek care than their female peers.[47] Given the potential protection conferred by service receipt, further research is needed to identify and understand the complex linkages between MST, mental illness, SUDs, service use rates, and housing. Moreover, though MST has gained increasing recognition within VA (with mandated screening at all VA facilities since 2004[46,47]), homeless Veterans with a history of MST would benefit from implementation work to tailor and embed relevant services within VA's housing programs. Additional information about MST among female Veterans can be found in Chapter 8.

## MENTAL ILLNESS AND SUBSTANCE USE DISORDERS AMONG HOMELESS VETERANS WHO SERVED IN OPERATION ENDURING FREEDOM (OEF), OPERATION IRAQI FREEDOM (OIF), OR OPERATION NEW DAWN (OND)

More than 2.2 million Veterans served in Afghanistan (OEF) and Iraq (OIF/OND).[50] Chapter 9 delves into the relationships between these military conflicts and Veteran homelessness; because OEF/OIF/OND Veterans have high rates of mental illness and traumatic brain injury (TBI),[2,51] we present mental illness and SUD prevalence data relevant to homeless Veterans who served during these conflicts.

The VA Office of the Inspector General (OIG) conducted the only population-based cohort study to estimate the prevalence of mental health diagnoses among homeless OEF/OIF/OND Veterans.[11] This study found that nearly half (52% of men and 48% of women) of homeless OEF/OIF/OND Veterans were diagnosed with at least one mental health disorder[11]; these rates are two-fold higher than their housed counterparts. Rates of TBI in homeless OEF/OIF/OND Veterans are higher than in their housed peers; among women, TBI rates are two-fold higher, compared with a three-fold difference among men.[11] Of note, rates of TBI in OEF/OIF/OND homeless Veterans are similar to those in homeless Veterans who served during other conflicts or eras. Across affective disorders, anxiety disorders (except PTSD), psychotic disorders, and SUDs, the percentage of OEF/OIF/OND Veterans with these diagnoses before military discharge is lower than their older counterparts. Yet, the percentages of these diagnoses among Veterans in the OEF/OIF/OND group who experience homelessness after military discharge rose higher than those of their counterparts shortly after military discharge, before the first episode of Veteran homelessness.[11] This disparity may reflect the potential protective effects of VA mental health services for these younger Veterans; alternatively, Veterans who served during OEF/OIF/OND may simply be disengaged from mental health care while on active duty. In the case of disengagement, secondary data underestimate the prevalence of mental health problems for active-duty service members.

Research from the National Center on Homelessness Among Veterans[52] extended the OIG study, assessing a broader range of factors (demographics, mental illness and SUD diagnoses, and military factors at the time of active-duty discharge) that could be associated with homelessness. These data showed that the 18% of OEF/OIF/OND Veterans who were diagnosed with a mental health problem at the time of active-duty discharge represented 44% of this era's Veterans who became homeless.[52] Moreover, this study suggested that socioeconomic status interplays with mental illness and SUDs to convey risk for homelessness.[52] Because most homeless Veterans served during the Vietnam era,[53] the literature remains sparse on homeless OEF/OIF/OND Veterans. Particularly given concerns about the emotional impacts of repeated and lengthy deployments for this newest cohort of Veterans,[2] additional study of the psychosocial consequences of OEF/OIF/OND deployments, including homelessness, is vital.

## SUICIDAL BEHAVIOR AMONG HOMELESS VETERANS

Suicidal ideation and attempts are highly prevalent among homeless adults, regardless of Veteran status.[36,54,55] Nearly 30 years ago, a survey of homeless adults in Los Angeles County shelters, food programs, and streets revealed that 22% reported a history of at least one lifetime suicide attempt and 25% reported suicidal ideation over the previous one year.[56] A more recent study of 330 homeless adults in Toronto found that 61% of the sample had a history of suicidal ideation; 34% had attempted suicide.[57] Suicidal behaviors were particularly pronounced in homeless adult women compared with men, with 78% versus 56% reporting suicidal ideation and 57% versus 28%, respectively, reporting an actual suicide attempt.[57] Given such striking rates of suicidal behavior, juxtaposed with suicide prevention as the VA's most salient clinical priority,[58] it is critically important to examine suicidal behavior among homeless Veterans.

Across the nation, in 2009–2010 there were 79,755 Veterans who received homeless services; secondary database analyses showed that the age-adjusted rate of suicide attempts among these Veterans was 3,808 per 100,000 unique Veterans (20 times higher than the rate of suicide attempts among all Veterans).[55] Further disparities were found between genders; homeless female Veterans had about 25% higher rates of suicide attempts (4,677/100,000) than homeless male Veterans (3,734/100,000).[55] Moreover, reattempt prevalence was high: 20.2% and 28.6% of homeless Veterans who attempted suicide reattempted suicide within one year or two years, respectively.[55] Similar to the general population, which has high rates of health care use before suicide attempts,[59] most homeless Veterans who attempted suicide received VA services within 30 days of their attempt.[55]

If we narrow our lens to homeless Veterans with mental illness, most (66.2% and 51.33%) reported a lifetime history of suicide attempts or suicidal ideation, respectively.[60] Given these very high prevalence rates, significant efforts are devoted to assessing and understanding predictors of suicide risk in homeless Veterans. Surveys with 3,595 homeless Veterans (without diagnostic exclusion criteria) were conducted in one VA regional network, aiming to identify risk for suicidal ideation and attempts associated with demographic factors, diagnoses, and self-reported psychological problems.[54] Self-reported serious depression or difficulties managing aggression or violence conferred notable (14-fold) increased risk for suicidal behaviors.[54] The linkages between depressive symptoms and suicidal behaviors were also seen in a study of older (55 years and older) homeless Veterans.[61] Of note, given studies' contrasting methodologies in identifying suicidal behaviors, prevalence rates vary, and it is challenging to identify whether subgroups of homeless Veterans, such as older individuals, are at particularly high risk.

The VA's suicide prevention initiative employs multiple modalities; Veterans with suicidal ideation or other behaviors can access services through a crisis line (available by telephone, text message, or instant messaging), services from designated suicide prevention coordinators, outreach efforts, and community training.[62] Given the VA's mission to end Veteran suicide[58] and the significant vulnerability toward suicidal behaviors seen among homeless Veterans, addressing homelessness among Veterans is well-aligned with the VA's salient suicide prevention efforts. Moreover, enhanced integration of suicide prevention and homeless services initiatives is vital. Clinicians working with homeless Veterans need to be cognizant of this population's elevated suicide risk and the potential value of linking this group to specialized suicide prevention efforts.

# Pathways to Homelessness Among Veterans with Mental Illness and Substance Use Disorders

Earlier in this chapter, in discussing risk factors for homelessness among Veterans with mental illness, SUDs, and CoD, we discussed the absence of a robust explanatory model for vulnerability to homelessness. Despite this gap in the literature, numerous researchers have used qualitative and quantitative methods to better describe the diverse pathways to homelessness among Veterans with mental health problems.

One of the earliest studies along these lines used structural equation modeling to map sequential steps in the pathway to homelessness among men who participated in a 1986–1987 national survey of Veterans of the Vietnam era.[18] Psychiatric disorders and SUDs experienced after military discharge, along with post-military social isolation, had the strongest effects on the incidence of homelessness.[18] Of note, many Vietnam-era Veterans were recruited by the draft; there is some debate if this group is less vulnerable than younger Veterans from the all-volunteer military (enlistment after 1953).[63] In a study of 4,488 homeless adults (28% Veterans) who enrolled in a national outreach program for persons with SMI in 18 communities across nine states, the younger, all-volunteer (vs. older) Veterans were found to have higher rates of symptoms consistent with childhood conduct disorder and instability in their family of origin, and they were disproportionately African American and never married.[63] However, many of these differences were also seen in the general, non-Veteran homeless population.[63] As such, while pathways to homelessness experienced by Vietnam Veterans are important to consider, the adult population experiencing homelessness has substantively changed over the time, necessitating the consideration of newer research.

Along these lines, some have queried whether the homeless Veterans from the all-volunteer eras have stronger personal resources than their homeless non-Veteran contemporaries, which could be protective in the pathway to homelessness.[63] In simply comparing these homeless Veterans with non-Veterans, the group with a history of military service is inherently more resourced by the training opportunities, pension, and health care (i.e., VA services) resources that are specific to Veterans.[63] Moreover, to join the military, the Veteran group passed entrance exams and navigated the processes required for military enlistment; these abilities often reflect lower levels of childhood adversity and family instability.[63] However, Veterans have more severe SUDs both during and subsequent to their time in the military, likely in part related to peer influences while enlisted, despite zero-tolerance policies enacted in the U.S. Armed Forces.[63] This disparity in SUD severity is inferred to be an important risk factor in the pathway to homelessness, perhaps negating the protection conferred by better personal resources seen in the homeless Veteran group.

Though mental illness and SUDs are recurrent themes in studies of pathways to homelessness,[18,23,63,64] little is known about differential pathways to homelessness for people with versus without mental health problems. Though we are unaware of studies along these lines in Veteran populations, this question was examined in the general adult homeless population, comparing mentally ill persons experiencing homelessness with homeless persons without mental illness, all drawn from RAND's Course of Homelessness (COH) study and the Epidemiological Catchment Area (ECA).[23]

In this study, regardless of mental health diagnoses, homeless adults had childhood factors that contributed to their path to homelessness, including financial and social vulnerabilities.[23] However, these adversities were compounded in homeless adults with mental health problems; in addition to poverty experienced in childhood, the group with mental illness had additional vulnerabilities rooted in their family of origin, including violence and other forms of instability.[23] In considering the pathways of homeless adults who have mental illness, the sequence of onset of homelessness versus mental illness was relevant: persons who experienced homelessness before the onset of mental health problems had the highest levels of childhood vulnerability, while those who became homeless after developing a mental health problem had higher rates of SUDs, particularly alcohol use disorder.[23] Of paramount importance, this study asserted that homeless persons with mental illness, overall, had similar pathways to homelessness to their peers without metal health problems. That is, homeless persons as a unified cohort had more in common, regardless of mental health diagnoses, than homeless versus housed persons with mental health problems.[23] Though this study was performed in a civilian population, it has important implications in considering pathways to homelessness among mentally ill Veterans. From a VA service planning perspective, these data suggest the value of treating homeless Veterans with mental illness within care systems tailored for persons with housing instability, such as homeless-focused patient-centered medical homes (branded as Homeless Patient-Aligned Care Teams [HPACTs, see Chapter 4] within VA),[65] as opposed to routing homeless Veterans with mental illness to specialty mental health clinics.

## PATHWAYS TO HOMELESSNESS FOR WOMEN VETERANS WITH MENTAL ILLNESS AND SUBSTANCE USE DISORDERS

Chapter 8 of this book describes the distinct needs and characteristics of homeless women Veterans; men and women have different vulnerabilities for SUDs and mental health problems as well as distinct interpersonal strengths and weaknesses with implications for housing status.[66] Women Veterans are up to four times as likely to be homeless than homeless non-Veteran women.[67] Here, we briefly describe pathways for homelessness for women Veterans with mental illness, SUDs, and CoD.

A civilian study that included 2,727 homeless women and 4,497 homeless men with mental illness asked participants to self-report factors that contributed to their path to homelessness.[66] Women were more likely than men to describe interpersonal conflicts and eviction as primary reasons for homelessness. Though both men and women in this study had mental health diagnoses, men were more likely to cite their mental illness and/or SUDs as important in their pathways to homelessness.[66]

In translating these findings to homeless women Veterans, it is important to consider this population's access to psychosocial services (both within and outside VA).[67] Focus groups with 29 homeless women Veterans in Los Angeles, who were mostly recruited from an annual VA-sponsored open house for homeless women Veterans, revealed three core barriers to care: (1) lack of education about available services for women Veterans; (2) lack of access to services due to geographic barriers or a frank dearth of services (particularly housing) for women Veterans experiencing homelessness; and (3) poor coordination of services, such as between screening for services and being linked for services deemed appropriate in that screening.[67] Moreover, SUDs were tightly linked with these women's experiences seeking care; profound care-seeking barriers led to feelings of isolation and abandonment, which often reinforced SUDs.[67]

These Los Angeles–based focus groups were also used to formulate a grounded description of pathways to homelessness among women Veterans.[64] Relevant to this discussion of homeless women Veterans with mental health problems, these data revealed a "web of vulnerability"[64] (Figure 3.2) that led to homelessness; five central themes comprised this web, all of which interplay with mental health problems. Post-military mental illness, SUDs, and/or medical issues represented one of these themes; the other themes, all of which have significant emotional ramifications, included pre-military adversity (e.g., childhood abuse, military trauma, and/or SUDs), post-military interpersonal violence (e.g., intimate partner violence [IPV]), and unemployment.[64] In considering ways to effectively address these themes, alongside stated pervasive barriers to access to care, these data suggest that primary and secondary homelessness prevention services for women Veterans must include robust mental health and SUD services, with a particular focus on trauma-informed care.[64]

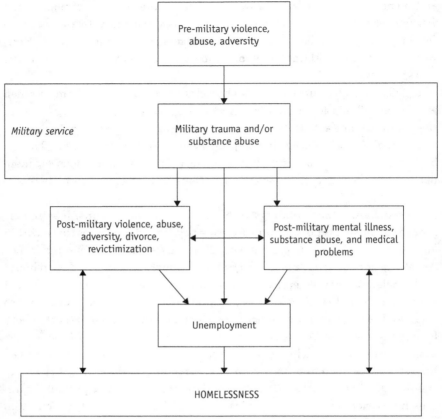

*Figure 3.2* Web of vulnerability into homelessness for women Veterans. Adapted from Hamilton AB, Poza I, Washington DL. "Homelessness and trauma go hand-in-hand": Pathways to homelessness among women Veterans. *Women's Health Issues.* 2011;21(suppl):S203–S209.

## PATHWAYS TO HOMELESSNESS FOR OEF/OIF/OND VETERANS WITH MENTAL ILLNESS AND SUBSTANCE USE DISORDERS

Chapter 9 of this book discusses risks for homelessness among Veterans who served during OEF/OIF/OND. Given the high prevalence of combat-related PTSD in this Veteran subpopulation, which may be associated with increased risk for experiencing homelessness,[52,68] we consider relevant data from a qualitative study of 17 male OEF/OIF/OND Veterans who received case management at any of four Philadelphia- and New Jersey–community agencies that provide homeless services to Veterans.[69] Participants who experienced combat linked their related mental health problems to their homelessness; PTSD was highly prevalent, as were depression, bipolar disorder, and TBI.[69] However, across the board, these Veterans felt that situational factors unrelated to their military service, such as unemployment or the end of romantic relationships, were of greater importance in their path to homelessness than their mental health.[69] The authors highlight the dichotomy between the diagnoses- and situational-based narratives that link personal characteristics to the experience of homelessness.[69] Health systems and clinicians tend to focus on Veterans' diagnoses, with hopes that decreased symptom burdens will improve overall functioning. However, Veterans' perceptions of the paramount importance of situational factors may impede engagement from at-risk OEF/OIF/OND Veterans with homeless service providers.[69]

Other than this small study, few have studied the intersections between mental health problems, SUDs, homelessness, and OEF/OIF/OND Veterans. Moreover, this study's focus on men, despite women Veterans totaling 12% of Veterans during these conflicts,[70] limits its generalizability. Additional qualitative and quantitative inquiry is needed to develop a richer understanding of pathways to homelessness for this newest cohort of Veterans, with particular focus on the mental health sequelae of Iraq and Afghanistan combat.

## Supported Housing Outcomes Among Veterans with Mental Illness and Substance Use

Supported housing programs provide permanent, community-based housing with supportive services for homeless consumers.[71,72] HUD-VASH is the linchpin of the VA's strategic plan to end Veteran homelessness[73] and is one of the nation's largest supported housing initiatives.[74] Prior research substantiates improved mental health outcomes of persons engaged in supported housing, including decreased substance use and increased perceived autonomy.[40,42,75]

Overall, persons with mental health problems (including SMI) do well in supported housing; in fact, this evidence-based practice to address homelessness[42] not only results in substantial reductions in homelessness among persons with SMI but also is associated with marked reductions in use of acute care and correctional facilities.[76] For chronically homeless Veterans, many of whom had psychiatric disorders and/or SUDs, a demonstration project in 2010 facilitated comparison of the HUD-VASH program with a traditional, "housing ready" program that required sobriety and treatment mandates.[77] HUD-VASH participants were housed more rapidly than the comparison group (35 vs. 223 days, respectively).[77] More important, the HUD-VASH group were more than eight times (odds ratio = 8.3) more likely than the comparison group to retain stable housing for one year.[77] These data suggest that, with the support of HUD-VASH or community-based supported housing initiatives, most homeless Veterans with mental illness or SUDs can live independently in their communities.[77]

Unfortunately, some Veterans who have experienced homelessness enroll in supported housing programs but disengage prematurely, before placement in permanent housing.[78] Other homeless Veterans attain but subsequently lose their supported housing, often returning to homelessness.[74,79,80] Several studies examine the role of mental illness and SUDs in these negative housing outcomes.

A study of HUD-VASH–enrolled Veterans at four locations across the country employed secondary data analyses ($N$ = 9,967) and in-person surveys ($n$ = 508) and used logistic regression analysis to identify predictors of housing receipt.[81] In this sample, 15% of participants exited the program before housing placement.[81] Having a schizophrenia spectrum or other psychotic disorder, serving during OEF/OIF/OND, having a service-connected disability, or having an emergency department visit in the 90 days after HUD-VASH admission significantly decreased the odds of becoming housed.[81] Receiving outpatient mental health care (including SUD treatment services) in the 90 days before HUD-VASH admission and use of outpatient care of any sort (including mental health care) in the 90 days after HUD-VASH significantly increased the odds of achieving housing.[81] This relationship between adherence to outpatient care and supportive housing receipt was supported by another HUD-VASH study in Los Angeles.[82] Overall, these data suggest that mental health problems closely interplay with service receipt to influence homeless Veterans' acquisition of supported housing. Particularly because the HUD-VASH program's fidelity to the Housing First approach is weak in the domain of supportive services,[83] these findings stress the importance of adequate pre-enrollment and post-enrollment care for vulnerable Veterans, particularly those with mental illness and/or SUDs.[81]

Considering Veterans who achieve HUD-VASH housing, a multisite, quantitative study identified several factors increasing homeless consumers' risk for premature exits from the HUD-VASH program.[74] Specifically, days intoxicated in the month before enrollment (a proxy for SUD intensity), lower income, and institutionalization history (in the mental health or criminal justice system) were associated with shorter program tenure.[74] A mixed methods study of HUD-VASH enrollees in Los Angeles researched a breadth of general medical, mental health, and psychosocial factors with potential implications for supported housing retention.[80] Nearly all variables relevant to HUD-VASH exits were linked to mental health problems; related themes were particularly prominent in this study's qualitative data.[80] A national mixed methods study corroborated these findings, suggesting that admissions to inpatient SUD treatment and mental health units, as well as emergency department visits, predicted exits from HUD-VASH into recidivistic homelessness.[79]

Of note, even for Veterans with mental illness or SUDs who achieve and retain supported housing, a fundamental problem remains: "recovery" from homelessness extends beyond the acquisition of permanent housing. Extrapolated from the mental health literature, recovery from homelessness for Veterans with psychiatric disorders or SUDs encompasses a deeper process of building a meaningful and fulfilling life, with autonomy and social relationships.[84,85] Yet, little is known about the social support and community involvement of formerly homeless Veterans with mental illness or SUDs who are engaged in HUD-VASH or other supported housing programs. Though several studies of the general homeless population show that consumers remain socially isolated even after achieving housing,[86,87] additional work is needed to conceptualize the construct of recovery for homeless Veterans with mental illness or SUDs who are engaged in supported housing.

Overall, studies of supported housing for Veterans with mental illness or SUDs endorse the use of this model to improve health and housing outcomes for this vulnerable population. However, despite substantive case management and other supports offered by HUD-VASH and comparable community-based supported housing programs, a subset of particularly vulnerable homeless Veterans struggle to attain and sustain housing; those who successfully use supported housing to exit homelessness likely struggle to attain deeper elements of recovery, such as social and community involvement. Mental illness and SUDs contribute to these vulnerabilities; additional services for persons with these diagnoses could improve HUD-VASH and community-based supported housing. Future research could tailor, implement, and evaluate effective interventions (e.g., motivational interviewing for SUDs, critical time interventions or assertive community treatment for persons with SMI or CoD, social skills training) adapted to the context of supported housing.[80]

## Conclusion

Mental illness, SUDs, and CoD confer profound risk for experiencing homelessness and are highly prevalent among homeless Veterans.[2,9] Military-specific experiences (e.g., combat exposure or MST) have significant emotional sequelae and may further predispose Veterans toward homelessness.[46,47] Though many homeless Veterans use the VA, which offers comprehensive mental health, SUD treatment, and psychosocial services, the challenges of transitioning from military to civilian life may supersede the benefits offered by VA care.[2] Moreover, some homeless Veterans experience significant barriers to accessing the VA or other available systems of care.[67] Though HUD-VASH, the center of the VA's strategic plan to end homelessness, employs an evidence-based practice to address homelessness among Veterans with psychiatric disorders and/or SUDs,[77]

Veterans with mental health problems are at increased risk for negative HUD-VASH outcomes.[79–81]

There are several key areas for future research on mental illness and SUDs among homeless Veterans. First, the field lacks a comprehensive explanatory model that explains the linkages between mental illness, SUDs, and homelessness; while established models elucidate the ties between SMI (e.g., schizophrenia) and other functional outcomes (vocational attainment, social relationships),[24–27] this work has yet to be translated to the outcome of housing. Moreover, an explanatory model could be expanded to examine the roles of social context in pathways to homelessness for Veterans with psychiatric disorders and/or SUDs, including adversities and life experiences that occur before, during, and after active duty. Pilot work to date highlights that these pathways differ between Veteran subgroups (e.g., women or OEF/OIF/OND Veterans)[64,69]; to strategically develop primary and secondary homelessness prevention services, additional mixed methods work is needed to understand core pathways to homelessness, along with ways that these pathways differ for special populations.

In addition, more research is needed to understand how and when to best provide mental health and SUD treatment in this era in which Housing First programs (e.g., HUD-VASH) dominate homeless services. Separating housing from treatment mandates is a core tenant of Housing First[88]; however, some Veterans with psychiatric disabilities and/or SUDs are failing these programs.[74,80–82] Some researchers have questioned whether Housing First is an adequate model for persons with active and recalcitrant SUDs.[43] There may be value in implementation work to adapt evidence-based practices for patients with mental health problems and/or SUDs (e.g., motivational interviewing, social skills training, financial management training, and/or critical time intervention) to the context and setting of Housing First. Moreover, for persons accustomed to the structure of military culture or those with significant institutionalization history, a hybrid housing and supportive services approach, valuing consumer choice but offering selected mandates for care, may prove useful.[89]

Also, with the advent of the U.S. opioid epidemic[90] and escalating use of synthetic drugs, such as synthetic cannabinoids ("K2" or "spice") or amphetamines, recognizing risks for SUDs among homeless Veterans and expanding treatment options for this group are a crucial part of homeless services. Moreover, innovations enhancing homeless Veterans' primary care engagement (e.g., the VA's population-tailored patient-centered medical home[91]) may hold promise to improve housing outcomes for Veterans with mental illness and/or SUDs. For homeless Veterans who do not live near a VA health center, telemedicine approaches encompassing medical services, mental health care, SUDs treatment, and psychosocial services hold promise to augment existing homeless services. Last, enhanced VA and community partnerships, including unique interventions like VA medical-legal partnerships,[92] may help support ongoing mental health services for homeless Veterans. Given the robust linkages between mental illness, SUDs, and homelessness, these directions hold great promise to substantively affect rates of Homelessness Among U.S. Veterans and to improve functional outcomes for homeless Veterans who use the VA and community-based housing services.

# References

1. Kuno E, Rothbard AB, Averyt J, Culhane D. Homelessness among persons with serious mental illness in an enhanced community-based mental health system. *Psychiatr Serv.* 2000;51(8):1012–1016.
2. Balshem H, Christensen V, Tuepker A, Kansagara D. A critical review of the literature regarding homelessness among veterans. *VA-ESP Project #05-225.* April 2011:1–64.
3. Petzel RA. *Re-Engaging Veterans with Serious Mental Illness in Treatment.* Washington, DC: Department of Veterans Affairs, Veterans Health Administration; 2012:1–5. http://www.va.gov/vhapublications/ViewPublication.asp?pub_ID=2476.
4. Lamb HR, Bachrach LL. Some perspectives on deinstitutionalization. *Psychiatr Serv.* 2001;52(8):1039–1045.
5. Lam JA, Rosenheck R. The effect of victimization on clinical outcomes of homeless persons with serious mental illness. *Psychiatr Serv.* 1998;49(5), 678–683.
6. Susser E, Moore R, Link B. Risk factors for homelessness. *Epidemiol Rev.* 1993;15(2):546–556.
7. Montgomery AE, Metraux S, Culhane D. Rethinking homelessness prevention among persons with serious mental illness. *Social Issues Policy Rev.* 2013;7(1):58–82. doi:10.1111/j.1751-2409.2012.01043.x.
8. Lincoln AK, Plachta-Elliott S, Espejo D. Coming in: An examination of people with co-occurring substance use and serious mental illness exiting chronic homelessness. *Am J Orthopsychiatry.* 2009;79(2):236–243. doi:10.1037/a0015624.
9. Tsai J, Rosenheck RA. Risk factors for Homelessness Among US Veterans. *Epidemiol Rev.* 2015;37:177–195. doi:10.1093/epirev/mxu004.
10. American Psychiatric Association. *Diagnostic and Statistical Manual of Mental Disorders.* 5th ed. Washington, DC: American Psychiatric Association; 2013.
11. VA Office of Inspector General. *Homeless Incidence and Risk Factors for Becoming Homeless in Veterans.* U.S. Department of Veterans Affairs, Washington, DC: 2012:1–61.
12. Elbogen EB, Sullivan CP, Wolfe J, Wagner HR, Beckham JC. Homelessness and money mismanagement in Iraq and Afghanistan veterans. *Am J Public Health.* 2013;103(suppl 2):S248–S254. doi:10.2105/AJPH.2013.301335.
13. O'Connell MJ, Kasprow W, Rosenheck RA. Rates and risk factors for homelessness after successful housing in a sample of formerly homeless veterans. *Psychiatr Serv.* 2008;59(3):268–275.
14. Edens EL, Kasprow W, Tsai J, Rosenheck RA. Association of substance use and VA service-connected disability benefits with risk of homelessness among Veterans. *Am J Addict.* 2011;20(5):412–419. doi:10.1111/j.1521-0391.2011.00166.x.
15. Teeters JB, Lancaster CL, Brown DG, Back SE. Substance use disorders in military veterans: Prevalence and treatment challenges. *Subst Abuse Rehabil.* 2017;8:69–77. doi:10.2147/SAR.S116720.
16. Rosenheck RA, Frisman L, Fontana A, Leda C. Combat exposure and posttraumatic stress disorder among homeless veterans of three wars. In: Ursano RJ, Fullterton CS, eds. *Posttraumatic Stress Disorder Acute and Long-Term Responses to Trauma and Disaster.* American Psychiatric Publishing, Inc., Washington, DC; 1997:191–207.
17. Washington DL, Yano EM, McGuire J, Hines V, Lee M, Gelberg L. Risk factors for homelessness among women veterans. *J Health Care Poor Underserved.* 2010;21(1):82–91. doi:10.1353/hpu.0.0237.

18. Rosenheck R, Fontana A. A model of homelessness among male veterans of the Vietnam War generation. *Am J Psychiatry*. 1994;151(3):421–427. doi:10.1176/ajp.151.3.421.

19. Perl L. (2015). *Veterans and Homelessness*. 2nd ed. CRS Report for Congress.

20. Murdoch M. Women veterans' experiences with domestic violence and with sexual harassment while in the military. *Arch Fam Med*. 1995;4(5):411–418. doi:10.1001/archfami.4.5.411.

21. Gabrielian S, Yuan AH, Andersen RM, Rubenstein LV, Gelberg L. VA health service utilization for homeless and low-income Veterans: A spotlight on the VA Supportive Housing (VASH) program in greater Los Angeles. *Med Care*. 2014;52(5):454–461.

22. Hermes E, Rosenheck R. Psychopharmacologic services for homeless Veterans: Comparing psychotropic prescription fills among homeless and non-homeless veterans with serious mental illness. *Commun Mental Health J*. 2016;52(2):142–147. doi:10.1007/s10597-015-9904-2.

23. Sullivan G, Burnam A, Koegel P. Pathways to homelessness among the mentally ill. *Soc Psychiatry Psychiatr Epidemiol*. 2000;35(10):444–450.

24. Green MF. What are the functional consequences of neurocognitive deficits in schizophrenia? *Am J Psychiatry*. 1996;153(3):321–330. doi:10.1176/ajp.153.3.321.

25. Bowie CR, Depp C, McGrath JA, et al. Prediction of real-world functional disability in chronic mental disorders: A comparison of schizophrenia and bipolar disorder. *Am J Psychiatry*. 2010;167(9):1116–1124. doi:10.1176/appi.ajp.2010.09101406.

26. Kaye JL, Dunlop BW, Iosifescu DV, Mathew SJ, Kelley ME, Harvey PD. Cognition, functional capacity, and self-reported disability in women with posttraumatic stress disorder: Examining the convergence of performance-based measures and self-reports. *J Psychiatr Res*. 2014;57:51–57. doi:10.1016/j.jpsychires.2014.06.002.

27. Goldberg JF, Chengappa KNR. Identifying and treating cognitive impairment in bipolar disorder. *Bipolar Disorders*. 2009;11(suppl 2):123–137. doi:10.1111/j.1399-5618.2009.00716.x.

28. Meyer MB, Kurtz MM. Elementary neurocognitive function, facial affect recognition and social-skills in schizophrenia. *Schizophr Res*. 2009;110(1-3):173–179. doi:10.1016/j.schres.2009.03.015.

29. Schmidt SJ, Mueller DR, Roder V. Social cognition as a mediator variable between neurocognition and functional outcome in schizophrenia: Empirical review and new results by structural equation modeling. *Schizophr Bull*. 2011;37(suppl 2):S41–S54. doi:10.1093/schbul/sbr079.

30. Janikowski T. Research on employment and substance abuse treatment. 2002:1–20. https://archives.drugabuse.gov/pdf/blending/Janikowski.pdf.

31. Jason LA, Ferrari JR. Oxford House Recovery Homes: Characteristics and effectiveness. *Psychol Serv*. 2010;7(2):92–102. doi:10.1037/a0017932.

32. Belyaev-Glantsman O, Jason LA, Ferrari JR. The relationship of gender and ethnicity to employment among adults residing in communal-living recovery homes. *J Groups Addict Recover*. 2009;4(1/2):92–99. doi:10.1080/15560350802712462.

33. Platt JJ. Vocational rehabilitation of drug abusers. *Psychol Bull*. 1995;117(3):416–433.

34. 100,000 Homes Campaign. *National Survey of Homeless Veterans in 100,000 Homes Campaign Communities*. Community Solutions, New York, 2011:1–12.

35. Folsom D, Jeste DV. Schizophrenia in homeless persons: A systematic review of the literature. *Acta Psychiatr Scand*. 2002;105(6):404–413.

36. Goldstein G, Luther JF, Jacoby AM, Haas GL, Gordon AJ. A preliminary classification system for homeless veterans with mental illness. *Psychol Serv*. 2008;5(1):36–48. doi:10.1037/1541-1559.5.1.36.

37. Folsom DP, Hawthorne W, Lindamer L, et al. Prevalence and risk factors for homelessness and utilization of mental health services among 10,340 patients with serious mental illness in a large public mental health system. *Am J Psychiatry*. 2005;162(2):370–376. doi:10.1176/appi.ajp.162.2.370.

38. O'Toole TP, Conde Martel A, Gibbon JL, Hanusa BH, Fine MJ. Health care of homeless veterans. *J Gen Intern Med*. 2003;18(11):929–933.

39. Tsai J, Kasprow WJ, Rosenheck RA. Alcohol and drug use disorders among homeless veterans: Prevalence and association with supported housing outcomes. *Addict Behav*. 2014;39(2):455–460. doi:10.1016/j.addbeh.2013.02.002.

40. Collins SE, Malone DK, Clifasefi SL, et al. Project-based Housing First for chronically homeless individuals with alcohol problems: Within-subjects analyses of 2-year alcohol trajectories. *Am J Public Health*. 2012;102(3):511–519. doi:10.2105/AJPH.2011.300403.

41. Tsemberis S, Gulcur L, Nakae M. Housing First, consumer choice, and harm reduction for homeless individuals with a dual diagnosis. *Am J Public Health*. 2004;94(4):651–656.

42. Fitzpatrick-Lewis D, Ganann R, Krishnaratne S, Ciliska D, Kouyoumdjian F, Hwang SW. Effectiveness of interventions to improve the health and housing status of homeless people: A rapid systematic review. *BMC Public Health*. 2011;11(1):638. doi:10.1186/1471-2458-11-638.

43. Kertesz SG, Crouch K, Milby JB, Cusimano RE, Schumacher JE. Housing First for homeless persons with active addiction: Are we overreaching? *Milbank Q*. 2009;87(2):495–534. doi:10.1111/j.1468-0009.2009.00565.x.

44. Urbanoski K, Veldhuizen S, Krausz M, et al. Effects of comorbid substance use disorders on outcomes in a Housing First intervention for homeless people with mental illness. *Addiction*. July 2017. doi:10.1111/add.13928.

45. Adams J, Rosenheck R, Gee L, Seibyl CL, Kushel M. Hospitalized younger: A comparison of a national sample of homeless and housed inpatient veterans. *J Health Care Poor Underserved*. 2007;18(1):173–184. doi:10.1353/hpu.2007.0000.

46. Pavao J, Turchik JA, Hyun JK, et al. Military sexual trauma among homeless veterans. *J Gen Intern Med*. 2013;28(suppl 2):S536–S541. doi:10.1007/s11606-013-2341-4.

47. Brignone E, Gundlapalli AV, Blais RK, et al. Differential risk for homelessness among US male and female Veterans with a positive screen for military sexual trauma. *JAMA Psychiatry*. 2016;73(6):582. doi:10.1001/jamapsychiatry.2016.0101.

48. Bell M. Homelessness and military sexual trauma. 2012:41.

49. RAINN. Scope of the problem: Statistics. https://www.rainn.org/statistics/scope-problem.

50. SAMHSA. *Behavioral Health Issues Among Afghanistan and Iraq U.S. War Veterans*. Vol 7. 2012:1–8. Rockville, MD.

51. Seal K, Metzler TJ, Gima KS, Bertenthal D, Maguen S, Marmar CR. Trends and risk factors for mental health diagnoses among Iraq and Afghanistan Veterans using Department of Veterans Affairs Health Care, 2002–2008. *Am J Public Health*. 2009;99(9):1651–1658. doi:10.2105/AJPH.2008.150284).

52. Metraux S, Clegg LX, Daigh JD, Culhane DP, Kane V. Risk factors for becoming homeless among a cohort of veterans who served in the era of the Iraq and Afghanistan conflicts. *Am J Public Health*. 2013;103(S2):S255–S261. doi:10.2105/ajph.2013.301432.

53. National Coalition for Homeless Veterans. FAQ about homeless Veterans. http://nchv.org/index.php/news/media/background_and_statistics/.

54. Goldstein G, Luther JF, Haas GL. Medical, psychiatric and demographic factors associated with suicidal behavior in homeless veterans. *Psychiatr Res*. 2012;199(1):37–43. doi:10.1016/j.psychres.2012.03.029.

55. Hill LL. Housing placement and suicide attempts among homeless veterans. 2012:1–36.

56. Gelberg L, Linn LS, Leake BD. Mental health, substance use, and criminal history among homeless adults. *Am J Psychiatry*. 1988;145(2):191–196.

57. Eynan R, Langley J, Tolomiczenko G, et al. The association between homelessness and suicidal ideation and behaviors: Results of a cross-sectional survey. *Suicide Life Threat Behav*. 2002;32(4):418–427.

58. US Department of Veterans Affairs. State of the VA fact sheet. 2017:1–4. Washington, DC.

59. Ahmedani BK, Stewart C, Simon GE, et al. Racial/ethnic differences in health care visits made before suicide attempt across the United States. *Med Care*. 2015;53(5):430–435. doi:10.1097/MLR.0000000000000335.

60. Desai RA, Liu-Mares W, Dausey DJ, Rosenheck RA. Suicidal ideation and suicide attempts in a sample of homeless people with mental illness. *J Nerv Mental Dis*. 2003;191(6):365–371. doi:10.1097/01.NMD.0000071584.88965.E1.

61. Schinka JA, Schinka KC, Casey RJ, Kasprow W, Bossarte RM. Suicidal behavior in a national sample of older homeless veterans. *Am J Public Health*. 2012;102(suppl 1):S147–S153. doi:10.2105/AJPH.2011.300436.

62. Thompson C. Suicide prevention and crisis intervention with Veterans. 2012:1–22.

63. Tessler R, Rosenheck R, Gamache G. Comparison of homeless veterans with other homeless men in a large clinical outreach program. *Psychiatr Q*. 2002;73(2):109–119.

64. Hamilton AB, Poza I, Washington DL. "Homelessness and trauma go hand-in-hand": Pathways to homelessness among women veterans. *Women's Health Issues*. 2011;21(S):S203–S209.

65. O'Toole TP, Johnson EE, Aiello R, Kane V, Pape L. Tailoring care to vulnerable populations by incorporating social determinants of health: The Veterans Health Administration's "Homeless Patient Aligned Care Team" program. *Prev Chronic Dis*. 2016;13:1–12. doi:10.5888/pcd13.150567.

66. Tessler R, Rosenheck R, Gamache G. Gender differences in self-reported reasons for homelessness. *J Soc Distress Homeless*. 2001;10(3):243–254. doi:10.1023/a:1016688707698.

67. Hamilton AB, Poza I, Hines V, Washington DL. Barriers to psychosocial services among homeless women veterans. *J Soc Work Pract Addict*. 2012;12(1):52–68. doi:10.1080/1533256X.2012.647584.

68. Tsai J, Pietrzak RH, Rosenheck RA. Homeless veterans who served in Iraq and Afghanistan: Gender differences, combat exposure, and comparisons with previous cohorts of homeless veterans. *Adm Policy Ment Health*. 2013;40(5):400–405. doi:10.1007/s10488-012-0431-y.

69. Metraux S, Cusack M, Byrne TH, Hunt-Johnson N, True G. Pathways into homelessness among post-9/11-era veterans. *Psychological Services*. 2017;14(2):229–237. doi:10.1037/ser0000136.

70. *Health and Homelessness Among Women Veterans*. 2012 ed. Nashville, TN: National Health Care for the Homeless Council; 2012:1–3. https://www.nhchc.org/wp-content/uploads/2012/07/Research-Update-Aug-2012-Women-Veterans.pdf.

71. Mares AS, Rosenheck RA. One-year housing arrangements among homeless adults with serious mental illness in the ACCESS program. *Psychiatr Serv*. 2004;55(5):566–574.

72. O'Connell MJ, Kasprow WJ, Rosenheck RA. Differential impact of supported housing on selected subgroups of homeless veterans with substance abuse histories. *Psychiatr Serv*. November 2012:1–11. doi:10.1176/appi.ps.201000229.

73. United States Interagency Council on Homelessness. *Opening Doors: Federal Strategic Plan to Prevent and End Homelessness*. June 2010:1–74. Washington, DC.

74. O'Connell M, Kasprow W, Rosenheck RA. National dissemination of supported housing in the VA: Model adherence versus model modification. *Psychiatr Rehabil J*. 2010;33(4):308–319. doi:10.2975/33.4.2010.308.319.

75. Stefancic A, Tsemberis S. Housing First for long-term shelter dwellers with psychiatric disabilities in a suburban county: A four-year study of housing access and retention. *J Primary Prevent*. 2007;28(3-4):265–279. doi:10.1007/s10935-007-0093-9.

76. Culhane DP, Metraux S, Hadley T. Public service reductions associated with placement of homeless persons with severe mental illness in supportive housing. *Housing Policy Debate*. 2002;13(1):107–163.

77. Montgomery AE, Hill LL, Kane V. Housing chronically homeless veterans: Evaluating the efficacy of a Housing First approach to HUD-VASH. *J Community Psychol*. 2013;41:505–514. doi:10.1002/jcop.21554.

78. Gabrielian S, Burns AV, Nanda N, Hellemann G, Kane V, Young AS. Factors associated with premature exits from supported housing. *Psychiatr Serv*. 2016;67(1):86–93. doi:10.1176/appi.ps.201400311.

79. Cusack M, Montgomer AE, Blonigen D, Gabrielian S, Marsh L, Fargo J. Factors that influence returns to homelessness following an exit from permanent supportive housing: Health and supportive services utilization proximal to program exit. *Families in Society*. 2016;97(3):221–229.

80. Gabrielian S, Hamilton AB, Alexandrino A Jr. "They're homeless in a home": Retaining homeless-experienced consumers in supported housing. *Psychol Serv*. 2017;14(2):154–166. doi:10.1037/ser0000119.supp.

81. Montgomery AE, Cusack M, Blonigen DM, Gabrielian S, Marsh L, Fargo J. Factors associated with Veterans' access to permanent supportive housing. *Psychiatr Serv*. 2016;67(8):870–877. doi:10.1176/appi.ps.201500248.

82. Gabrielian S, Bromley E, Hellemann GS, et al. Factors affecting exits from homelessness among persons with serious mental illness and substance use disorders. *J Clin Psychiatry*. 2015;76(4):e469–e476. doi:10.4088/JCP.14m09229.

83. Kertesz SG, Austin EL, Holmes SK, DeRussy AJ, Van Deusen Lukas C, Pollio DE. Housing First on a large scale: Fidelity strengths and challenges in the VA's HUD-VASH program. *Psychol Serv*. 2017;14(2):118–128. doi:10.1037/ser0000123.

84. Andresen R, Oades L, Caputi P. The experience of recovery from schizophrenia: Towards an empirically validated stage model. *Aust N Z J Psychiatry*. 2003;37(5):586–594. doi:10.1046/j.1440-1614.2003.01234.x.

85. Lloyd C, Waghorn G. Conceptualising recovery in mental health rehabilitation. *The British Journal of Occupational Therapy*. 2008;71(8):321–328. doi:10.1177/030802260807100804.

86. Stergiopoulos V, Hwang SW, Gozdzik A, et al. Effect of scattered-site housing using rent supplements and intensive case management on housing stability among homeless adults with mental illness. *JAMA*. 2015;313(9):905. doi:10.1001/jama.2015.1163.

87. Tsai J, Mares AS, Rosenheck RA. Does housing chronically homeless adults lead to social integration? *Psychiatr Serv*. 2012;63(5):427–434. doi:10.1176/appi.ps.201100047.

88. Greenwood RM, Schaefer-McDaniel NJ, Winkel G, Tsemberis SJ. Decreasing psychiatric symptoms by increasing choice in services for adults with histories of homelessness. *Am J Commun Psychol*. 2005;36(3–4):223–238. doi:10.1007/s10464-005-8617-z.

89. Waegemakers Schiff J, Schiff RAL. Housing First: Paradigm or program? *J Soc Distress Homeless*. 2014;23(2):80–104. doi:10.1179/1573658X14Y.0000000007.

90. *About the Epidemic*. https://www.hhs.gov/opioids/about-the-epidemic/index.html.

91. O'Toole TP, Pape L. Innovative efforts to address homelessness among veterans. *N C Med J*. 2015;76(5):311–314. doi:10.2307/3070692?ref=search-gateway:35c663507716b18fc23ae793349ecbd7.

92. Tsai J, Middleton M, Retkin R, et al. Partnerships between health care and legal providers in the Veterans Health Administration. *Psychiatr Serv*. 2017;68(4):321–323. doi:10.1176/appi.ps.201600486.

# 4

# Primary Care for Homeless Veterans

THOMAS P. O'TOOLE

> . . . [T]he question of who got sick, why they got sick, and
> what happened to them—these were not just biological
> phenomena, but social, racial, economic, and political
> phenomena. That was the beginning of my sense that
> medicine can be an instrument of social change.
> —H. Jack Geiger, *MD, Founding member and past president of*
> *Physicians for Human Rights*

## Engaging Homeless Veterans in Health Care

Homelessness often defines both the health and the health care of people without a permanent, secure, and safe place to live. In many ways homelessness itself is a health issue as well as a reflection of the viability of our social safety net and the economic and environmental realities of lower socioeconomic populations. It is also sometimes a consequence of drug and alcohol abuse, the relative paucity of addiction treatment services, and underresourced mental health services. The disproportionate use of emergency department and other acute care services by homeless persons has come to define some of those care settings. This can also serve as one of the most frequent points of first contact for people in a housing crisis.[1] Homeless Veterans have garnered specific attention over the past several years in acknowledgement of their national service and the long-standing commitment to their needs following military service as well as the unique capacities within the U.S. Department of Veterans Affairs (VA) to meet those needs.

In this chapter we present a brief synopsis of health services research on homeless persons, including the health care needs and service use of both Veteran and non-Veteran homeless. This synopsis is followed by a brief historical overview of how health services have been organized and care systems developed for homeless persons over the past 30-plus years. This includes the original Robert Wood Johnson and Pew Charitable Trust–funded Health Care for the Homeless Clinics as well as the VA-based Homeless Patient-Aligned Care Team (HPACT) program. We then discuss primary care for homeless persons within a larger context that includes challenges and opportunities for treatment engagement, the role of identification and stabilization of precipitating and exacerbating health conditions that are associated with homelessness, and the unique role the health care system has in helping homeless persons engage in broader social and housing services.

## Health Care Needs and Access Issues Among People Experiencing Homelessness

In 1988, the Institute of Medicine (IOM) released a report on homelessness that succinctly described the relationship between health and homelessness in three contexts.[2] First, some health problems precede and causally contribute to homelessness. For example, mental illnesses such as depression, schizophrenia, and bipolar disorder have long been reported as precipitants of homelessness.[3] Similarly, drug and alcohol addiction, accelerated with the readier availability of crack cocaine in the 1990s, has also been described as a pathway to homelessness for many.[4] Second, some health problems are consequences of homelessness. Frostbite, trench foot, hypothermia, and hyperthermia from exposure to the elements can frequently be seen among people who are homeless.[3] Infestations from scabies, bed bugs, and fleas are extremely common and may serve as vectors for more serious diseases.[5] Overcrowding of shelters, especially during inclement weather, makes transmission of airborne illnesses such as tuberculosis much easier, particularly when the immune system of homeless persons is already often weakened. Trauma is also much more common among homeless persons, with women being most vulnerable to this reality.[6] Finally, as noted in the IOM report, homelessness itself complicates the care of many illnesses, especially chronic conditions. Managing insulin-dependent diabetes while living in a dusk-to-dawn emergency shelter presents significant obstacles, not only to storing and securing medications, but also to managing multiple injections in the context of an unstable, erratic, and usually suboptimal supply of food and unstable sheltering arrangements. Similarly, wound care is seriously compromised by the dependent edema that results from prolonged standing and walking that unsheltered and emergency-sheltered homeless persons often face along with inadequate hygiene in many of these sheltering arrangements.

Research documenting the prevalence of specific health conditions among homeless persons is often subject to selection bias depending on who are being surveyed, where they reside, and the context for how they are identified. What is consistent in all of this research, however, is not only the high prevalence of mental health conditions, substance use disorders, and chronic medical conditions but also the co-occurrence of multiple acute and chronic conditions at the same time in the same person—often referenced as "tri-morbidity."

Prevalence of disease in a study of almost 20,000 homeless Veterans enrolled in the HPACT program[7] is surprisingly consistent with other samples[8] despite being limited to Veterans who were engaged in a care system and somewhat older and more likely male. In that study, the majority had at least one medical condition, with musculoskeletal disorders and associated pain syndromes the most commonly diagnosed, followed by lower rates of other common medical conditions. The most common mental health conditions were depression, anxiety disorders, and post-traumatic stress disorder, and alcohol abuse was the most common substance use disorder other than tobacco abuse (Table 4.1). Additionally, research on homeless adults in Canada found that the prevalence of traumatic brain injury (TBI) was substantially higher among homeless individuals than the general population, and the precipitating event more often preceded the onset of homelessness.[9]

Several studies have compared homeless Veterans to homeless non-Veterans over the past 30 years. In a systemic review of the literature, Tsai and Rosenheck found homeless Veterans to be older, better educated, male, married or to have been married, and to have health insurance than non-Veteran homeless adults.[10] They have higher rates of substance abuse, mental illness, and physical illness preceding their homelessness,[11] with mental health problems and substance use more likely to be self-reported causes of homelessness.[12] Additionally, they have a higher overall disease burden. In a cross-sectional two-community sample, two-thirds of homeless Veterans had at least one chronic medical problem, with most having three or more, and 33% had two or more mental health problems; both rates were significantly higher than for the non-Veteran homeless people in the sample.[8]

These findings help explain some of the difficulties and challenges associated with providing care to homeless persons in traditional settings. Both TBI and chronic pain disorders can distort clinical presentations and challenge treatment engagement and compliance. The concurrent presentation of chronic and acute medical, behavioral, and substance use disorders can make triage and coordination difficult—dynamics that further fragment care and make navigating the care system more untenable. Individuals lacking shelter or in unstable sheltering arrangements also face several homeless-specific barriers to care that need to be considered in any model or systems design. Additional factors, including long-term homelessness (>2 years); competing needs such as food, clothing, finding shelter; and social isolation are also all associated with not having a regular source of care.[13]

From a patient perspective, competing sustenance needs often dilute the relative importance of accessing health care, particularly for health maintenance and

*Table 4.1* **Prevalence of disease among veterans in HPACT**

| Diagnosis | % |
| --- | --- |
| Chronic medical | 50.6% |
| Hypertension without complications | 27.8% |
| Chronic pulmonary disease | 11.6% |
| Diabetes without complications | 10.9% |
| Liver disease | 10.3% |
| Fluid and electrolyte disorders | 9.5% |
| Cardiac arrhythmias | 6.8% |
| Congestive heart failure | 4.5% |
| Other neurological disorders | 4.5% |
| Renal failure | 4.1% |
| Obesity | 3.9% |
| Mental health | 57.6% |
| Depression | 43.1% |
| Post-traumatic stress disorder | 21.5% |
| Suicide/self-harm | 17.7% |
| Psychoses | 12.7% |
| Substance use | 50.8% |
| Drug abuse | 36.9% |
| Alcohol abuse | 36% |
| Tri-morbidity | 24% |

Szymkowiak, et al. Persistent super-utilizwation of acute care services among subgroups of veterans experiencing homelessness. Medical Care.

monitoring of chronic, asymptomatic conditions.[14] Further, the social environment of homelessness, including perceived stigma and past negative experiences seeking care, have all been shown to impede access.[15] One's perception of both the need for health care and anticipated outcomes also plays a role. Homeless adults who reported "not caring what happens" were significantly less likely to have received any health care, independent of self-identified comorbidities.[16] In another study, patterns of health care avoidance were identified in more than half of homeless persons with a self-described (and subsequently confirmed) acute health need. This cohort identified a pessimistic and fatalistic expectation of their outcome and lacked confidence in the health care system to address their concerns.[17]

# Health Services Utilization and Outcomes Among People Experiencing Homelessness

It is with this backdrop that health outcomes among persons experiencing homelessness need to be critically assessed. Despite the hundreds of millions of dollars spent on homeless programming in the United States, the advances made in our understanding of how to best provide care and assist homeless persons and in the overall increase in numbers served, significant health disparities persist. Homeless adults have age-adjusted mortality 3.5 times higher than their domiciled counterparts.[18] More alarming, in a study of Boston Health Care for the Homeless patients in the 1990s, the average age at death for a homeless person was 47 years; younger age groups were more likely to die from infections such as HIV/AIDS and trauma, while cancer and heart disease were the most common causes of death for the 45- to 64-year age group, three-fold higher than the general population.[19] This has significant implications when considering the type of health care, social services, and interventions needed by homeless persons as well as the importance of strategies that ensure compliance and continuity of care being provided.

Given the high risk for and rate of multiple morbidities, it is not surprising that homeless persons also use acute-level health services at very high rates. In a survey of homeless adults, more than 40% used the emergency department at least once for care in the previous year, and more disturbingly, 7.9% of those surveyed accounted for 54.5% of visits.[20] In a national survey of homeless persons, one out of four was hospitalized annually,[21] and in a study of homeless persons accessing New York City hospitals, the average length of stay was 36% longer per admission than for nonhomeless persons.[22] Homeless adults in more unstable sheltering arrangements (unsheltered and emergency sheltered) were more likely to go to emergency departments for care than those living in more stable or structured settings.[23] Substance abuse, trauma, mental illness, and exacerbations of chronic disease conditions were the most common reasons for seeking care in that study.

Research on non-Veteran homeless consistently identifies the role of health insurance as a significant determinant of how and where care is accessed.[13,23] For Veterans experiencing homelessness, those seeking care at a VA facility do not need health insurance, and their copays are waived based on income, removing these factors as barriers to care. However, several studies have also found an overreliance on emergency departments for care among these individuals.[24-26] Tsai and colleagues reported that homeless Veterans have four times the odds of using an emergency department compared with nonhomeless Veterans. This may be related to the higher rates of psychiatric and medical conditions among homeless Veterans compared with non-Veterans. It is also often for conditions that had been delayed and deferred until they were much more serious. This suggests that other factors related to how care is organized and delivered,[25] including the capacity to address underlying and perceived stigma, access challenges, and competing needs, may be playing a significant role.[14,15]

# The Role of Primary Care in Homeless Health Care

Primary care, and specifically primary care tailored to the needs of homeless persons, provides a unique opportunity to address some of the service gaps and vulnerabilities in homeless health care. It also provides the platform on which to engage homeless persons in an array of services over a continuum of time and needs. The role for primary care in caring for homeless persons has been described and discussed extensively in the literature. Shortt et al., in a policy analysis of care models in Canada, found that traditional primary care approaches performed poorly compared with targeted clinic for homeless persons, fixed outreach site-based care, and mobile outreach services for homeless persons.[27] This is also reflected in a survey of homeless persons, of whom 84% preferred specialized homeless service for their primary care needs.[28] In contrast, primary care models specifically oriented to homeless persons have been linked with reductions in acute care service use,[29-31] increases in use of ambulatory services,[31] high rates of engagement in ancillary and referral services,[32] improved chronic disease management,[30] and expedited housing placements.[32]

There is a long tradition and notable history of health professionals caring for the poor, with communities adapting and developing care approaches that reflect local needs, resources, and capacity. Public hospitals, free clinics, street and soup kitchen–based outreach programs, inebriate centers, respite programs, and others have long served as a venerable safety net and primary care hub for the most needy and destitute, many of whom were homeless.[2,3] The following are descriptions of the two largest networks in the country and common features associated with both.

## HEALTH RESOURCES AND SERVICES ADMINISTRATION HEALTH CARE FOR THE HOMELESS PROGRAM

In 1983 the first national effort to organize health services for homeless persons was undertaken by the Robert Wood Johnson Foundation, Pew Charitable Trusts, and the U.S. Conference of Mayors with the launching of the Health Care for the Homeless (HCH) demonstration project. In all, 19 projects were initially funded and operating by 1985 with an initial focus on primary medical care and service coordination. This was followed by efforts to improve mental health and substance abuse treatment, provide dental care, and treat HIV/AIDS and tuberculosis. In July 1987, Congress passed the Stewart B. McKinney Homeless Assistance Act, which assumed the funding for HCH programs under Section 340 of the Public Health Service Act and grew the program exponentially. There are currently 295 grantees/clinics serving more than 900,000 patients each year.[33]

The program is built around an approach that encompasses four principles: (1) the services provided must be comprehensive and encompass the global needs of homeless persons; (2) the care must be accessible to homeless persons and work around their needs and limits; (3) the attitudes of the providers must reflect a sensitivity to cultural and ethnic diversity along with dignity and respect to the clients; and (4) the philosophy of the clinics is ultimately the goal to help people escape homelessness.[34] The HCH program has also served as the platform for additional programming and services from organized street outreach and street medicine to medical respite care that now serve across the continuum of needs and settings where homeless persons are encountered.[35]

## HOMELESS PATIENT-ALIGNED CARE TEAMS: HOMELESS PRIMARY CARE MEDICAL HOME MODELING

The VA is the largest integrated health system model, with a universal electronic health record and single-payer comprehensive coverage in which issues of insurance eligibility are negated. Most important, it is a model that incorporates social determinants of health, including housing and income security into care delivery. However, even with these attributes, the challenges of getting homeless Veterans into care and sustaining that care has been problematic.[8] HPACT was developed in 2010 as part of the larger initiative of Ending Veteran Homelessness spearheaded by the Obama Administration. HPACT is a multidisciplinary, population-based medical home model organized around the unique challenges that homeless Veterans face accessing and engaging in care. It builds on the core principles outlined earlier for the HCH model but adapted and organized within the VA integrated health system platform. As of 2017, the model has been adopted in 65 VA medical centers and provides ongoing care to about 20,000 Veterans during their highest risk periods of homelessness and clinical instability. The goal is to addresses the multiple medical and social needs of these Veterans in one setting by incorporating five organizational approaches that complement and align with the four tenets of the HCH model and that distinguish it from traditional primary care approaches:

1. *Reducing barriers to receiving care.* HPACTs provide open-access, walk-in care as well as outreach to the community to engage those Veterans disconnected from VA services. This open-access/care-on-demand/noncontingent model

for seeking health care is coupled with scheduled appointments so that on-going continuity of care is concurrently provided.

2. *Providing one-stop, wrap-around services* that are integrated and coordinated. Mental health, housing programs, and primary care staff are colocated to create a continuum of care and an integrated care team. Several HPACTs also provide food and clothing assistance, hygiene items, showers, and laundry facilities and other services on site to meet a fuller continuum of Veteran needs. The intent is to emphasize a whole-person approach while minimizing the off-site referrals.

3. *Engaging Veterans in intensive, community-linked case management.* This recognizes the importance of the community social service network in ef-fective care and care management. It includes routinely schedule care coor-dination meetings with local community agencies, outreach, cohosted health fairs, and other events.

4. *Providing high-quality, evidence-based, and culturally sensitive care.* Critical to the model are deliberate efforts to engage the Veteran in care and foster a therapeutic relationship with that Veteran's care team. This is intended to destigmatize seeking care while supporting professionalism among the providers delivering that care. This includes hosting a curriculum emphasizing cultural competency specific to the needs of homeless Veterans and those at-risk for homelessness, as well as monthly national community of practice calls intended to keep the provider community from being profes-sionally isolated.

5. *Being performance-based and accountable* with real-time data and predictive analytic applications that assist teams in targeting those most in-need, while providing ongoing technical assistance and personalized feedback that in-form team performance. Availing of the national electronic medical record within VA, the reporting has focused on performance metrics on how well teams are outreaching to and engaging in care of those homeless Veterans with the highest clinical complexities, metrics reflecting sustained care across the continuum (primary care, mental health substance use disorders, specialty care, homeless programming), and metrics that assist a team in identifying who is at highest risk for acute care use ("hot-spotting").

Critical to the HPACT model is a consideration of how it organization-ally fits within the continuum of programming and needs of the homeless Veteran. This includes consideration of the evolving needs of the person experiencing homelessness and what services can best address those needs. This is conceptualized into three phases (Figure 4.1). In phase 1, the indi-vidual has just become homeless or is experiencing health complications exacerbated or precipitated by homelessness and is unable to access care through traditional venues. This may be because shelter locations make it

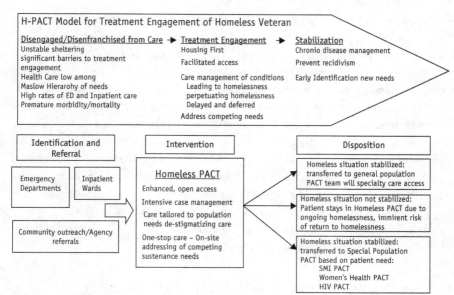

*Figure 4.1* Process map of evolving care needs of homeless Veterans in the HPACT model. From O'Toole TP, Johnson EE, Aiello R, Kane V, Pape L. Tailoring care to vulnerable populations by incorporating social determinants of health: The Veterans Health Administration's "Homeless Patient Aligned Care Team" program. *Prev Chronic Dis*, 2016;13:e44.

difficult to physically or logistically get to a clinic appointment, because their appearance or presentation is stigmatizing and causing them to avoid care, or because their competing sustenance needs force them to deprioritize health care. It is in this phase that the HPACT model is best suited for engaging the Veteran by having partnered outreach into the community, an open-access/ care-on-demand program with no preconditions to that care, and a provider team that understands and is considerate of the unique challenges facing this population. Phase 2 reflects a stabilization and treatment stage of care in which the focus is on addressing root causes of homelessness (addiction, mental illness, disability) and securing housing, food security, and income security—necessary elements for their recovery and capacity to leave home-lessness. This is also the stage during which chronic disease management and self-care practices are introduced and the patients can become empowered in better managing their health needs outside of urgent and emergent contexts and settings. This may include diabetes education, pain management, assisting in medication compliance, and transitioning to more scheduled appointments. Finally, after the Veteran has been able to demonstrate effec-tive self-care and chronic disease management skills and secure and main-tain permanent housing, phase 3 is marked by a transition or "graduation" to a traditional primary care practice within the VA. On average these three phases take anywhere between 9 and 18 months to accomplish, and in our experience upward of 70% of Veterans transition successfully.

The "graduation" element has been an important aspect of the care model for three reasons: First, for practical purposes, it allows the team to maintain capacity to add new patients to the panel who may need an intensive level of care in order to stabilize; second, it operationalizes homelessness as a state and not a disease or permanent affliction and models the care delivery approach around a recovery paradigm; and finally, from an individual perspective, it facilitates goal setting and a "graduation" that is intended to be empowering and discourage any permanent labeling. The caveat of course is that this needs to be individually applied with a flexible approach to when each phase can occur. It also requires patient care planning that is not typically afforded in traditional care settings but is critical to a population-based approach.

## PROGRAM EVALUATIONS AND QUALITY IMPROVEMENT

The HPACT model has benefited from and is informed by an extensive and rigorous evaluation effort supported by VA Health Services Research and Development funding and other sources. Evaluations to date have focused on health services use, cost of care, treatment engagement, housing outcomes, use of peers in this setting, and impact on non-VA payers and community providers (e.g., Medicare). Emerging from these efforts is a growing literature base applicable to both Veteran and non-Veteran homeless populations that has allowed us to consider the role of how health systems are organized for this population relative to distinct engagement, treatment, and homeless recovery outcomes:

### H-PACT Enrollment Is Associated with Lower Rates of Emergency Department Use and Hospitalizations

- Six-month patterns of acute-care use before and after enrollment, controlling for sheltering status for 3,543 consecutively enrolled patients, showed a 19% reduction in emergency department use and a 34.7% reduction in hospitalizations.[36]
- In a national case-control study, the monthly mean number of emergency encounters for all HPACT enrollees decreased from 0.26 to 0.19 from the six months before enrollment to the six months after enrollment ($P < 0.001$). This decrease was most pronounced among HPACT enrollees with two or more emergency department visits in the baseline period.[37]
- In a prospective, single blinded, multicenter quasi-experimental trial, homeless Veterans in HPACTs were hospitalized less often than those in general Patient-Aligned Care Teams (PACTs; 23.1% vs. 35.4%, $P = 0.04$).[38]

**HPACTs Are More Effective at Engaging Homeless Veterans in Ambulatory Care Services**

- HPACT-enrolled Veterans averaged three to five primary care visits per year, which was substantially higher than both homeless and nonhomeless Veterans seen in traditional primary care settings.[31,38]
- They also received more social work support than in a nonhomeless/general PACT, averaging 4.6 visits per year compared with 2.7 visits per year ($P < 0.01$).[32]
- They averaged almost two specialty visits per year; more than 80% were actively engaged in mental health care, and more than 90% were enrolled in a VA homeless program.[36]
- In a single-blinded, multicenter prospective comparison study, the average HPACT-enrolled Veteran cost $9,379/year less to care for than a homeless Veteran enrolled in a nonhomeless/general PACT (primary care) VA clinic, driven largely by fewer hospitalizations in VA and community centers.[38]

**Intensive Engagement in HPACTs Was Associated with Identification of Undiagnosed Conditions**

- Homeless Veterans newly enrolled in an HPACT who received high-intensity outpatient primary and specialty care had a mean of 4.1 new diagnoses of chronic conditions during their first six months of care compared with 0.9 new diagnoses in a matched control group of nonhomeless veterans enrolled in general VA primary care services.[31]

**Veterans Enrolled in HPACTs Were Housed Faster and at Higher Rates**

- Veterans enrolled in HPACT gained housing 81.1 days faster than those not enrolled in an HPACT.[32]

# Using Primary Care as an Expanded Platform to Address Homeless Persons' Needs

One of the challenges we confront when considering population-tailored primary care models such as Health Care for the Homeless or HPACTs is whether the intent and focus should be on making homeless persons healthier or assuming a more ambitious goal of contributing to their leaving homelessness. Securing better health care and hopefully health for homeless Veterans is clearly important, especially in the context of their substantial chronic disease burden and premature mortality. There are also the public health considerations—screening and treatment of communicable diseases such as tuberculosis and vaccinations for influenza and hepatitis A and B, for example—that have both individual and societal benefit. There is also substantial appeal for the financial benefits from redirecting care away from high-cost emergency departments to less costly ambulatory settings. However, if the goal of population-tailored primary care for homeless Veterans is more ambitiously aligned with that person's exit from homelessness, then more must be assumed and expected from the model.

The role of health care, and especially primary health care, in exiting homelessness may not be obvious. Unlike treatment for a debilitating addiction or mental illness that is causing one's homelessness, managing hypertension or diabetes may not have the same urgency or immediacy to this outcome. To reconcile this with the observations, both anecdotally among providers and in the literature, that suggest a more substantive contributing role, it is useful to look at primary care for homeless persons in a somewhat different context. Gelberg and Anderson developed the Behavioral Model for Vulnerable Populations that posited three drivers or domains for health-seeking behavior among homeless persons.[39] The *predisposing vulnerable domain* includes age, gender, marital status, as well as residential status, acculturation, and literacy; the *enabling vulnerable domain* includes personal and family resources such as receipt of public assistance, competing needs, and access to and use of information sources; and the *need vulnerable domain* includes both evaluated and perceived health condition needs. This framing of health care–seeking behavior helps explain why someone with a clear need for physical or mental health care may or may not pursue treatment, even if barriers like health insurance are removed.

Primary care provides a vehicle for addressing health care needs prioritized by the Veteran while also addressing many of the *predisposing* and *enabling* vulnerable factors and barriers identified in this model. The VA HPACT and Health Resources and Services Administration HCH models described provide a low-intensity entry to health care whereby Veterans do not need to commit to an intensive treatment regimen or behavior plan at the outset but instead are provided the opportunity to expand their perception of what their needs may actually include and an understanding of how they can address them. This is while getting their immediate needs addressed and being socialized to a health care model and health care team. This facilitates a treatment engagement process during which trust can be developed, autonomy is protected, and relationship-based care can be established. It is from this foundational starting point that the Veterans' readiness for change can be cultivated and barriers addressed that can enable them to accept a referral and participate in the essential care and treatment needed to assist them in existing homelessness. The research on the HPACT program supports this premise because the low-threshold/low-barrier care model was associated with higher rates of use and parallel engagement in other services, including specialty and mental health care and homeless programming and services. Within this framework, social determinants of health also play an important role as drivers of both access and utilization.

Finally, primary care for homeless Veterans becomes an opportunity to use the process of treatment engagement as a gateway to address other needs, such as tobacco cessation, chronic disease management, and treatment readiness for addiction services.[17,40] It also serves as a platform for introducing specialized services, including use of mobile technologies and peer support specialists to assist in care delivery, medication-assisted treatment for opioid dependence, hepatitis C and HIV testing and treatment, housing support, and food insecurity.[27,32,41–45] More work in both systems design and evaluation is needed to fully explore these opportunities and the feasibility of interventions.

The challenge, then, is how to engage homeless persons in primary care programming. How do we keep them engaged so that they can benefit fully from the services offered? And if they have a setback, how do we avail of the open-access/noncontingent nature of care delivery to intervene early before they experience a return to homelessness? It may be that the models described in this chapter are more unique in their approach and capacity to engage and retain homeless persons in care and it is this dynamic that ultimately facilitates recovery and exiting homelessness.

In summary, primary care needs to be seen and considered as more than a service reserved for those individuals capable of and with the resources to navigate our byzantine health system. The benefits of primary care extend beyond providing subacute, chronic disease management and age-specific preventive health care. Primary care is a service that can be tailored and modified to meet the unique access and clinical needs of the homeless Veteran and non-Veteran alike with substantive potential benefits on the personal, societal, and health systems levels. Primary care needs to be seen as a point of first contact and early engagement that can serves as an entree to the continuum of programs and services needed to exit homelessness. However, it will not happen without deliberate planning and organization relating to how we deliver care and services to those most in need and a commitment to the capacity in order to bring the services to scale.

# References

1. O'Toole TP, Conde-Martel A, Gibbon JL, Hanusa BH, Freyder PJ, Fine MJ. Where do people go when they first become homeless? *Health Soc Care Community* 2007;15(5):446–453.
2. Institute of Medicine/Committee on Health Care for Homeless People. *Homelessness, Health, and Human Needs.* Washington, DC: National Academy Press; 1988.
3. Brickner PW, Scharer LK, Conanan BA, Savarese M, Scanlan BC, eds. *Under the Safety Net.* New York, NY: W. W. Norton; 1990.
4. Jencks C. *The Homeless.* Cambridge, MA: Harvard University Press; 1995.
5. Bonilla DL, Kabeya H, Henn J, Karamer VL, Kosoy MY. *Bartonella quintana* in body lice and head lice from homeless persons, San Francisco, California, USA. *Emerg Infect Dis.* 2009;15(6):912–915.

6. Kushel MB, Evans JL, Perry S, Robertson MJ, Moss AR. No door to lock: Victimization among homeless and marginally housed persons. *Arch Intern Med*. 2003;163(20):2492–2499.

7. Szymkowiak D, Montgomery AE, Johnson EE, Manning T, O'Toole TP. Persistent super-utilization of acute care services among subgroups of veterans experiencing homelessness. *Med Care*. 2017 Oct;55(10):893–900.

8. O'Toole TP, Conde-Martel A, Gibbon JL, Hanusa BH, Fine MJ. Health care for homeless veterans: Why do some individuals fall through the safety net? *J Gen Intern Med*. 2003;18 (11):929–933

9. Topolovec-Vranic J, Ennis N, Colantonio A, Cusimano MD, Hwang SW, Kontos P, Ouchterlony D, Stergiopoulos V. Traumatic brain injury among people who are homeless: A systemic review. *BMC Public Health*. 2012;12:1059.

10. Tsai J, Roseheck RA. Risk factors for Homelessness Among US Veterans. *Epidemiol Rev*. 2015;37:177–195.

11. Winkleby MA, Fleshin D. Physical, addictive, and psychiatric disorders among homeless veterans and nonveterans. *Public Health Rep*. 1993;108(1):30–36.

12. Dunne EM, Burrell, Diggine AD, Whitehead NE, Latimer WW. Increased risk for substance use and health-related problems among homeless veterans. *Am J Addict*. 2015; 24(7): 676–680.

13. Gallagher TC, Andersen RM, Koegel P, Gelberg L. Determinants of regular source of care among homeless adults in Los Angeles. *Med Care*. 1997;35(8):814–830.

14. Gelberg L, Gallagher TC, Andersen RM, Koegl P. Competing priorities as a barrier to medical care among homeless adults in Los Angeles. *Am J Public Health*. 1997;87:217–220.

15. O'Toole TP, Johnson EE, Redihan S, Borgia M, Rose J. Needing primary care but not getting it: The role of trust, stigma and organizational obstacles reported by homeless Veterans. *J Health Care Poor Underserved*. 2015;26(3):1019–1031.

16. O'Toole TP, Gibbon JL, Hanusa BH, Fine MJ. Preferences for site of care among homeless adults. *J Gen Intern Med*. 1999;14:599–605.

17. O'Toole TP, Buckel L, Bourgault C, Blumen J Redihan S, Jan L, Friedmann P. Applying the chronic care model to homeless veterans: Can a tailored primary care model reduce emergency department use and improve clinical outcomes? *Am J Public Health*. 2010;100(12):2493–2499.

18. Hibbs JR, Benner L, Klugman L, et al. Mortality in a cohort of homeless adults in Philadelphia. *N Engl J Med*. 1994;331:301–309.

19. Hwang SW, Orav J, O'Connell JJ, Lebow JM, Brennan TA. Causes of death in homeless adults in Boston. *Ann Intern Med*. 1997;126(8):625–628.

20. Kushel MB, Perry S, Bangsberg D, Clark R, Moss AR. Emergency department use among the homeless and marginally housed: Results from a community-based study. *Am J Public Health*. 2002;92(5):778–784.

21. Kushel MB, Vittinghoff E, Haas JS. Factors associated with the health care utilization of homeless persons. *JAMA*. 2001;285(2):200–206.

22. Salit SA, Kuhn EM, Hartz AJ, Vu JM, Mosso AL. Hospitalization costs associated with homelessness in New York City. *N Engl J Med*. 1998;338:1734–1740.

23. O'Toole TP, Gibbon JL, Hanusa BH, Fine MJ. Utilization of health care services among subgroups of urban homeless. *J Health Politics Policy Law*. 1999; 24(1):91–114

24. Tsai J, Rosenheck RA. Risk factors for ED use among homeless veterans. *Am J Emerg Med*. 2013; 31(5):855–858.

25. Tsai J, Doran KM, Rosenheck RA. When health insurance is not a factor: National comparison of homeless and nonhomeless US veterans who use Veterans Affairs Emergency Departments. *Am J Public Health*. 2013;103(suppl 2):S225–S231.

26. Doran KM, Raven MC, Rosenheck RA. What drives frequent emergency department use in an integrated health system? National data from the Veterans Health Administration. *Ann Emerg Med*. 2013;62(2):151–159.

27. Shortt SE, Hwang S, Stuart H, Bedore M, Zurba M, Darling M. Delivering primary care to homeless persons: A policy analysis approach to evaluating the options. *Health Policy*. 2008;4(1):108–122.

28. Hewett NC. How to provide for the primary health care needs of homeless people: What do homeless people in Leicester think? *Br J Gen Pract*. 1999;49(447):819.

29. Han B, Wells BL. Inappropriate emergency department visits and use of the Health Care for the Homeless Program services by homeless adults in the northeastern United States. *J Public Health Manag Pract*. 2003;9(6):530–537.

30. McGuire J, Gelberg L, Blue-Howell J, Rosenheck RA. Access to primary care for homeless veterans with serious mental illness or substance abuse: A follow-up evaluation of co-located primary care and homeless social services. *Adm Policy Ment Health*. 2009;36(4):255–264.

31. O'Toole TP, Bourgault C, Johnson EE, et al. New to care: Demands on a health system when homeless veterans are enrolled in a medical home model. *Am J Public Health*. 2013;103(suppl 2):s374–s379.

32. Johnson EE, Borgia M, Rose J, O'Toole TP. No wrong door: Can clinical care facilitate veteran engagement in housing services? *Psychol Serv*. 2017;14(2):167–173.

33. https:www.bphc.hrsa.gov. Accessed December 6, 2017.

34. McMurray-Avilla M. *Organizing Health Services for Homeless People*. Nashville, TN: National Health Care for the Homeless Council; 1997.

35. https://www.nhchc.org. Accessed December 6, 2017.

36. O'Toole TP, Johnson EE, Aiello R, Kane V, Pape L. Tailoring care to vulnerable populations by incorporating social determinants of health: The Veterans Health Administration's "Homeless Patient Aligned Care Team" program. *Prev Chronic Dis*. 2016;13:e44.

37. Gundlapalli A, Petty W, Fargo J, Johnson EE, O'Toole TP. Patient aligned care team engagement to connect veterans experiencing homelessness with appropriate healthcare. *Med Care*. 2017;55(suppl 9/suppl 2):s104–s110.

38. O'Toole TP, Johnson EE, Borgia M, Yoon J, Lo J, Gelhert EH. Does population-tailored care for homeless veterans impact acute care use, cost, and satisfaction? Results from a prospective quasi-experimental trial. *Prev Chronic Dis*. 2018;15:E23.

39. Gelberg L, Anderson RM, Leake BD. The Behavioral Model for Vulnerable Populations: Application to medical care use and outcomes for homeless people. *Health Serv Res*. 2000;34(6):1273–1302.

40. O'Toole TP, Pollini RA, Ford D, Bigelow G. Physical health as a motivator for substance abuse treatment: is it enough to keep them in treatment? *J Subst Abuse Treat*. 2006;31(2):143–150.

41. McInnes DK, Petrakis BA, Gifford AL, et al. Retaining homeless veterans in outpatient care: A pilot study of mobile phone text message appointment reminders. *Am J Public Health*. 2014;104(suppl 4):s588–s594.

42. Yoon J, Lo J, Gelhert EH, Johnson EE, O'Toole TP. Homeless veterans use of peer mentors and effects on costs and utilization in VA clinics. *Psychiatr Serv*. 2017;68(6):628–631.

43. Alford DP, LaBelle CT, Richardson JM, et al. Treating homeless opioid dependent patients with buprenorphine in an office-based setting. *J Gen Intern Med*. 2007;22(2):171–176.

44. Noska A, Loomis T, Belperio P, O'Toole TP, Backus L. Engagement in hepatitis C care cascade among homeless veterans, 2015. *Public Health Rep*. 2017;132(2):136–139.

45. O'Toole TP, Roberts CB, Johnson EE. Screening for food insecurity in clinical settings: More than getting food. Findings from a clinical screener piloted in six national Veterans Affairs clinics, June–December 2015. *Prev Chronic Dis*. 2017;14:E04.

# 5

# Supported Housing

## Twenty-Five Years of the Housing and Urban Development–Veterans Affairs Supported Housing (HUD-VASH) Program

MARIA J. O'CONNELL AND ROBERT A. ROSENHECK

A decent provision for the poor is the true test of civilization.
—Samuel Johnson, *Boswell: Life of Johnson*

## Introduction

Supportive housing, in which housing rent subsidies are combined with clinical case management, has emerged in recent years as one of the most effective and most valued treatment approaches for helping homeless adults with psychiatric and/or addictive disorders to exit from homelessness and join mainstream community life. Jointly initiated by the U.S. Department of Housing and Urban Development (HUD) and the Veterans Health Administration (VHA) in the early 1990s, the Housing and Urban Development and Veterans Affairs Supportive Housing (HUD-VASH) program is, by far, the largest supportive housing initiative, anywhere, for any group of homeless persons worldwide. Now a major VHA vehicle for ending homelessness among Veterans, HUD-VASH has been implemented across the United States to further the public health goal of ending homelessness among Veterans. The HUD-VASH program now provides Housing Choice rental subsidies and supportive case management services to more than 80,000 Veterans nationwide each year and has assisted more than 146,000 Veterans since a major expansion of the program was initiated in 2008. It has been estimated that since 2010, homelessness among Veterans has declined by more than 50% (U.S. Department of Veterans Affairs, 2016; https://www.va.gov/opa/pressrel/pressrelease.cfm?id=2805), a decline that federal officials have attributed to the success of the HUD-VASH program.

In this chapter, we begin with a brief review of the policy history surrounding the development and evolution of the HUD-VASH program, review major findings from more than 25 years of HUD-VASH research, and conclude with a discussion of possible future initiatives for the HUD-VASH program and the Veterans it serves.

## Policy and Program Origins

The roots of HUD-VASH can be traced back to three developments in the 1980s: (1) a growing recognition and visibility of homelessness among Americans and specifically among Veterans, at a time of especially strong concern about hardships among Vietnam-era Veterans; (2) an ongoing movement that viewed housing as a critical social service for people with serious mental illness, particularly those who are homeless; and (3) recognition that there was a need to strengthen community-based and rehabilitative services provided by the VHA. In 1987, Congress passed the McKinney Act (later renamed the McKinney-Vento Act), which created the Interagency Council on Homelessness charged with overseeing major federal initiatives to fund emergency and temporary homeless assistance programs (http://www.nationalhomeless.org/publications/facts/McKinney.pdf). Simultaneously, through congressional legislation, the VHA launched two national initiatives to address the needs of homeless Veterans: the 43-site Homeless Chronically Mentally Ill (HCMI) Veterans program and the 23-site Domiciliary Care for Homeless Veterans (DCHV) program. These programs, designed to offer diverse clinical services and time-limited transitional residential treatment, assisted more than 40,000 homeless Veterans during the first four years of operation (Rosenheck, 1992). Yet, as with other programs under the McKinney-Vento Act, permanent supportive housing to which Veterans could transition had not been developed and thus was not included.

After the first set of HCMI and DCHV evaluation results were compiled, a meeting of VA and non-VA experts was convened to plan the next steps in program development. Consultants from the Robert Wood Johnson Foundation program on Chronic Mental Illness and the HUD Special Needs Assistance Programs (SNAPS) office met with VA leaders and program evaluators to consider ways of furthering their efforts to assist homeless Veterans (Personal communication from RR). Strong recommendations were made to combine VHA outreach and case management efforts with HUD housing rental subsidies. In the spring of 1992, the HUD-VASH program emerged as a demonstration project to be implemented at 19 HCMI and DCHV sites nationwide—all of which participated in a national program evaluation and four of which participated in a randomized clinical trial (RCT). HUD set aside 750 Housing Choice housing vouchers, administered through the Local Public Housing Authorities, to cover the portion of the local fair market rent that exceeded 30% of the Veteran's income (Kasprow et al., 2000). The VA's Health Care for Homeless Veterans (HCHV) program provided intensive case management (ICM), along with housing development and procurement assistance, to support Veterans receiving the vouchers. Using a modified Assertive Community Treatment (ACT) model, case managers delivered community-based care and provided linkages to VA and non-VA services, including employment and substance abuse counseling, to a targeted caseload of 25 Veterans, and weekly face-to-face contact was encouraged (Kasprow, Rosenheck, Frisman, & DiLella, 2000).

HUD-VASH differed from the clinic-based staged or transitional housing models that were common at the time, through which individuals proceeded toward independent housing conditional on completion of more structured or supervised time-limited residential or skills-training programs after which they were presumed to have demonstrated "housing readiness." HUD-VASH, in contrast, emphasized *direct and rapid placement* into permanent housing of the Veteran's *choice*, offered the availability of *sustained ICM* and other rehabilitation services as long as needed while Veterans were in independent housing (or if they lost their housing and needed help finding a new place to live), and there were *no formal requirements at the national programmatic level to maintain sobriety* before or after being housed or to participate in clinical programs other than basic involvement with case managers, except as required by HUD regulations. Some local programs, nevertheless, added some restrictive policies, reflecting caution about adopting new approaches to Veteran care.

To be eligible for HUD-VASH, a Veteran needed to meet the McKinney-Vento definition of homelessness: "lacking a fixed, regular, adequate nighttime residence or identifying his/her primary residence as a shelter, hotel, temporary or transitional housing, or public or private placement" (Public Law 100-77) for at least one month and have a documented mental health or substance abuse problem (Kasprow et al., 2000). However, by agreement with HUD, preference was given to Veterans living on the street rather than in shelters. Over the next several years, the HUD Housing Choice allocation increased through additional congressional legislation, and HUD-VASH developed a capacity to provide nearly 1,800 Veterans with supportive housing services at any given time.

An RCT of HUD-VASH, designed and implemented by the VA Northeast Program Evaluation Center, which was responsible for evaluating all VA homeless programs at the time, provided rigorous scientific data on the program's effectiveness and cost. Experimental data came from 460 homeless Veterans with psychiatric and/or substance abuse disorders who were randomly assigned to one of three groups: (1) HUD-VASH, consisting of access to Housing Choice housing vouchers and ICM ($n = 182$); (2) ICM only (without access to housing vouchers, $n = 90$); and (3) standard VA care ($n = 188$) (Rosenheck, Kasprow,

Frisman, & Liu-Mares, 2003). The RCT sought to evaluate the overall cost-effectiveness of the program and the housing, clinical, and social outcomes associated with the voucher and the ICM services provided. Findings from the RCT and observational program evaluation on all participants during the first decade of program operation (O'Connell et al., 2010) demonstrated that providing housing through rental subsidies was more effective and had many other benefits than usual care and ICM without rental subsidies. In the experimental trial, 78.6% of HUD-VASH participants received their housing voucher (vs. less than 5% in the comparison conditions), and HUD-VASH participants were housed an average of 140 days earlier than those assigned to ICM only and 100 days before those assigned to standard care (Rosenheck et al., 2003). Nationally, 87.5% of Veterans who were enrolled in the program and 85% of Veterans who obtained a Housing Choice housing voucher through HUD-VASH were eventually housed (Kasprow et al., 2000; O'Connell, Kasprow, & Rosenheck, 2008, 2010; O'Connell, Rosenheck, Kasprow, & Frisman, 2006). Approximately 84% of Veterans housed through HUD-VASH were housed within the first year of enrollment (Kasprow et al., 2000), and 66% were housed within the first three months of the program (O'Connell et al., 2010; O'Connell, Kasprow, & Rosenheck, 2013). Although modestly more expensive, the benefits were such that when they were compared with the costs of the program, HUD-VASH not only was cost-effective (i.e., benefits in days housed justified additional costs) but also was superior to other interventions that did not include rental subsidies in reducing homelessness, increasing social support, therapeutic alliance, and reducing substance use (Cheng, Lin, Kasprow, & Rosenheck, 2007; Rosenheck et al., 2003). By 2003, these original housing vouchers had assisted 2,950 homeless Veterans in accessing safe, affordable, and permanent housing at 36 sites nationwide, many of whom had moved on to permanent unsubsidized housing (O'Connell et al., 2008, 2010).

Analysis of entry data showed that out of 65,424 Veterans screened for the HCHV program nationally during the period of program implementation, more than 60% ($n$ = 39,752) met HUD-VASH eligibility criteria (Kasprow et al., 2000). Yet only 1,750 Housing Choice housing vouchers had been allocated to the HUD-VASH program, and as a result, only 7% of eligible Veterans could be referred to HUD-VASH ($n$ = 2,798). Although no new housing vouchers had been allocated to the program in nearly 10 years, the story of HUD-VASH was far from over.

In the early 2000s, Congress was revisiting the problem of homelessness in America with a renewed interest in a finding a permanent solution to ending and preventing homelessness. Twenty federal agencies of the U.S. Interagency Council on Homelessness, with the VA prominent among them, launched research, policy, and budget initiatives to advance the goal of ending chronic homelessness. Among other initiatives, 11 awardees were funded in a demonstration program called the Collaborative Initiative on Chronic Homelessness (CICH) with VA leadership at all levels and active participation at all sites. CICH funded the development of integrated community partnerships of VA and non-VA programs to provide permanent housing and mainstream supports to homeless Veterans. After 12 months, CICH achieved an 85% housing retention rate (Mares & Rosenheck, 2007), and a substudy comparing CICH programs at four sites with comparable community programs found robust benefits in housing outcomes at little additional cost (Mares & Rosenheck, 2011).

In 2008, partially in response to broad-based concern about the well-being of returning Veterans of the Iraq and Afghanistan conflicts, a commitment was made to a major expansion of services for homeless Veterans. The VHA announced its determination to end homelessness among Veterans within five years, and HUD-VASH was central to the plan. By expanding the HUD-VASH program, with new allocations of vouchers and staff over several years, the target level of services rose to more than 80,000 Veterans each year. A three-phased strategy focused on (1) identifying Veterans who are homeless or at risk for becoming homeless through universal screening procedures, (2) addressing and preventing homelessness among families through the VA's Supportive Services for Veteran Families [SSVF] program (a grant program to community-based nonprofit organizations to provide temporary, immediate housing resources for Veterans and their families), and (3) providing permanent supportive housing to chronically homeless Veterans through HUD-VASH (Montgomery, 2016). In 2009, Congress passed the Homeless Emergency Assistance and Rapid Transition to Housing (HEARTH) Act, which broadened the McKinney-Vento definition of homelessness to include individuals who were living in transitional housing or were in imminent threat of losing their housing.

In 2010, *Opening Doors*, the first Federal Strategic Plan to Prevent and End Homelessness (U.S. Interagency Council on Homelessness, 2010), was published and influenced the VA's five-year plan to end Veteran homelessness by 2015. Several years later, HUD published the outcomes of its three-city, 12-month nonexperimental study of Housing First programs, reporting an 84% housing retention rate for 12 months (Henwood et al., 2015). And by July 2014, the 100K Homes Campaign, an initiative aiming 100,000 chronically homeless individuals into permanent housing, had achieved its goal through community collaboration to implement a Housing First approach. As researchers and policymakers watched the emergence of additional evidence for rapid-placement approaches to supportive housing among non-Veteran homeless adults, and specifically the Housing First program (Tsemberis, Gulcur, & Nakae, 2004), VHA leaders remained focused on HUD-VASH and its impact on the Veterans served.

# The VA Data Management and Performance Monitoring System

The evolution of HUD-VASH from what began as a pilot demonstration in 1992 to what has become the single largest and longest standing collaborative federal initiative to end homelessness has been shaped and informed by a wealth of national data from the VA's extensive and comprehensive data management and performance monitoring system. One of the unusual strengths of this system is the careful documentation and collection of outcome data beginning from the first point of contact with a Veteran and continuing through every step of housing procurement, retention, and discharge. These data extended beyond the initial timeframe of the RCT and included information about living situation, psychiatric symptoms, alcohol and drug use, quality of life, employment, income, criminal activity, and more, collected as frequently as every three months on every Veteran HUD-VASH participant during the implementation of the program and in the ensuing years. These data served to inform regular performance evaluations and feedback and would become one of the largest sources of longitudinal data on supportive housing. Since the initial publication of the HUD-VASH RCT, HUD-VASH researchers published 16 more outcome studies that demonstrated the value of HUD-VASH for Veterans with varied life experiences, clinical profiles, and networks of support, with equally positive housing outcomes for those with the most severe psychiatric illnesses, alcohol and/or drug use dependencies, and incarceration histories (see references). This body of research has both confirmed the original experimental findings published in 2003 and, with the inclusion of longitudinal data available beyond the original three-year study period and closer examination of specific vulnerable subgroups, has contributed new findings that have shed light on various aspects of supportive housing services generally, and researchers have been able to trace the paths of different trajectories in housing and socio-clinical outcomes, according to distinct characteristics of Veterans and programs. The evidence strongly supports the view that on average supportive housing was and is the most effective service model for assisting homeless Veterans and, more generally, homeless adults, although many individuals benefit from other intervention approaches as well. These positive results have also been observed in experimental studies of the Pathways to Housing program in New York (Tsemberis & Eisenberg, 2014; Tsemberis et al., 2004) and the At Home/Chez Soi program in Canada (Adair et al., 2016; Aubry et al., 2015, 2016; Goering & Streiner, 2015).

# HUD-VASH Officially Adopts Housing First

Although many HUD-VASH programs already employed a model similar to Housing First (Tsai, 2014), in 2012, VA officially adopted Housing First as its guiding model for HUD-VASH. The transition to Housing First, as reported by qualitative research efforts, was not easy. Philosophical and attitudinal barriers, operational issues, resource issues, and tight rental markets were observed to pose significant challenges to meeting both the goal of implementing Housing First and the VA's larger goal of ending Veteran homelessness by 2015 (Austin et al., 2014; Austin, Pollio, & Kertesz, 2016). Although funds were available from the housing vouchers to pay rent, resources were not formally provided for the inevitable move-in costs and, in some cases, for enough case managers to support Veterans in their transition. Staff-to-client ratios were reported to be high, and researchers reported that many sites struggled to meet client needs when a crisis occurred. Achieving fidelity to the Housing First principles was reported to be modest at best (Kertesz et al., 2017). As opposed to the ideal Housing First model, which relies strongly on a team-based approach whereby intensity can be adjusted and shared according to client needs, qualitative research suggested the predominance of an approach largely based on individual responsibility (Austin et al., 2016). Some have suggested that with such "intensive focus on housing veterans, case management and follow-up support for veterans may have fallen to the wayside" after they were housed (Tsai, 2014).

In some ways, the current qualitative research on HUD-VASH presents itself as addressing a different set of issues than the original HUD-VASH research agenda, which was focused on measurement of process, outcomes, and cost-effectiveness. This more recent research has sought to evaluate the match between the capacity of the housing market, the health service system, and needs of Veterans. As noted earlier, a qualitative evaluation suggested that the large-scale Housing First implementation project may require significant additional resources "to assure that results are concordant with those found in previous research" (Kertesz et al., 2017).

Despite the implementation challenges identified through qualitative research, by expanding both HUD-VASH and the VA's transitional housing programs and implementing new programs dedicated to preventing and ending homelessness, the VA reported a 35% decrease in the number of homeless Veterans between 2009 and 2015 (U.S. Department of Housing and Urban Development, 2015), which then increased by nearly 47% by 2017 (U.S. Department of Housing and Urban Development, 2017).

In the remainder of this chapter, we briefly review some of the major findings from the HUD-VASH program, including (1) data on service delivery and housing, social, and clinical outcomes; (2) outcomes among particular vulnerable subgroups; and (3) variation in fidelity to and outcomes associated with four key HUD-VASH and Housing First principles (i.e., rapid and direct housing, choice in housing, availability of flexible and comprehensive supports, and no preconditions for sobriety). Although there have been several other studies that similarly demonstrated the effectiveness of supported housing (Adair et al., 2016; Aubry et al., 2015, 2016; Goering & Streiner, 2015; Tsemberis & Eisenberg, 2014; Tsemberis et al., 2004), they do not pertain to Veterans in particular and thus are not reviewed here.

## HUD-VASH Outcomes

### HOUSING OUTCOMES

In addition to the more rapid procurement of housing through HUD-VASH (as noted earlier), HUD-VASH participants have demonstrated greater stability in housing. Results from the experimental trial show that, at the three-year follow-up, HUD-VASH participants in the RCT had been housed altogether for 16% more days than those assigned to ICM only and for 25% more days than those assigned to standard care (Rosenheck et al., 2003). HUD-VASH Veterans also experienced 35% fewer days homeless than participants in both groups (Rosenheck et al., 2003) (Figures 5.1 and 5.2) and had significantly longer periods of continuous housing (approximately 200 more days) compared with ICM and treatment as usual (TAU) (O'Connell et al., 2008).

Once housed, participants were documented to have continued in the program for an average of 940 days (2.6 years) (O'Connell et al., 2010), and 78% remained housed throughout the study. Over a five-year follow-up period, 172 (44%) of those Veterans who had been housed had lost their housing for a period of at least one day (most of whom were rehoused by the program), commonly within the first 6 months of housing (O'Connell et al., 2008). Predictors of continuous housing without any interruption included having a psychiatric disorder at intake and more psychiatric symptoms at the time of housing, perhaps reflecting the fact that psychological distress can strengthen motivation for continued program participation.

In 2014, a study was published on the use of vouchers, with varying levels of case management (as contrasted with the HUD-VASH experimental trial, in which rental subsidies varied and case management was held constant in two groups), with a comparison to standard care as a third condition. This study compared HUD-VASH voucher holders who received ICM services with voucher holders who did not receive additional ICM (Patterson, Nochajski, & Wu, 2014). Results suggest that voucher holders with ICM lived in better neighborhoods and that white voucher holders, in general, found housing in higher quality neighborhoods than African Americans. But for African Americans, being in the

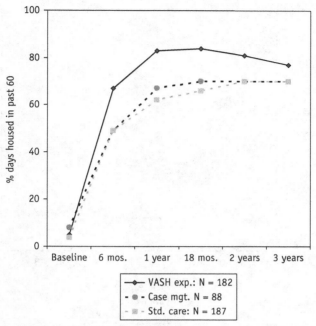

*Figure 5.1* Outcomes in the HUD-VASH program: percentage of days housed in the past 60 days. From Rosenheck, R. A., Kasprow, W., Frisman, L., & Liu-Mares, W. (2003). Cost-effectiveness of supported housing for homeless persons with mental illness. *Arch Gen Psychiatry, 60*(9), 940–951.

HUD-VASH program increased the likelihood of being housed in a higher quality neighborhood.

Not only did HUD-VASH significantly improve the likelihood of exiting from homeless, but it also reduced the risk for loss of housing after it was obtained. A separate study of the risk of losing housing after exiting from homelessness in the RCT showed that HUD-VASH participants were at 87% lower risk for loss of housing after they had obtained it than Veterans assigned to the ICM-only group and at 76% lower risk for losing housing than those assigned to standard care. The strongest predictors of loss of housing/discontinuous housing were drug use and a diagnosis of post-traumatic stress disorder (O'Connell et al., 2008).

HUD-VASH was not intended to foster lifelong program participation but rather, in the long run, to foster independent program-free living. At the five-year follow-up, three-fourths of the Veterans who had entered HUD-VASH had terminated their involvement in the program, at a rate of approximately 25% a year. However, 82% of those who terminated were reported to have been housed at the time of program exit. Thus, it appears that most of these Veterans had transitioned to other, potentially more independent housing (O'Connell et al., 2010). Twenty-nine percent of Veterans retained their Housing Choice housing

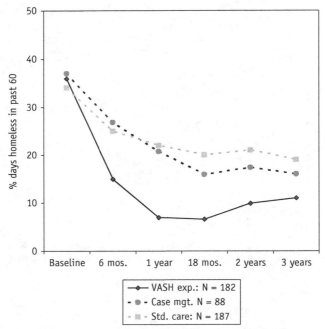

*Figure 5.2* Outcomes in the HUD-VASH program: percentage of days housed in past 60 days. From Rosenheck, R. A., Kasprow, W., Frisman, L., & Liu-Mares, W. (2003). Cost-effectiveness of supported housing for homeless persons with mental illness. *Arch Gen Psychiatry, 60*(9), 940–951.

voucher after leaving the HUD-VASH program, 45% lost their voucher, and only 19% returned to homelessness or to an unknown type of housing after exiting HUD-VASH (O'Connell et al., 2010). The most frequent reasons for termination were active substance use (31%) and losing the voucher due to having income that exceeded program limits (45%) (O'Connell et al., 2010). Most episodes of recurrent homelessness happened within the first year of housing.

Rates of housing retention among HUD-VASH participants in more recent studies are similar to those found in the program from the 1990s. The most recent published information reports that 45,834 Veterans have exited HUD-VASH after becoming housed, and 85% of them moved into permanent housing (Montgomery et al., 2016). The most common single reason for exiting the program was having accomplished both housing and service goals (*n* = 15,462, 33%). Approximately 10% of Veterans left the program because of an eviction. Veterans who exited HUD-VASH for more positive reasons stayed in the program an average of 40% longer than those who were evicted from their housing (an average of 27 months compared with 19 months) (Montgomery, Cusack, Szymkowiak, Fargo, & O'Toole, 2017). Exiting because of goal accomplishment was associated with greater use of primary care and more case manager contact before exit (Montgomery et al., 2017). Those who were evicted from their HUD-VASH housing appeared to have had more serious recent problems of various types and were more likely to be male and younger; received more acute care for medical, mental health, and substance use problems in the 90 days before exit; were more likely to have had a mental health and/or substance use inpatient admission in the 30 days before eviction, and were more likely to have used acute care of any type in the period before exiting (Montgomery et al., 2017). Having a substance use disorder raised the odds of eviction by 150%. The use of outpatient care, with the exception of substance use treatment, was a protective factor against eviction.

In an earlier study restricted to four sites, 87% of Veterans retained their housing for at least one year, and 60% retained housing for at least two years. More than 50% of those who left the program did so successfully, and 93% of Veterans who left housing did not access a VA homeless program within the next year (Montgomery & Cusack, 2017). Veterans who left HUD-VASH generally did not return to homelessness within one year, and only 11.3% accessed a VA homeless program within the first 360 days after leaving. Among evictees, 33.6% returned to homelessness compared with only 8.8% of those who left their housing for other reasons, with nearly half of these accessing a transitional residential program. Veterans who exited because of eviction also returned to homelessness more quickly (average of 122 days) than those who exited for other reasons (average of 139 days). Time to return to homelessness was predicted by eviction, mental health, and substance use inpatient admissions and emergency department use in the first 90 days after exiting. Receipt of outpatient substance use treatment, mental health inpatient treatment, emergency department visits, and a diagnosis of schizophrenia were associated with increased risk for returning to homelessness, while greater age and receipt of outpatient medical services in the 91 to 180 days after exiting were protective factors (Cusack & Montgomery, 2017). Thus, eviction appears to be a negative outcome associated with diverse indications of serious health and mental health problems.

## CLINICAL OUTCOMES

HUD-VASH has been associated with significant reductions in substance and alcohol use. A secondary analysis that examined more extensive data on five-year outcomes from experimental and observational samples, using multiple imputation techniques to address the potential bias introduced by greater rate of study attrition among substance users, found specifically that they reported drinking alcohol and using drugs on significantly fewer days than ICM-only and standard care participants (Cheng et al., 2007).

## COMMUNITY ADJUSTMENT OUTCOMES

The results pertaining to employment suggest that having a housing subsidy may reduce incentive for employment, as has been found in other public support programs, including the VA service–connected compensation program (Drew et al., 2001; Greenberg & Rosenheck, 2007; Rosenheck, Frisman, & Sindelar, 1995). Being housed *without* a voucher (i.e., among controls in the RCT) at three months was associated with significantly more days worked and greater likelihood of being employed than Veterans housed with a voucher or not yet housed (Drew et al., 2001; Greenberg & Rosenheck, 2007; Rosenheck et al., 1995; Tsai, Kasprow, & Rosenheck, 2011).

## SOCIOEMOTIONAL OUTCOMES

There is also evidence that the voucher, in and of itself, may be a key contributor to enhanced quality of life and greater social support among homeless Veterans. In the RCT, HUD-VASH participants reported higher overall quality of life than ICM-only participants across the three-year period (O'Connell et al., 2008; Rosenheck et al., 2003). HUD-VASH participants also reported significantly higher satisfaction with their living situation, with their family relations, and with finances, health, and social relationships than those assigned to ICM over the three-year period (Rosenheck et al., 2003). Being housed with a voucher, regardless of condition, was associated with significantly higher quality of life, greater satisfaction with their living situation, and a greater sense of safety than being housed without a voucher or not housed at all (Tsai, Kasprow, et al., 2011). Quality of life was further enhanced for Veterans who obtained their desired features in the housing procured (O'Connell et al., 2006).

In the RCT, HUD-VASH Veterans reported having more social contacts and higher overall social support than ICM-only participants and larger social networks than ICM-only and standard care participants over the three-year observation period (Rosenheck et al., 2003). Greater social support was also associated with having more positive housing features obtained in housing at one year (O'Connell et al., 2006) and not reporting a history of abuse as a child at three months (Tsai & Rosenheck, 2013).

Although no significant differences were found in the RCT between HUD-VASH and comparison groups on psychiatric symptoms, medical issues, or community adjustment outcomes (Rosenheck et al., 2003), subsequent subgroup analyses did reveal some improvements in these areas among certain subgroups of individuals. These and other key findings among vulnerable subgroups are examined next.

## VULNERABLE SUBGROUPS

While HUD-VASH has empirically demonstrated success in helping homeless Veterans achieve positive housing and socio-clinical outcomes, these data do not address the experience of specific, potentially vulnerable subgroups of Veterans enrolled in the program.

The extensive data available on Veterans enrolled in HUD-VASH over the past 25 years have allowed researchers to examine multiple subgroups of Veterans who may be particularly vulnerable to experiencing poorer outcomes. Potentially vulnerable subgroups were identified based on previous research on sociodemographic disparities in treatment and outcomes (e.g., race, ethnicity), differences in philosophical viewpoints on supported housing (i.e., treatment first or housing first for persons with substance use disorders), growing segments of the Veteran population (e.g., females and older adults), differences in severity or type of illnesses (e.g., Veterans with severe mental illness or co-occurring substance and mental health disorders), and other factors that may lead an individual to be excluded from mainstream public housing or otherwise considered "high risk" (i.e., criminal justice history, length of time homeless, having limited social support).

Post hoc subgroup analysis of data from the experimental trial revealed that HUD-VASH had an equally positive impact on housing outcomes for all enrolled Veterans, regardless of severity of mental illness, co-occurring substance use disorders, length of time homeless, race or ethnicity, or level of social support (Rosenheck et al., 2003). Thus, for Veterans in each of the subpopulations examined, housing outcomes in HUD-VASH were superior to the comparison conditions, as was found for the larger sample.

Since this initial study, several secondary analytic studies have contributed further to our understanding of the differential impact HUD-VASH may have on specific vulnerable subgroups of Veterans using both interactional subgroup analyses and separate subgroup comparisons. These findings, along with specific vulnerabilities associated with each subgroup, are described next.

### Race

African Americans in the HUD-VASH program may experience slightly better social, clinical, and functional outcomes than Whites and may reside in higher quality neighborhoods, although both groups experience similar improvements in housing tenure. Research on the general population of people with mental illness has shown that in many studies compared with Whites, African Americans experience poorer access to health care, have greater unmet needs for mental health and substance abuse treatment, and most important in the context of HUD-VASH, have been subject to housing discrimination (Alegria, Canino, & Rios, 2004; Alegria et al., 2002; Wells, Klap, Koike, & Sherbourne, 2001).

A subgroup analysis of national observational data from Veterans enrolled in HUD-VASH in the 1990s found that, after controlling for significant baseline differences, African Americans experienced significantly less severe psychiatric symptoms, less alcohol use, and fewer days of drug use than Whites enrolled in HUD-VASH over a two-year follow-up period (O'Connell, Kasprow, & Rosenheck, 2012). Compared with Whites, HUD-VASH appeared to have slightly less impact on reducing days of homelessness over time for African Americans but had a significantly greater positive impact on reducing days spent in institutions, reductions in drug use, increases in employment, and improvements in quality of life. Another recent study suggests that African Americans housed through HUD-VASH may be housed in higher quality, more desirable neighborhoods than African Americans housed through traditional Housing Choice housing vouchers (Patterson et al., 2014).

## Gender
Subgroup analyses of male versus female Veterans enrolled in HUD-VASH in 2012 found no differences in attrition or main housing outcomes, although females were more rapidly admitted into the program and case managers provided more services related to employment and income than male Veterans (Tsai, Rosenheck, & Kane, 2014). Women are the fastest growing segment of the Veteran population (Blackstock, Haskell, Brandt, & Desai, 2012; Meehan, 2006), and female Veterans are twice as likely to be homeless as non-Veteran females (Gamache, Rosenheck, & Tessler, 2003). In a system that historically serves a predominantly male population of Veterans, a high value has been placed on the goal that the VA should understand and attend to the specific needs and concerns of female Veterans. HUD-VASH research has contributed to this understanding. Although additional data are needed to further our understanding of how and why employment and income may be more of a focus for female Veterans, as well as the impact this may have on longitudinal outcomes, observational data suggest that one factor may be related to the fact that a significant portion of female Veterans have children in their custody (Tsai, Rosenheck, Kasprow, & Kane, 2015).

## Age
HUD-VASH research has not identified disparities in housing or clinical outcomes among older versus younger Veterans (O'Connell et al., 2012). Both groups experience similar benefits of HUD-VASH. Surprisingly, despite expected increases in medical comorbidities among older Veterans, an evaluation of service use and cost data associated with HUD-VASH in FY 2010 did not reveal patterns of service use or cost that differed from the larger population of HUD-VASH Veterans (Byrne, Roberts, Culhane, & Kane, 2014). The population of Veterans is diverse not only in terms of gender but also in terms of age. It is

estimated that 42% of Veterans treated by the VHA are now older than 65 years. Older adults may be at high risk for homelessness because of reductions in social support due to death of spouses and friends, increased isolation, lack of availability of appropriate medical and social services, and increases in comorbid medical conditions (Crane & Warnes, 2010).

## Incarceration History

While it is well established that past incarceration is a major risk factor for homelessness (Greenberg & Rosenheck, 2008), history of incarceration has not been found to have significant impact on housing outcomes in HUD-VASH. In a study conducted on Veterans who entered the HUD-VASH program in 2008 and 2009 (Greenberg & Rosenheck, 2008; Tsai, Kasprow, & Rosenheck, 2014), a majority of Veterans (65%) had a history of incarceration. Although Veterans with incarceration histories were more likely to experience a host of additional difficulties, including greater alcohol and drug use, chronic homelessness, and psychotic disorders at the time of program entry, subgroup analysis has found that Veterans with incarceration histories are housed at only slightly lower rates than those without incarceration histories. Although having a longer incarceration history (more than one year of incarceration) was associated with a two-week delay in moving into housing, the total mean days from admission to move-in and one-year housing outcomes were similar across groups. Another HUD-VASH study found that after adjusting for baseline characteristics and site, history of incarceration did not appear to adversely affect therapeutic alliance, progression through the housing procurement process, or eventually obtaining housing (Tejani, Rosenheck, Tsai, Kasprow, & McGuire, 2014).

## Co-occurring Mental Health and Substance Use Disorders

Despite significant comorbidity of mental health and substance use disorders among persons who are homeless, as well as poorer outcomes associated with comorbidity, HUD-VASH research has found that individuals with co-occurring disorders benefit significantly *more* from HUD-VASH in reductions in homelessness. Early models of supportive housing were geared toward addressing behavioral health needs, with significant demarcations between mental health and substance use treatment. Fortunately, today's systems of care are more integrated and offer more holistic, coordinated treatment for individuals with co-occurring mental health and substance use disorders. However, most supportive housing research to date has not examined differential effects on persons living with co-occurring disorders compared with those living with a singular mental health or substance use disorder. A widely read commentary on supportive housing suggested that individuals with addictive disorders may have more positive housing outcomes in housing models that emphasize rapid placement into housing regardless of continued substance use, but they may have more positive clinical outcomes in models that address treatment issues before housing is secure (Kertesz, 2009). Again, extensive data on Veterans enrolled in HUD-VASH over the years have allowed researchers to begin exploring differential effects that may occur.

In particular, one study of Veterans enrolled in HUD-VASH in the 1990s observational sample compared Veterans with co-occurring disorders to Veterans with a substance use disorder only (O'Connell et al., 2012). This research found that for individuals with co-occurring disorders (i.e., mental health and substance use disorders), HUD-VASH had a more positive impact on reducing days homeless compared with HUD-VASH enrollees without a co-occurring disorder, despite fewer days housed, greater psychiatric symptoms, and lower quality of life than their counterpart without co-occurring disorders.

The evaluation of the HUD-VASH supportive housing program has thus systematically evaluated outcomes for diverse vulnerable subgroups and found that all have shown improvements in housing and many clinical outcomes during the period of their participation in the program. Interactional subgroup analyses shows significantly greater benefits for some subgroups, particularly active alcohol or drug users, on some key clinical outcomes. We now turn our attention to an examination of four key principals of HUD-VASH and Housing First models of housing.

## PRINCIPLE 1: DIRECT AND RAPID PLACEMENT INTO PERMANENT HOUSING

Although a key feature of HUD-VASH has been an emphasis on rapid placement into community housing, recent expansion efforts and the formal adoption of Housing First as the HUD-VASH program's guiding model have made rapid placement into permanent housing an even higher priority. Results of a demonstration project at a single site compared processing times and outcomes between two HUD-VASH programs—one that was implementing a Housing First model and one that was providing standard HUD-VASH treatment as usual—suggest that the Housing First model may be associated with shorter housing procurement times and better housing retention rates than standard HUD-VASH programming (Montgomery, Hill, Kane, & Culhane, 2013). This observational study found that Veterans in the Housing First program were housed, on average, six months sooner and were eight times more likely to retain their housing for 12 months (98% vs. 86%) than Veterans in the standard HUD-VASH model of care program.

Although these findings suggest strong support in favor of the VA's transition to the Housing First model as policy, a comparison of these limited data with those from national HUD-VASH programming over three different HUD-VASH implementation periods (Figure 5.3) suggests that these dramatic findings may

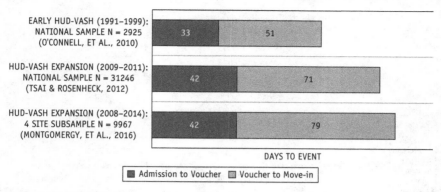

EARLY HUD-VASH (1991–1999):
NATIONAL SAMPLE N = 2925
(O'CONNELL, ET AL., 2010)

33    51

HUD-VASH EXPANSION (2009–2011):
NATIONAL SAMPLE N = 31246
(TSAI & ROSENHECK, 2012)

42    71

HUD-VASH EXPANSION (2008–2014):
4 SITE SUBSAMPLE N = 9967
(MONTGOMERGY, ET AL., 2016)

42    79

DAYS TO EVENT

■ Admission to Voucher  ▨ Voucher to Move-in

*Figure 5.3* HUD-VASH processing times.

not be representative of the operation of the program more widely. Despite the shift in policy toward more immediate placement with few preconditions, the average time to placement appears to have expanded by almost 50% from an average of 84 days during the 1990s to more than 120 days in subsequent years.

One aspect that seems to have changed since the initial implementation of HUD-VASH is the amount of time it takes from initial point of contact of a homeless Veteran with the VHA to admission into the program. Figure 5.4 shows that in early HUD-VASH, this was the longest period of the procurement process, averaging between five and six months. Time to enrollment was hindered by the limited number of available vouchers and local tendencies to place Veterans with needs for substance abuse treatment in residential treatment before housing (O'Connell, Kasprow, & Rosenheck, 2009). Evaluation of data from selected HUD-VASH expansion sites suggests that this time period has been cut to less than two weeks (Montgomery et al., 2016). Research from all periods of HUD-VASH implementation suggests individual predictors of more rapid placement in housing, including not having a service-connected disability, having a drug use disorder, having more numerous case management contacts between admission and public housing referral, and more case manager contacts between receipt of the voucher and moving in to an apartment (Montgomery et al., 2016).

However, above and beyond any Veteran or service characteristics, researchers have found that the single greatest contributor to variance in time to housing is program site (O'Connell et al., 2010; Tsai, O'Connell, Kasprow, & Rosenheck, 2011). Fastest procurement rates were found, at the time of a 2010 review of recent experience, at relatively newer program sites or those that have been in existence the longest (Tsai, O'Connell, et al., 2011). Recent qualitative research on HUD-VASH's adoption of Housing First at eight sites suggests that site- and location-specific factors such as the availability of suitable housing, relationships with Public Housing Authorities, and the availability of move-in

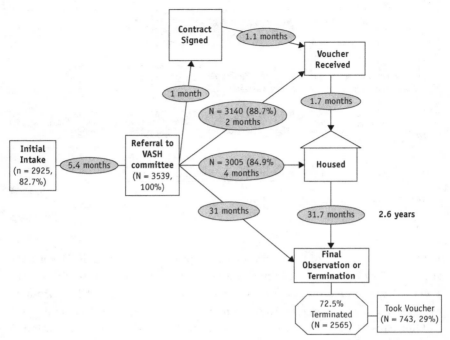

*Figure 5.4* Time through the housing procurement process. From O'Connell, M. J., Kasprow, W. J., & Rosenheck, R. A. (2010). National dissemination of supported housing in the VA: Model adherence versus model modification. *Psychiatric Rehabil J, 33*(4), 308–319.

funds may contribute to these site-level differences (Austin et al., 2014, 2016; Kertesz et al., 2017; Kertesz et al., 2014).

## Residential Treatment Before Housing

In an analysis of observational data from the early HUD-VASH implementation period, out of 589 Veterans who had been housed through HUD-VASH nationally, 31% (*n* = 183) had spent the majority of the 90-day period before being housed exclusively in a VA residential treatment program, and 24% (*n* = 139) had spent the majority of the 90-day period before housing in literally homeless conditions; that is, they went straight from the street to housing as in Housing First (O'Connell et al., 2009) with other Veterans residing in a mixtures of settings. It had been decided that although the program was designed to take Veterans directly from the street to their own apartments, it would be unfair to exclude those who had been admitted to residential treatment. The comparison of Housing First and "housing second" approaches showed that individuals who went directly into an apartment from homelessness (Housing First) were significantly older, had more income, were more likely to have public support, spent fewer days intoxicated in the 30 days before intake, used more VA services in the 6 months before intake, and had more serious psychiatric problems than those who spent time in residential treatment settings before being housed ("housing second"). Those who were in residential treatment were more likely to have a recent history of substance use but were also more likely to report abstinence from alcohol and drugs just before housing (i.e., after residential treatment) (O'Connell et al., 2013).

In terms of outcomes, psychiatric symptoms and quality of life improved over time for both direct placement and treatment-first conditions, although Veterans entering housing directly from homelessness experienced smaller improvements in quality of life (O'Connell et al., 2009). Veterans going directly into housing from homelessness also had less improvement in social contacts over time than those who were housed from a residential treatment setting (O'Connell et al., 2009). Veterans who went into housing from a residential treatment facility continued to use significantly more inpatient services than those being housed directly from the homeless condition on the street (223 days vs. 48 days) (O'Connell et al., 2009). Veterans who went directly into housing from homelessness used more outpatient services before and after intake into the program than those who spent time in residential treatment settings before housing (O'Connell et al., 2009).

## PRINCIPLE 2: NO FORMAL REQUIREMENTS TO MAINTAIN SOBRIETY BEFORE OR AFTER BEING HOUSED

Perhaps one of the most controversial differences between HUD-VASH and more traditional, staged models of supportive housing is the absence of absolute requirements for abstinence from alcohol and drugs before and during independent, community-based housing (Kertesz, Austin, Holmes, Pollio, & VanDeusen Lukas, 2015; Tsemberis & Asmussen, 1999; Tsemberis et al., 2004; Westermeyer, Lee, & Y Carr, 2015). In 2012, when HUD-VASH formally adopted Housing First as its guiding model, the VA made explicit its long-held value that HUD-VASH should provide individualized "low-demand" housing—meaning that there are limited preconditions for sobriety and participation in services, beyond a minimum level of case management. Although HUD-VASH will not exclude a Veteran from the program if he or she is actively using substances, the needs of individual Veterans are taken into consideration, and residential or inpatient substance use treatment may be recommended or encouraged if deemed necessary. Anecdotal observations from early HUD-VASH implementation data suggested that HUD-VASH committees were more likely to award vouchers to Veterans with some income and those who had recently completed substance use residential treatment (Kasprow et al., 2000). These data suggest that case managers, given the limited number of vouchers available at each site and faced with a large comprehensive set of VHA programs with a broad mandate, were reluctant to penalize Veterans who had entered residential treatment or domiciliary care because they were successfully pursuing recovery and employment.

The goal of "low-demand" or "harm-reduction" programs is to minimize the negative social, psychological, and physical consequences associated with alcohol or drug use. For some, this may be achieved through abstinence, but others may continue to use alcohol or drugs in a "safer," less harmful manner. A critical review of the research suggests that individuals with addictive disorders may have positive housing outcomes in Housing First models, but these programs may inadequately address substance use (Kertesz, 2009). One study of HUD-VASH Veterans suggests similar findings—those with substance use disorders experienced similar housing outcomes to those without substance use disorders, despite higher rates of continued substance use and related problems (Tsai, Kasprow, et al., 2014). However, this research does not take into account the impact that degree of substance or alcohol use (ranging from abstinence to daily use) may have on housing or clinical outcomes among those diagnosed with substance use disorders. The VA's philosophical decision not to exclude Veterans from housing because of substance use, combined with its rigorous and methodical data collection procedures, allowed researchers to examine, for the first time, whether active substance use impaired housing outcomes.

Research on subgroups of Veterans who were actively using substances at the time of entry into housing in the CICH and HUD-VASH supportive housing programs has demonstrated convincingly that active substance use, in and of itself, does not impede successful housing outcomes (Edens, Kasprow, Tsai, & Rosenheck, 2011; O'Connell et al., 2012, 2013). The first study (Edens et al., 2011) compared abstainers to high-frequency substance users (those who reported using alcohol or substances for more than 15 of the previous 30 days) in the CICH program. Edens and colleagues found no differences in the proportion of clients successfully housed or the duration of their maintenance of housing, despite higher rates of continued substance use and more severe psychiatric symptoms across a 24-month follow-up period. Thus, active substance users appear to have worse clinical outcomes, by several measures, than other Veterans, but have no worse long-term housing outcomes after entering a supported housing program. An additional study of CICH participants did find, however, that extensive users of amphetamines or cocaine, in particular, had poorer housing outcomes than other Veterans with active substance use (Edens, Tsai, & Rosenheck, 2014).

In 2012, O'Connell et al. examined two subgroups of HUD-VASH Veterans who reported active substance use—those reporting less than 15 days of alcohol or drug use out of the 30 days before baseline and those reporting more than 15 days of substance use (O'Connell et al., 2012). Veterans who used alcohol or drugs more than 15 days out of the 30 before intake (active substance users) had no worse outcomes on any housing or clinical outcomes over a three-year follow-up period than Veterans with no active substance use. Interaction analyses revealed, however, that active substance users in HUD-VASH had significantly *more* days housed and *fewer* days homeless than less active substance users compared with those enrolled in ICM. Active substance users in HUD-VASH also had significantly more social contacts than less active users in HUD-VASH compared with differences observed among those in the treatment-as-usual group. Thus, this highly vulnerable group seems to have benefited more from HUD-VASH than other Veterans on several outcomes, indicating that the extra assistance provided by HUD-VASH was especially helpful to these highly vulnerable Veterans.

A final study of substance use, published in 2013, found that moderate (1–14 days out of the past 30 days) and high-frequency users (15 or more days out of the past 30 days) *at the time of housing* had slightly more days homeless across a three-year follow-up period than abstainers (effect sizes 0.06 and 0.19, respectively), but no differences in days housed over time (O'Connell et al., 2013). Subsequent analyses found that active substance or alcohol users *who had spent time in residential treatment before entering supportive housing but were still using addictive substances after discharge* had the poorest housing outcomes, yet those who did not spend time in residential treatment before housing had similar outcomes as abstainers. These findings suggest that the most vulnerable population may be Veterans who continue to use alcohol or drugs even after intensive residential substance abuse treatment.

These findings broadly suggest that use of substances or alcohol at the time of housing or beforehand does not seem to negatively affect housing outcomes. Yet considering that substance use is a significant predictor of subsequent loss of housing (O'Connell et al., 2008), more research is needed to identify specific subgroups, such as those making extensive use of stimulants identified by Edens et al. (2014), that may be most at risk. It is worth reiterating here that, apart from the issue of admitting active users into supported housing, HUD-VASH is the only supportive housing program to have shown significant improvements for supportive housing on alcohol and drug use outcomes in an RCT. As noted earlier, five-year outcomes from the experimental study using multiple imputation techniques found HUD-VASH to be associated with significant reductions in alcohol and drug use compared with a control group receiving usual care (Cheng et al., 2007).

## PRINCIPAL 3: CHOICE IN HOUSING

Elements of choice are central to HUD-VASH and Housing First supportive housing models. One of the important questions about supportive housing concerns which housing features are most important to Veterans because an important goal of the program is to honor their preferences. The housing features considered most important to Veterans were cleanliness/upkeep, low cost, preferred location, safety, and privacy (O'Connell et al., 2006). In general, apartments largely met Veteran's expectations, with approximately 84% receiving their top three desired characteristics. Less valued features were being in a neighborhood where they had formerly resided, being allowed to have a pet, and having access to a garage.

Looking at data from the RCT, quality of housing was rated significantly higher among HUD-VASH Veterans compared with those housed under standard care, and HUD-VASH Veterans reported fewer problems with their housing than those housed under either ICM or standard care (Rosenheck et al., 2003).

## PRINCIPAL 4: AVAILABILITY OF A FLEXIBLE ARRAY OF SUPPORTIVE AND REHABILITATIVE SERVICES FOR AS LONG AS NEEDED

An essential feature of the HUD-VASH program design was the supportive case management offered to Veterans throughout the housing process. Although continued interactions with case managers was not required in the early phase of the program (i.e., keeping the voucher was not contingent on such contact), they were encouraged. As expected, the most intensive period of service use was during the early housing process and focused largely on housing-related activities (O'Connell et al., 2010; Rosenheck et al., 2003). Over the course of three years, only 17% of clients had help with employment and 19% had help obtaining other income. Interestingly, despite the high prevalence of substance and alcohol use disorders among HUD-VASH enrollees, only 5.4% to 8.7% of Veterans' case managers reported activities related to substance use counseling during the program. Nevertheless, significant improvements were observed in substance use outcomes with access to general case management service and housing vouchers (Cheng et al., 2007).

In the larger observational outcome monitoring effort, the frequency of contacts with case managers decreased progressively over time (O'Connell et al., 2010). By the final observation period, case managers described their relationship with Veterans as being primarily supportive in nature (O'Connell et al., 2010). Only 6% to 11% at any point in time described the relationship as being rehabilitative, and only 5% to 9% of Veterans indicated that the most important service provided was substance abuse treatment or counseling, despite 64% having a primary substance abuse disorder at the time of housing (O'Connell et al., 2010).

In the experimental trial, HUD-VASH Veterans had significantly more interactions with their case managers than those receiving ICM and standard care across a three-year follow-up period. Case managers of HUD-VASH Veterans also reported significantly higher therapeutic alliance ratings throughout the follow-up period (Rosenheck et al., 2003). Thus, having vouchers to offer significantly improved the therapeutic relationship.

More recent HUD-VASH research has found that program participants who were successfully housed received more intensive assistance finding apartments, had fewer monthly meetings with case managers, were more likely to feel that their case managers could help them, and were more engaged in services than those who were not housed (Montgomery et al., 2016). While this study does not allow causal interpretation, it does suggest that more intensive service is associated with better housing outcomes.

## OVERALL COST-EFFECTIVENESS

Although convincing, the evidence of enhanced housing and socio-clinical outcomes associated with HUD-VASH is only one part of the equation in determining the potential sustainability of such resource-intensive programming. Key questions related to cost and cost-effectiveness of such programming must also be evaluated. The VHA's extensive quality and data management program has allowed researchers to answer some of these questions. Data from the experimental trial revealed that HUD-VASH costs approximately 15% more than standard care from the perspective of the VA health care system, largely owing to greater use of outpatient mental health and homeless case management services (Figure 5.5). These cost data reflect a high level of validity because they are based on three years of outcome data from a RCT (Figure 5.6).The benefits in days housed were estimated to be worth this modest additional cost and were judged to be at least equivalent in value to the additional costs of services (Rosenheck et al., 2003). These findings are consistent with findings from a recent review of Housing First program cost-effectiveness, which found that the most rigorous experimental studies, like the HUD-VASH study, reported a net increase in overall costs associated with Housing First, while studies using much weaker pre-post comparisons reported a net decrease in overall Housing First costs (Ly & Latimer, 2015).

More recent data from a nonexperimental evaluation of VA health care costs among tenants who moved into HUD-VASH during FY 2010 and stayed in housing for two years found that HUD-VASH was associated with a 34% reduction in cost compared with the year prior to move-in (Byrne et al., 2014) based on a pre-post nonexperimental evaluation. However, these savings were significantly greater than cost savings in other VA residential programs before and after move-in and were largely attributable to reductions in inpatient services, although the groups cannot be considered equivalent. It is important to note that the decrease in inpatient costs associated with HUD-VASH in this study is likely to be a function of regression to the mean (i.e., people typically enter

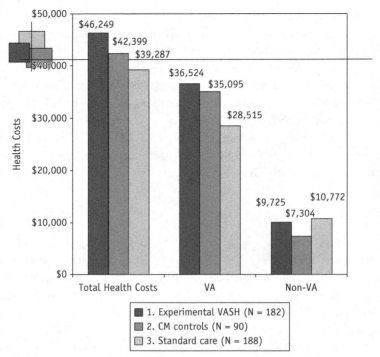

*Figure 5.5* Three-year health care costs by randomized treatment groups. From Rosenheck, R. A., Kasprow, W., Frisman, L., & Liu-Mares, W. (2003). Cost-effectiveness of supported housing for homeless persons with mental illness. *Arch Gen Psychiatry, 60*(9), 940–951.

housing programs at a time when they may rely on costlier temporary or transitional services such as inpatient care or residential treatment programs) and thus does not reflect the true program impact on costs.

## ADDING PEER SUPPORT TO HUD-VASH

In addition to the core HUD-VASH program, several program modifications have been developed and appear to be promising ways to meet Veteran needs. Data pertaining to three models that involve adding an element of peer support have been published in the literature.

The model with the most published research to date is the Group Intensive Peer-Support (GIPS) model of case management developed in 2009 by researchers at the VA New England Mental Illness Research, Education, and Clinical Center (Tsai, Reddy, & Rosenheck, 2014; Tsai & Rosenheck, 2012; Tsai, Rosenheck, Sullivan, & Harkness, 2011; Tsai, Stefanovics, & Rosenheck, 2014). GIPS is designed to be an alternative to individual ICM services for Veterans

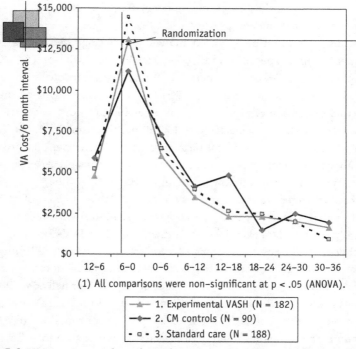

*Figure 5.6* VA inpatient and residential treatment costs one year before and three years after randomization by six-month interval. Data from Rosenheck, R. A., Kasprow, W., Frisman, L., & Liu-Mares, W. (2003). Cost-effectiveness of supported housing for homeless persons with mental illness. *Arch Gen Psychiatry, 60*(9), 940–951.

entering HUD-VASH. Although individual case managers are still assigned and available to each HUD-VASH Veteran, Veterans are encouraged to attend groups facilitated by case managers for clinical, practical, and emotional support within a context in which peers play an active role in helping one another. Research suggests that GIPS is associated with greater increases in social integration, increased contact with case managers, and faster acquisition of housing vouchers (Tsai & Rosenheck, 2012). Case managers are able to provide support to a greater number of clients at once through the group intervention, which may also free up time to assist individual Veterans with more intensive needs (Tsai & Rosenheck, 2013). At one site, 42% of HUD-VASH Veterans attended at least one group, with an average attendance of three groups per month (Tsai, Stefanovics et al., 2014). No Veteran characteristics distinguished group attenders from nongroup attenders, although among group attenders, those with more severe mental health symptoms and more days homeless at program entry attended groups more frequently. However, another study found that 77% of Veterans enrolled in HUD-VASH at this site attended GIPS (Tsai, Reddy et al., 2014). Qualitative research from this same study suggests that Veterans are typically satisfied with the groups and, in particular, like the social interactions and peer support that the groups offer.

The second intervention involved individual meetings between a trained Veteran peer support specialist and HUD-VASH Veterans (Ellison et al., 2016). Peer support was offered over the period of 9 months and involved a balance of structured and unstructured meetings. Structured meetings involved the presentation and discussion of preplanned topics related to recovery, questions for discussion, and worksheets. Researchers found that the number of peer-Veteran contacts ranged from zero to 39 contacts over a nine-month period, with an average of about one meeting per month. Most peer sessions occurred within the first six months and dropped off considerably after that. Although comparison data on case manager–Veteran contacts are not available, the rate of contact is slightly less than the average of 1.21 contacts per month with case managers that was reported in data examined from the national HUD-VASH sample (Tsai & Rosenheck, 2012), and the pattern of a reduction in contact following what is presumably the most intensive engagement time of housing procurement is similar to what has been reported in previous studies (O'Connell et al., 2010).

A final study tested the augmentation of HUD-VASH care with a Care Coordination Home Telehealth that uses health information technology (HIT) and nurse care management, with peer support, to promote illness self-management (Gabrielian et al., 2013). Results from this small exploratory study of 14 participating HUD-VASH Veterans (10 of whom used auxiliary peer support and four of whom did not) indicate that HIT-driven care management may be valuable in addressing chronic physical illnesses and that peer support generally was not required for using the HIT, but Veterans who felt particularly isolated especially valued the personal connection with peers (Gabrielian et al., 2013).

## Conclusion

The HUD-VASH program evaluation of the 1990s can be viewed as the prototype for the much more expansive dissemination of supported housing that would come about 20 years later. Several lessons/themes can be taken from this large body of research: (1) HUD-VASH was carefully evaluated during the decade after its initial implementation through a rigorous cost-effectiveness evaluation, which showed it to be effective at reducing homelessness at acceptable cost, significantly increasing social support, and reducing substance use and abuse. (2) The study showed that a key feature of supportive housing is the rental subsidy, although other factors also contribute to successful exit from homelessness. For some people, particularly those with substance use problems, more intensive supports through residential treatment may be required to address the substance use issues. (3) The experimental study was accompanied by a large-scale observational monitoring effort, which has documented that the program benefitted thousands of homeless Veterans in much the same way as those participating in the RCT. Thus, the positive findings from the RCT were shown to be generalizable to the thousands of other Veterans who participated in HUD-VASH. (4) The overall process of achieving housing can be lengthy and requires patience and much work on the part of both Veterans and case managers. In the VA, there was a deliberate decision not to disadvantage Veterans who were doing well in traditional VA programs for homeless Veterans. Thus, many Veterans with extensive prior treatment benefited from participation in HUD-VASH (albeit with longer time to entering housing), although the program was also shown to be effective in helping Veterans coming right off the street or out of a shelter. (5) Finally, further data analysis shows that many homeless Veterans are closely linked with family members and peers, and these ties may be an underused source of support that can help Veterans in achieving permanent housing and improving their quality of life (O'Connell, Kasprow, & Rosenheck, 2017; O'Connell & Rosenheck, 2016).

## Acknowledgment

We would like to acknowledge unpublished data and comments from Jesse Vazzano, National Director of the HUD-VASH Veterans Health Administration Homeless Programs.

## References

Adair, C. E., Kopp, B., Distasio, J., Hwang, S. W., Lavoie, J., Veldhuizen, S., . . . Goering, P. (2016). Housing quality in a randomized controlled trial of Housing First for homeless individuals with mental illness: Correlates and associations with outcomes. *Journal of Urban Health, 93*(4), 682–697. doi:10.1007/s11524-016-0062-9

Alegria, M., Canino, G., & Rios, R. (2004). Inequalities in use of specialty mental health services among Latinos, African Americans, and non-Latino Whites. *Year Book of Psychiatry & Applied Mental Health, 2004*(1), 184–185.

Alegria, M., Canino, G., Ríos, R., Vera, M., Calderon, J., Rusch, D., & Ortega, A. N. (2002). Mental health care for Latinos: Inequalities in use of specialty mental health services among Latinos, African Americans, and non-Latino Whites. *Psychiatric Services, 53*(12), 1547–1555.

Aubry, T., Goering, P., Veldhuizen, S., Adair, C. E., Bourque, J., Distasio, J., . . . Tsemberis, S. J. (2016). A multiple-city RCT of Housing First with assertive community treatment for homeless Canadians with serious mental illness. *Psychiatric Services, 67*(3), 275–281. doi:doi:10.1176/appi.ps.201400587

Aubry, T., Tsemberis, S. J., Adair, C. E., Veldhuizen, S., Streiner, D., Latimer, E., . . . Goering, P. (2015). One-year outcomes of a randomized controlled trial of housing first with ACT in five Canadian cities. *Psychiatric Services*, 66(5), 463–469. doi:10.1176/appi.ps.201400167

Austin, E. L., Pollio, D. E., Holmes, S., Schumacher, J., White, B., Lukas, C. V., & Kertesz, S. (2014). VA's expansion of supportive housing: Successes and challenges on the path toward Housing First. *Psychiatric Services*, 65(5), 641–647. doi:10.1176/appi.ps.201300073

Austin, E. L., Pollio, D. E., & Kertesz, S. G. (2016). Ethnographic observation of a Housing First approach to case management at four VA medical centers. *Psychiatric Services*, 67(12), 1384–1385. doi:10.1176/appi.ps.201600382

Blackstock, O. J., Haskell, S. G., Brandt, C. A., & Desai, R. A. (2012). Gender and the use of Veterans Health Administration homeless services programs among Iraq/Afghanistan veterans. *Medical Care*, 50(4), 347–352.

Brookes, S. T., Whitley, E., Peters, T. J., Mulheran, P. A., Egger, M., & Davey Smith, G. (2001). Subgroup analyses in randomised controlled trials: Quantifying the risks of false-positives and false-negatives. *Health Technology Assessment*, 5(33), 1–56.

Byrne, T., Roberts, C. B., Culhane, D. P., & Kane, V. (2014). *Estimating Cost Savings Associated with HUD-VASH Placement*. Retrieved from https://www.va.gov/HOMELESS/Estimating_Cost_Savings_Associated_With_HUD_VASH_Placement.pdf

Cheng, A.-L., Lin, H., Kasprow, W., & Rosenheck, R. A. (2007). Impact of supported housing on clinical outcomes analysis of a randomized trial using multiple imputation technique. *Journal of Nervous and Mental Disease*, 195(1), 83. doi:10.1097/01.nmd.0000252313.49043.f2

Crane, M., & Warnes, A. M. (2010). Homelessness among older people and service responses. *Reviews in Clinical Gerontology*, 20(4), 354–363.

Cusack, M., & Montgomery, A. E. (2017). The role of eviction in veteran's homelessness recidivism. *Journal of Social Distress and the Homeless*, 26(1).

Drew, D., Drebing, C. E., Van Ormer, A., Losardo, M., Krebs, C., Penk, W., & Rosenheck, R. A. (2001). Effects of disability compensation on participation in and outcomes of vocational rehabilitation. *Psychiatric Services*, 52(11), 1479–1484.

Edens, E. L., Kasprow, W., Tsai, J., & Rosenheck, R. A. (2011). Association of substance use and VA service-connected disability benefits with risk of homelessness among Veterans. *American Journal on Addictions*, 20(5), 412–419.

Edens, E. L., Tsai, J., & Rosenheck, R. A. (2014). Does stimulant use impair housing outcomes in low-demand supportive housing for chronically homeless adults? *American Journal on Addictions*, 23(3), 243–248.

Ellison, M. L., Schutt, R. K., Glickman, M. E., Schultz, M. R., Chinman, M., Jensen, K., . . . Eisen, S. (2016). Patterns and predictors of engagement in peer support among homeless veterans with mental health conditions and substance use histories. *Psychiatric Rehabilitation Journal*, 39(3), 266–273. doi:10.1037/prj0000221

Gabrielian, S., Yuan, A., Andersen, R. M., McGuire, J., Rubenstein, L., Sapir, N., & Gelberg, L. (2013). Chronic disease management for recently homeless veterans: A clinical practice improvement program to apply home telehealth technology to a vulnerable population. *Medical Care*, 51(3 suppl 1), S44–S51. doi:10.1097/MLR.0b013e31827808f6

Gamache, G., Rosenheck, R. A., & Tessler, R. (2003). Overrepresentation of women Veterans among homeless women. *American Journal of Public Health*, 93(7), 1132–1136.

Goering, P. N., & Streiner, D. L. (2015). Putting housing first: The evidence and impact. *Canadian Journal of Psychiatry*, 60(11), 465–466.

Greenberg, G. A., & Rosenheck, R. A. (2007). Compensation of veterans with psychiatric or substance abuse disorders and employment and earnings. *Military Medicine*, 172(2), 162–168.

Greenberg, G. A., & Rosenheck, R. A. (2008). Jail incarceration, homelessness, and mental health: A national study. *Psychiatric Services*, 59(2), 170–177.

Henwood, B., Wenzel, S. L., Mangano, P. F., Hombs, M. E., Padgett, D. K., Byrne, T., . . . Uretsky, M. C. (2015). *The Grand Challenge of Ending Homelessness*. https://pdxscholar.library.pdx.edu/socwork_fac/136/

Kasprow, W. J., Rosenheck, R. A., Frisman, L., & DiLella, D. (2000). Referral and housing processes in a long-term supported housing program for homeless veterans. *Psychiatric Services*, *51*(8), 1017–1023.

Kertesz, S. G. (2009). Housing First for homeless persons with active addiction—Are we overreaching? *Milbank Quarterly*, *87*(2), 495–534.

Kertesz, S. G., Austin, E. L., Holmes, S. K., DeRussy, A. J., Van Deusen Lukas, C., & Pollio, D. E. (2017). Housing First on a large scale: Fidelity strengths and challenges in the VA's HUD-VASH program. *Psychological Services*, *14*(2), 118–128. doi:10.1037/ser0000123

Kertesz, S. G., Austin, E. L., Holmes, S. K., Pollio, D. E., Schumacher, J. E., White, B., & Lukas, C. V. (2014). Making Housing First happen: Organizational leadership in VA's expansion of permanent supportive housing. *Journal of General Internal Medicine*, *29*(suppl 4), 835–844. doi:10.1007/s11606-014-3025-4

Kertesz, S. G., Austin, E. L., Holmes, S. K., Pollio, D. E., & VanDeusen Lukas, C. (2015). Housing First and the risk of failure: A comment on Westermeyer and Lee (2013). *Journal of Nervous and Mental Disease*, *203*(7), 559–562. doi:10.1097/NMD.0000000000000328

Lagakos, S. W. (2006). The challenge of subgroup analyses-reporting without distorting. *New England Journal of Medicine*, *354*(16), 1667.

Ly, A., & Latimer, E. (2015). Housing First impact on costs and associated cost offsets: A review of the literature. *Canadian Journal of Psychiatry*, *60*(11), 475–487. doi:10.1177/070674371506001103

Mares, A. S., & Rosenheck, R. A. (2007). HUD/HHS/VA Collaborative Initiative to Help End Chronic Homelessness: Preliminary Client Outcomes Report. Northeast Program Evaluation Center, West Haven, CT. https://aspe.hhs.gov/report/hudhhsva-collaborative-initiative-help-end-chronic-homelessness-preliminary-client-outcomes-report.

Mares, A. S., & Rosenheck, R. A. (2011). A comparison of treatment outcomes among chronically homelessness adults receiving comprehensive housing and health care services versus usual local care. *Administration and Policy in Mental Health*, *38*(6), 459–475. doi:10.1007/s10488-011-0333-4

Meehan, S. (2006). Improving health care for women veterans. *Journal of General Internal Medicine*, *21*(S3).

Montgomery, A. E. (2016). Presentation at "Reckoning with Homelessness in New York City" conference. New York, New York. May 10–11, 2016.

Montgomery, A. E., & Cusack, M. (2017). HUD-VASH Exit Study: Final Report. Prepared for US Department of Housing and Urban Development. September, 2017.

Montgomery, A. E., Cusack, M., Blonigen, D. M., Gabrielian, S., Marsh, L., & Fargo, J. (2016). Factors associated with Veterans' access to permanent supportive housing. *Psychiatric Services*, *67*(8), 870–877. doi:10.1176/appi.ps.201500248

Montgomery, A. E., Cusack, M., Szymkowiak, D., Fargo, J., & O'Toole, T. (2017). Factors contributing to eviction from permanent supportive housing: Lessons from HUD-VASH. *Evaluation and Program Planning*, *61*, 55–63. doi:10.1016/j.evalprogplan.2016.11.014

Montgomery, A. E., Hill, L. L., Kane, V., & Culhane, D. P. (2013). Housing chronically homeless veterans: Evaluating the efficacy of a Housing First approach to HUD-VASH. *Journal of Community Psychology*, *41*(4), 505–514. doi:10.1002/jcop.21554

O'Connell, M. J., Kasprow, W., & Rosenheck, R. A. (2008). Rates and risk factors for homelessness after successful housing in a sample of formerly homeless veterans. *Psychiatric Services*, *59*(3), 268–275. doi:10.1176/appi.ps.59.3.268

O'Connell, M. J., Kasprow, W. J., & Rosenheck, R. A. (2009). Direct placement versus multistage models of supported housing in a population of veterans who are homeless. *Psychological Services*, *6*(3), 190–201. doi:10.1037/a0014921

O'Connell, M. J., Kasprow, W. J., & Rosenheck, R. A. (2010). National dissemination of supported housing in the VA: Model adherence versus model modification. *Psychiatric Rehabilitation Journal*, *33*(4), 308–319. doi:10.2975/33.4.2010.308.319

O'Connell, M. J., Kasprow, W. J., & Rosenheck, R. A. (2012). Differential impact of supported housing on selected subgroups of homeless veterans with substance abuse histories. *Psychiatric Services*, *63*(12), 1195–1205. doi:10.1176/appi.ps.201000229

O'Connell, M. J., Kasprow, W. J., & Rosenheck, R. A. (2013). The impact of current alcohol and drug use on outcomes among homeless veterans entering supported housing. *Psychological Services, 10*(2), 241–249. doi:10.1037/a0030816

O'Connell, M. J., Kasprow, W. J., & Rosenheck, R. A. (2017). Impact of supported housing on social relationships among homeless veterans. *Psychiatric Services, 68*(2), 203–206. doi:10.1176/appi.ps.201500276

O'Connell, M. J., Rosenheck, R. A., Kasprow, W. J., & Frisman, L. (2006). An examination of fulfilled housing preferences . . . homeless persons with mental illness and-or substance use disorders. *Journal of Behavioral Health Services & Research, 33*(3), 354–365.

O'Connell, M. J., & Rosenheck, R. A. (2016). The family ties that bind: Tangible, instrumental, and emotional support among homeless Veterans. In S. M. Wadsworth & D. S. Riggs (Eds.), *War and Family Life* (pp. 281–319): Springer International Publishing.

Patterson, K. L., Nochajski, T., & Wu, L. (2014). Neighborhood outcomes of formally homeless veterans participating in the HUD-VASH program. *Journal of Community Practice, 22*(3), 324–341. doi:10.1080/10705422.2014.929605

Rosenheck, R., Leda, C. A., & Gallup, P. (1992). Program design and clinical operation of two national VA initiatives for homeless mentally ill veterans. *New England Journal of Public Policy, 8*(1), 315–337.

Rosenheck, R. A., Frisman, L., & Sindelar, J. (1995). Disability compensation and work among veterans with psychiatric and nonpsychiatric impairments. *Psychiatric Services, 46*(4), 359–365.

Rosenheck, R. A., Kasprow, W., Frisman, L., & Liu-Mares, W. (2003). Cost-effectiveness of supported housing for homeless persons with mental illness. *Archives of General Psychiatry, 60*(9), 940–951. doi:10.1001/archpsyc.60.9.940

Tejani, N., Rosenheck, R. A., Tsai, J., Kasprow, W., & McGuire, J. F. (2014). Incarceration histories of homeless veterans and progression through a national supported housing program. *Community Mental Health Journal, 50*(5), 514–519. doi:10.1007/s10597-013-9611-9

Tsai, J. (2014). Letter to the editor: Timing and momentum in VA's path toward Housing First. *Psychiatric Services, 65*(6), 836.

Tsai, J., Kasprow, W., & Rosenheck, R. A. (2011). Exiting homelessness without a voucher: A comparison of independently housed and other homeless veterans. *Psychological Services, 8*(2), 114. doi:10.1037/a0023189

Tsai, J., Kasprow, W. J., & Rosenheck, R. A. (2014). Alcohol and drug use disorders among homeless veterans: Prevalence and association with supported housing outcomes. *Addictive Behaviors, 39*(2), 455–460. doi:10.1016/j.addbeh.2013.02.002

Tsai, J., O'Connell, M. J., Kasprow, W. J., & Rosenheck, R. A. (2011). Factors related to rapidity of housing placement in housing and Urban Development–Department of Veterans Affairs supportive housing program of 1990s. *Journal of Rehabilitation Research and Development, 48*(7), 755–762.

Tsai, J., Reddy, N., & Rosenheck, R. A. (2014). Client satisfaction with a new group-based model of case management for supported housing services. *Evaluation and Program Planning, 43*, 118–123. doi:10.1016/j.evalprogplan.2013.12.004

Tsai, J., & Rosenheck, R. A. (2012). Outcomes of a group intensive peer-support model of case management for supported housing. *Psychiatric Services, 63*(12), 1186–1194. doi:10.1176/appi.ps.201200100

Tsai, J., & Rosenheck, R. A. (2013). Conduct disorder behaviors, childhood family instability, and childhood abuse as predictors of severity of adult homelessness among American veterans. *Social Psychiatry and Psychiatric Epidemiology, 48*(3), 477–486. doi:10.1007/s00127-012-0551-4

Tsai, J., & Rosenheck, R. A. (2013). Use of group treatment among case managers in Department of Veterans Affairs supported housing program. *Journal of Rehabilitation Research and Development, 50*(4), 471. doi:10.1682/Jrrd.2012.04.0073

Tsai, J., & Rosenheck, R. A. (2016). Psychosis, lack of job skills, and criminal history: Associations with employment in two samples of homeless men. *Psychiatric Services, 67*(6), 671–675. doi:10.1176/appi.ps.201500145

Tsai, J., Rosenheck, R. A., & Kane, V. (2014). Homeless female US Veterans in a national supported housing program: Comparison of individual characteristics and outcomes with male veterans. *Psychological Services, 11*(3), 309–316. doi:10.1037/a0036323

Tsai, J., Rosenheck, R. A., Kasprow, W. J., & Kane, V. (2015). Characteristics and use of services among literally homeless and unstably housed US veterans with custody of minor children. *Psychiatric Services, 66*(10), 1083–1090. doi:10.1176/appi.ps.201400300

Tsai, J., Rosenheck, R. A., Sullivan, J., & Harkness, L. (2011). A group-intensive peer support model of case management for supported housing. *Psychological Services, 8*(3), 251–259. doi:10.1037/a0024837

Tsai, J., Stefanovics, E., & Rosenheck, R. A. (2014). Predictors of attendance in a group-based model of case management for supported housing. *Psychiatric Rehabilitation Journal, 37*(4), 324–328. doi:10.1037/prj0000059

Tsemberis, S. J., & Asmussen, S. (1999). From streets to homes: The pathways to housing consumer preference supported housing model. *Alcoholism Treatment Quarterly, 17*(1-2), 113–131.

Tsemberis, S. J., & Eisenberg, R. F. (2014). Pathways to housing: Supported housing for street-dwelling homeless individuals with psychiatric disabilities. *Psychiatric Services, 51*(4), 487–493.

Tsemberis, S. J., Gulcur, L., & Nakae, M. (2004). Housing First, consumer choice, and harm reduction for homeless individuals with a dual diagnosis. *American Journal of Public Health, 94*(4), 651–656. doi:10.2105/ajph.94.4.651

US Department of Housing and Urban Development. (2017). *The 2017 Annual Homeless Assessment Report (AHAR) to Congress: Part 1 Point-in-Time Estimates of Homelessness.* Retrieved from Washington, DC: https://www.hudexchange.info/resources/documents/2017-AHAR-Part-1.pdf

US Interagency Council on Homelessness. (2010). *Opening Doors: Federal Strategic Plan To Prevent and End Homelessness.* Washington, DC: US Interagency Council on Homelessness.

Wells, K., Klap, R., Koike, A., & Sherbourne, C. (2001). Ethnic disparities in unmet need for alcoholism, drug abuse, and mental health care. *American Journal of Psychiatry, 158*(12), 2027–2032.

Westermeyer, J., Lee, K., & Y Carr, T. B. (2015). Housing First/HUD-VASH: Importance, flaws, and potential for transformation. Response to Commentary. *Journal of Nervous and Mental Disease, 203*(7), 563–567. doi:10.1097/NMD.0000000000000329

# 6

## Criminal Justice Issues Among Homeless Veterans

JESSICA BLUE-HOWELLS, CHRISTINE TIMKO,
SEAN CLARK, AND ANDREA K. FINLAY

> Every justice-involved Veteran will have access to care,
> services and other benefits to help him or her maximize their
> potential for success and stability in the community, including
> by avoiding homelessness and ending their involvement in the
> justice system.
> —*Vision for the VA's Veterans Justice Programs*

## Introduction

Starting in the 1980s, literature emerged indicating that people being incarcerated had histories of homelessness, that people who were homeless had histories of incarceration, and that there seemed to be a "revolving door" between living on the street and being sentenced to jail or prison.[1] A significant proportion of people in the United States who are homeless and involved in the criminal justice system (i.e., "criminal justice involved") are U.S. military Veterans. In this chapter, we explore the intersection of homelessness and criminal justice involvement among Veterans. First, we briefly explain how we define homelessness and criminal justice involvement and how criminal justice involvement differs from but is related to civil legal involvement. Next, we discuss the prevalence of and risk factors for criminal justice involvement among homeless Veterans. We also address the prevalence of and risk factors for homelessness among criminal justice–involved Veterans. Then, we describe how we view the structure of the criminal justice system and the role the U.S. Department of Veterans Affairs (VA) has in partnering with criminal justice agencies to address homelessness and criminal justice involvement among Veterans. Finally, we identify opportunities to develop further knowledge about strategies to address the needs of this population and improve their health and housing.

# VA Definition of Homelessness

The VA defines homelessness using the same criteria as the U.S. Department of Housing and Urban Development, defined in the McKinney-Vento Homeless Assistance Act, and amended by the Homeless Emergency Assistance and Rapid Transition to Housing Act. Briefly, a homeless person is defined as a person without a regular nighttime residence that is fixed and adequate. Individuals who live in nighttime residences that are not regularly used as sleeping accommodations, such as cars, train or bus stations, campgrounds, and abandoned buildings; who live in temporary shelters or hotels/motels; who reside in places not meant for human habitation; or who are in imminent danger of losing their accommodations and have no subsequent permanent housing identified meet criteria for homelessness. The studies reviewed in this chapter have different definitions of homelessness, both in defining homeless samples and in measuring the prevalence of homelessness. For the purposes of this chapter, we broadly define homelessness to encapsulate the various definitions used across prior studies.

# What Is Criminal Justice Involvement?

We broadly define criminal justice involvement to include contact with any aspect of the criminal justice system, regardless of the specific acts or circumstances that initiated contact. Criminal offenses are defined in federal and state statutes, which lay out the specific elements that must be proved in order for an individual to be found guilty of each offense, and set the penalties that may be imposed on those who are. Criminal statutes address a wide range of acts, which can be broadly categorized as public order offenses (e.g., disorderly conduct, public intoxication), property offenses (e.g., burglary, arson, motor vehicle theft), drug offenses (e.g., possession, trafficking), violent offenses (e.g., rape, murder, domestic violence), and parole or probation violations (e.g., missing an appointment with a parole officer, failing a urine test). Crimes punishable by incarceration for one year or less are generally referred to as misdemeanors, while those carrying a maximum potential sentence of more than one year are referred to as felonies.

The Sequential Intercept Model[2] depicts the criminal justice system in simplified form, as a continuum with five distinct components (called "intercepts," reflecting the model's intended function as a planning tool for integrating mental health services in criminal justice settings): (1) law enforcement and emergency services; (2) initial detention (when an individual has been arrested and is held in jail before his or her first appearance in court) and initial court hearings; (3) jails (when an individual is held in jail before trial) and courts, including specialty courts (e.g., drug court, Veterans Treatment Court); (4) community re-entry from jail or prison; and (5) community corrections and community support (e.g., probation or parole). Jails and prisons are often referred to collectively in discussions of incarceration in the United States; however, they are functionally distinct and therefore appear in different levels of the Sequential Intercept Model. People incarcerated in jails are generally held on the authority of local governments, and their cases may be at one of several different procedural stages—initial detention, pretrial detention, or serving a sentence after being convicted of more minor crimes, usually misdemeanors with a sentence of one year or less. People who are incarcerated in prisons are generally held by the state or federal government following conviction for more major crimes, usually felonies with a sentence of more than one year. Incarcerated persons' longer lengths of stay mean that prison populations are generally much more stable than jail populations. The research studies reviewed in the current chapter measured criminal justice involvement in a variety of ways.

## Criminal Justice Involvement as a Risk Factor for Homelessness

The link between criminal justice involvement and homelessness is influenced by person-level demographic and clinical factors as well as structural-level policy factors. A cycle of homelessness and incarceration, particularly among people with mental illness or addiction problems, has been observed among the general U.S. population. Greenberg and Rosenheck[3] examined a national data set of persons incarcerated in jails collected by the U.S. Department of Justice to understand interactions between jail incarceration, homelessness, and mental health issues. They found that 15.3% of jail-incarcerated adults had been homeless either immediately preceding arrest or in the previous year. Compared with jail-incarcerated adults who were not homeless, homeless adults in jail were more likely to be incarcerated for a property crime, had higher levels of substance use and mental health disorders, were more likely to have trauma exposure, and had lower employment rates.

Approximately 10% of people coming into prisons have a history of homelessness, and at least 10% of people experience homelessness after exiting prison.[1] Older age and mental illness increased the risk for homelessness after release from prison. Greenberg and Rosenheck[3] also examined a national data set collected by the U.S. Department of Justice to understand contributing factors of homelessness among the prison population. They found that 9% of prison-incarcerated adults had experienced homelessness in the year before arrest. This study compared homeless and nonhomeless individuals and, similar to findings for jailed adults,[3] found that prison-incarcerated adults with a history of homelessness were more likely to be incarcerated for a property crime; had higher levels of substance use and mental health disorders; were more likely to have a history of trauma exposure, including physical and sexual abuse; and had lower employment rates. Homeless prison-incarcerated adults were also older than their nonhomeless counterparts.

Structural policy factors in the United States influence vulnerability for becoming homeless and other collateral consequences of criminal justice involvement such as accessing voting, employment, or education (see the National Inventory of Collateral Consequences for details by state: https://niccc. csgjusticecenter.org/). For example, federal, state, and local policies restrict where someone with a criminal record may live. People with a sexual offense history face the most restrictions on their residences. Prisons are mostly located in rural areas, far distant from the urban centers where a majority of incarcerated persons both commit crimes and are released back to the community. This distance during incarceration both reduces the natural social supports that could assist a re-entering person from becoming homeless and reduces the effectiveness of re-entry planning among prison staff because they are not proximate to and cannot develop relationships with housing supports in the communities where prison-incarcerated adults will release. Additionally, responsibility for housing resources for people exiting incarceration exists in a policy gap. Correctional agencies are not seen as responsible for helping people leaving incarceration to obtain secure housing, but the definition of who is homeless often excludes people with lengthy incarcerations (i.e., 90 days or greater), making it difficult for them to access housing supports developed for homeless populations on exiting incarceration.

# Prevalence of Criminal Justice Involvement Among Homeless Veterans

Beginning in the 1990s, studies on homeless Veterans in VA addiction treatment programs or VA supportive housing programs emerged. Although not their primary focus, these studies shed light on the prevalence of criminal justice involvement among samples of homeless Veterans. Table 6.1 displays studies of homeless Veterans and the prevalence of criminal justice involvement.

Summarizing this literature is difficult for two reasons. First, although all the studies are of Veterans seeking treatment at Veterans Health Administration (VHA) facilities—most often in VA supportive housing programs (e.g., Housing and Urban Development–Veterans Affairs Supportive Housing [HUD-VASH]),

Table 6.1 Prevalence of Criminal Justice Involvement Among Homeless Veterans

| Authors | Study Design | Sample Size | Prevalence of Criminal Justice Involvement |
|---|---|---|---|
| Benda et al.[4,5] | Random sample of military Veterans in a VA domiciliary substance use disorder treatment program for homeless Veterans | 188 homeless Veterans | Adapted from the Addiction Severity Index—How many times persons have committed crimes in the past year: 27% committed nuisance offenses, and 41% committed felonies in the past year |
| Buchholz et al.[6] | Secondary data analysis of a prospective, randomized controlled trial of patients seeking addiction treatment who were randomized to receive primary care in the Addiction Treatment Clinic or the General Internal Medicine Clinic | 622 Veterans seeking addiction treatment: 168 consistently homeless across 12-month follow-up 51 housed at baseline, homeless at 12-month follow-up 148 homeless at baseline, housed at 12-month follow-up 255 consistently housed across 12-month follow-up | Addiction Severity Index—Legal problems; lifetime months incarcerated Consistently homeless group: 38% had lifetime incarceration <10 months; 37% had lifetime incarceration ≤10 months; 0.07 ± 0.15 on legal problems scale Housed baseline, homeless at follow-up: 53% had <10 months lifetime incarceration, 22% had ≤10 months lifetime incarceration; 0.12 ± 0.15 on legal problems scale Homeless baseline, housed follow-up: 32% had <10 months lifetime incarceration; 29% had ≥10 months lifetime incarceration; 0.13 ± 0.20 on legal problems scale |

(continued)

*Table 6.1* Continued

| Authors | Study Design | Sample Size | Prevalence of Criminal Justice Involvement |
|---|---|---|---|
| Cheung et al.[7] | Observational study of homeless Veterans in a VA domiciliary program | 829 homeless Veterans | 69% were previously imprisoned |
| Douyon et al.[8] | Observational study of consecutive Veterans who entered acute inpatient Psychiatric Services | 33 homeless Veterans: 18 acutely homeless (duration of homelessness was less than one month) 15 chronically homeless (duration of homelessness exceeded three months) | History of legal history from Homelessness Questionnaire—Childhood criminal activity and chart review of first- and second-degree criminal charges: 83.3% of acute homeless group had a legal history 46.7% of chronic homeless group had a legal history |
| Gabrielian et al.[9] | Observational study of homeless Veterans in VA supportive housing in 2011–2012 | 102 homeless Veterans in VA supportive housing | At baseline, 41% of the sample had past criminal justice involvement but were not on parole or probation, and 21.5% of the sample were currently on parole or probation |
| Kashner et al.[10] | Randomized control trial of Veterans who were homeless, eligible for VA care, had a substance use disorder, and were willing to enter a therapeutic program | 142 homeless Veterans with substance use disorders | 6.3% of intervention group and 3.2% of control group were incarcerated in the prior three months at baseline |

| Study | Description | Sample | Findings |
|---|---|---|---|
| Schaffer[11] | Observational study of homeless Veterans who were screened for domestic violence | 507 homeless Veterans in homeless shelters or transitional housing | 23.6% had been charged and convicted of domestic violence post-military; 16% were on supervised parole or probation; 11% had juvenile records |
| Seidner et al.[12] | Observational study of Veterans who applied for a VA residential rehabilitation program for homeless Veterans | 163 homeless Veterans | All measures were lifetime history of charged/arrested: 71.15% any crime 42.31% driving under the influence 29.49% disorderly conduct, public intoxication, vagrancy 13.46% narcotics charges 8.33% assault 5.13% weapons offense 1.92% rape 1.28% robbery 0.64% homicide or manslaughter 8.33% burglary, larceny, breaking and entering 6.41% shoplifting 1.28% arson 7.05% parole or probation violation 2.56% forgery 5.77% other |
| Tejani et al.[13] | National observational study of homeless Veterans in VA supportive housing | 14,557 homeless Veterans | 43.4% of Veterans had a lifetime incarceration history of ≤ one year 22.1% of Veterans had a lifetime incarceration history of >one year |

(continued)

Table 6.1 Continued

| Authors | Study Design | Sample Size | Prevalence of Criminal Justice Involvement |
|---|---|---|---|
| Tsai et al.[14] | National observational study of homeless Veterans in VA supportive housing | 627 homeless Veterans | Average incarceration in months 9.8 ± 20.3 |
| | | | Average number of convictions 2 ± 3.2 |
| | | | Last conviction: minor crime |
| | | | 2.9% shoplifting |
| | | | 9.9% disorderly conduct |
| | | | 3.5% major driving violation |
| | | | 13.2% driving while intoxicated |
| | | | 4.8% parole/probation violation |
| | | | Last conviction: major crime |
| | | | 8.8% drug charge |
| | | | 1.8% weapons offense |
| | | | 4% burglary/larceny |
| | | | 5.9% assault |
| | | | Last conviction: Serious crime |
| | | | 0.2% arson |
| | | | 2.2% robbery |
| | | | 0.3% rape |
| | | | 0.8% homicide/manslaughter |
| | | | Average length of last incarceration 4.3 ± 11.3 |
| | | | 2.4% current awaiting charges, trial, or sentence |

| Tsai & Rosenheck[15] | National observational study of homeless Veterans in VA supportive housing | 1,160 homeless Veterans | History of (charges related to most recent incarceration): |
|---|---|---|---|
| | | | 17.8% (4.3%) shoplifting/vandalism |
| | | | 41.7% (13.4%) disorderly conduct/vagrancy/public intoxication |
| | | | 41.4% (18%) driving while intoxicated |
| | | | 24.1% (4.3%) major driving violation |
| | | | 13.8% (5.6%) parole/probation violation |
| | | | 5.7% (2.1%) forgery |
| | | | 13.8% (14.3%) other minor crimes |
| | | | 26.8% (14.1%) drug charge |
| | | | 12.7% (2.4%) weapons offense |
| | | | 14.1% (6.9%) burglary/larceny |
| | | | 24% (8.8%) assault |
| | | | 7.2% (3.9%) robbery |
| | | | 1.1% (0.3%) arson |
| | | | 1% (0.5%) rape |
| | | | 1.7% (0.8%) homicide, manslaughter |
| | | | Mean number of: |
| | | | Minor crimes 1.6 ± 1.4 |
| | | | Major crimes 0.8 ± 1 |
| | | | Serious crimes 0.1 ± 0.3 |
| Tsai & Rosenheck[16] | Observational study of homeless male Veterans in VA supportive housing | 1,101 homeless male Veterans | 79% criminal history |

*(continued)*

*Table 6.1* **Continued**

| Authors | Study Design | Sample Size | Prevalence of Criminal Justice Involvement |
|---|---|---|---|
| Tsai et al.[17] | National observational study of homeless Veterans in VA supportive housing | 43,853 homeless Veterans | 42.61% one year or less of lifetime incarceration 22.72% more than one year of lifetime incarceration |
| Wenzel et al.[18] | Observational study of homeless male Veterans in a VA residential treatment program for homeless Veterans | 429 homeless male Veterans | 33.9% had ≥ one conviction for a criminal offense |
| Wenzel et al.[19] | Observational study of homeless male Veterans in a VA residential treatment program for homeless Veterans | Sample 1: 67 short-term homeless (homeless <12 months) and 58 long-term homeless (homeless ≥12 months male Veterans Sample 2: 96 short-term and 122 long-term homeless male Veterans | Sample 1: 13.4% of short-term and 33.3% of long-term homeless Veterans were ever charged with major driving violations; 28.8% of short-term and 50.9% of long-term homeless Veterans were ever charged with disorder conduct, vagrancy, or public intoxication Sample 2: 12.6% of short-term and 20.7% of long-term homeless Veterans were ever charged with major driving violations; 31.3% of short-term and 38% of long-term homeless Veterans were ever charged with disorder conduct, vagrancy, or public intoxication |
| Westermeyer & Lee[20] | Observational study of Veterans who were referred to supportive housing addiction specialty treatment | 8 male Veterans in VA | 37.5% of men were convicted of felonies |

residential treatment programs, or addiction treatment settings—the samples differ in terms of patient characteristics (e.g., mental health or substance use disorder was an inclusion criterion) and study design (e.g., randomized controlled trial vs. observational study). Furthermore, most studies do not include the definition of homelessness used to select the sample. Second, there was variation in the definition of criminal justice involvement used in each study. Four studies used legal questions from the Addiction Severity Index—a semi-structured interview tool used to gather information on seven areas of a person's life that may contribute to addiction problems, including medical status, psychiatric status, alcohol use, drug use, legal status, family/social status, and employment/support.[21] Other studies measured lifetime incarceration, previous imprisonment, legal history, being on probation or parole, specific crimes committed (e.g., driving under the influence, assault), and criminal history. However, we attempt to broadly summarize the literature.

## LIFETIME CRIMINAL JUSTICE INVOLVEMENT

The majority of homeless Veterans seeking or receiving mental health or addiction treatment or other services had experienced lifetime incarceration or had a legal history. The prevalence of criminal justice involvement, defined as a legal history of childhood criminal convictions or significant first- or second-degree criminal convictions, in a sample of patients in VA inpatient mental health treatment, was 83.3% of the acutely homeless group (homeless less than one month) and 46.7% of the chronically homeless group (homeless more than three months).[8] Another study with 622 Veterans entering addiction treatment found that 75% of Veterans who were consistently homeless across a 12-month follow-up period had experienced incarceration (jail or prison not specified) in their lifetime, 75% of Veterans who were housed at baseline and homeless at follow-up had experienced lifetime incarceration, and 61% of Veterans who were homeless at baseline and housed at follow-up experienced incarceration.[6] However, one study of male homeless Veterans in the Domiciliary Care for Homeless Veterans program that compared Veterans who had been homeless 12 months or less (short-term homeless) with Veterans who had been homeless longer than 12 months (long-term homeless) found mixed results. The first sample of 125 Veterans found that a significantly higher percentage of long-term homeless Veterans (33.3%) had ever been charged with a major driving violation compared with short-term homeless Veterans (13.4%). However, the second sample of 218 homeless Veterans found no significant difference in major driving violations (long-term homeless = 20.7%; short-term homeless = 12.7%) or ever being charged with disorderly conduct, vagrancy, or public intoxication (long-term homeless = 38%; short-term homeless = 31.3%).[19]

Veterans in residential treatment programs and VA supportive housing programs, which is an indicator of homelessness, also had a high prevalence of criminal justice involvement. A prior incarceration was reported among 69% of homeless Veterans in a VA domiciliary program—a time-limited residential treatment program for homeless Veterans.[7] A sample of 163 homeless Veterans in a VHA residential rehabilitation program indicated that 71.15% had been charged and arrested with any crime[12]; and in another study of 429 male homeless Veterans in a VHA domiciliary program, one-third had been convicted of a criminal offense and 21% had been charged or arrested for a crime against another person.[18] Finally, national samples of Veterans in VA supportive housing found that in 2008–2009, 65% had a history of incarceration,[13] and in 1992–2003, 79% had a criminal history, including criminal charges, convictions, and incarcerations.[15] Gender differences in criminal justice involvement have also been observed. A large national sample of Veterans in VA supportive housing found that 41% of female Veterans ($n$ = 1857 of 4686) and 68% of male Veterans ($n$ = 25,400 of 39,167) had a history of lifetime incarceration.[17]

## RECENT CRIMINAL JUSTICE INVOLVEMENT

A few studies measured more recent criminal justice involvement. Among a sample of 188 homeless males in a VA addiction treatment program, 27% committed nuisance offenses and 41% committed felonies in the past year.[4] Among Veterans in transitional housing or homeless shelters in Cincinnati, 16% were on supervised parole or probation.[11] Among a sample of 142 homeless Veterans with substance use disorders who were in a randomized controlled trial testing a VA compensated work therapy program, relatively few patients (6.3% of the work group and 3.2% in the control group) were incarcerated (jail or prison not specified) in the three months before the baseline interview.[10]

The research on homeless Veterans suggests that criminal justice involvement is a common life experience for these Veterans and that for a substantial minority, criminal justice involvement is a current issue in their lives while they are receiving treatment at VHA facilities. Many of the crimes committed by Veterans were minor crimes or crimes that were substance use or homeless related. For example, 27% of homeless Veterans in a residential treatment program had committed nuisance offenses, such as public intoxication or vagrancy.[4] Another study of homeless Veterans in a residential program indicated that 42% had driven under the influence; 29.5% had been arrested for disorderly conduct, vagrancy, or public drunkenness; and 13.5% had been arrested for narcotics charges.[12] Other studies of Veterans in supportive housing also found these minor crimes to be common among homeless Veterans with a criminal justice history.[22]

The lack of consistent definitions for homelessness and criminal justice involvement, as well as the lack of attention to the relationship between these two factors, other than reporting prevalence rates, limits our ability to discern trends in these studies. Furthermore, although criminal justice involvement is clearly something experienced by many homeless Veterans at some point in their lives, most studies lack nonhomeless comparison groups, so general statements of how common criminal justice involvement is for homeless Veterans are hard to place into the context of the broader population of Veterans. These studies are also limited in that all used self-report criminal justice data, which may or may not be accurate for this population, and many of the measures used were crude estimations of lifetime criminal justice contact or any incarceration. Along with other sources of criminal justice data, such as arrest records or convictions from law enforcement or judicial sources, fine-tuned measures of criminal justice involvement in relation to the timing of homelessness are needed to understand the interplay between these factors. Prospective studies following Veterans for years as they transition in and out of homelessness and criminal justice involvement may help answer these questions.

# Risk Factors for Criminal Justice Involvement Among Homeless Veterans

A variety of risk factors have been associated with criminal justice involvement among homeless Veterans. We organize these factors into (1) dynamic risk factors that could be altered through health care treatment or other interventions and (2) static risk factors that are not changeable. Among homeless Veterans in VHA addiction treatment or supportive housing, dynamic risk factors, including current alcohol or drug use, comorbid conditions, and living with a person who had a substance use disorder, were associated with higher odds of criminal behavior.[4] Treatment offered by the VA may help attenuate risk for criminal justice involvement among homeless Veterans; however, it is unknown whether addiction, mental health, or medical treatment is effective at reducing criminal justice involvement. For Veterans who may become criminal justice involved owing to factors related to homelessness, such as arrests for panhandling and vagrancy or stealing to make money, supportive housing may directly decrease their risk for criminal justice involvement. This assumption, however, is also largely untested. Static risk factors for criminal justice–involved people included childhood factors of experiencing abuse (physical or sexual) before age 18 years and conduct disorders in childhood, as well as having a prior hospitalization.[4,22] Although these static factors are less amenable to intervention to prevent criminal justice involvement among homeless Veterans, trauma-informed care or other mental health treatment may help address long-term traumatic experiences or other mental health issues that may still be affecting Veterans' health. Studies that directly test the effects of mental health treatment on homeless Veterans will help identify evidence-based practices for this population.

## Prevalence of and Risk Factors for Homelessness Among Criminal Justice–Involved Veterans

### PREVALENCE

A growing body of literature has examined the prevalence of homelessness among criminal justice–involved Veterans, primarily focused on Veterans who received VA outreach services. Almost all studies employed were observational studies of VA electronic health records, but patient characteristics differed across studies, as did the definitions of criminal justice involvement and homelessness used in each study. Table 6.2 displays studies on criminal justice–involved Veterans and the prevalence of homelessness observed.

Most studies examined a history of homelessness among Veterans, with Veterans self-reporting on their history of homelessness or looking back in VHA electronic health records for receipt of VA's homeless services. A national sample of Veterans in prison who received Health Care for Re-entry Veterans (HCRV) outreach services found that 30% had a homeless history: 11% were chronically homeless (homeless at the time of incarceration for one year or more or homeless more than three times in the past three years), 11% were episodically homeless (homeless at the time of incarceration for one month or more and less than one year and/or homeless three times or less in the past three years), and 8% were transiently homeless (homeless at the time of incarceration for less than one month or homeless only once in the past three years).[40] A nationally representative survey of incarcerated people found that among 142 Veterans 55 years or older who were exiting prison, 10% had a history of homelessness, including being homeless at the time of arrest (2.5%) or in the year before arrest (8.7%) or being marginally housed at the time of arrest (3.5%).[39] Homelessness was also more common among transgender Veterans who had a history of justice involvement (80%) compared with nontransgender Veterans with justice involvement (67%), although criminal justice involvement was quite prevalent in both groups.[23]

Two studies have examined homelessness among Veterans in Veterans Treatment Courts, which are specialized courts designed to divert Veterans from jail and prison and support their engagement in mental health and substance use disorder treatment. Veterans Treatment Court participants had the

*Table 6.2* **Prevalence of Homelessness Among Criminal Justice Involved Veterans**

| Authors | Study Design | Sample Size | Prevalence of Homelessness |
|---|---|---|---|
| Brown & Jones[23] | National sample of transgender Veterans and a matched control group of nontransgender Veterans who used VHA health care from 2007–2013 | 138 transgender Veterans and 188 nontransgender Veterans with criminal justice involvement | History of homelessness: ICD-9-CM diagnosis code V60.0 or clinical stop code indicting receipt of homeless services: 79.7% of transgender Veterans and 67% of nontransgender Veterans had a history of homelessness |
| Clark et al[24] | National observational study of Veterans in Veterans Treatment Courts from September 2008–February 2013 | 3,166 Veterans total 1,168 Veteran parents of minor children 1,998 Veterans without minor children | 16% were literally homeless; 5% were in imminent risk of losing housing; 15% were unstably housed; 64% were stably housed

Among Veterans who were homeless, 15% were homeless at least one night, less than one month; 28% were homeless at least one month, less than 6 months; 15% were homeless at least six months, less than one year; 13% were homeless at least one year, less than two years; 29% were homeless two years or more

21% had one homeless episode, 8% had two homeless episodes, 5% had three homeless episodes, 2% had four homeless episodes, and 5% had five homeless episodes in the past three years |

(continued)

*Table 6.2* **Continued**

| Authors | Study Design | Sample Size | Prevalence of Homelessness |
|---|---|---|---|
| Finlay et al.[25] | National observational study of Veterans who received VA outreach services in jail or court from FY 2010–FY 2012 | 37,542 criminal justice–involved Veterans | Received VA homeless indicator variable, clinic stop codes for VA services for homeless Veterans, ICD-9-CM diagnosis code for homelessness in the year after they received a justice outreach visit: 23% of criminal justice–involved Veterans were homeless in the one year after they received a justice outreach visit |
| Finlay, Binswanger et al.[26] | National observational study of Veterans who received VA outreach services in jail or court from FY 2010–FY 2012 | 1,535 female Veterans and 30,478 male Veterans | Received VA homeless indicator variable, clinic stop codes for VA services for homeless Veterans, ICD-9-CM diagnosis code for homelessness in the year after they received a criminal justice outreach visit: 19% of criminal justice–involved women Veterans and 24% of criminal justice–involved men Veterans were homeless in the one year after they received a VA criminal justice outreach visit |
| Finlay, Stimmel et al.[27] | National observational study of Veterans who received VA outreach services in prison from FY 2008–FY 2013 | 32,155 criminal justice–involved Veterans | Received VA homeless indicator variable, clinic stop codes for VA services for homeless Veterans, ICD-9-CM diagnosis code for homelessness the day they entered VA face-to-face care after their outreach visit: 5% of Veterans who received outreach services in prison were homeless the day of their first face-to-face visit |
| Hamilton et al.[28] | Focus groups of homeless women Veterans | 29 homeless women Veterans | 47% were on probation or parole |

| Study | Description | Sample | Findings |
|---|---|---|---|
| McGuire et al.[29] | Observational study of Veterans who received outreach services while in jail between May 1997 and October 1999 | 1,676 Veterans in jail | 21% had experienced homelessness for 6 months or more |
| Schaffer[30] | Observational study of Veterans who received VA outreach services in prison from 2004–2008 | 42 criminal justice–involved male Veterans | 59.4% had experienced one homeless episode; 56.7% had experience two or more homeless episodes |
| Schaffer[31] | Observational study of women Veterans who received VA outreach services in prison from 2003–2011 | 91 criminal justice–involved women Veterans | 60% had a history of homelessness. Average of 1.6 times homeless |
| Schaffer[32] | Observational study of Veterans who received outreach services while in jail probation and parole settings | 282 Veterans in jail probation and parole settings | 58% had homeless episodes before criminal justice involvement. 20% were homeless at jail release. 15.9% were unsure if they were homeless at jail release. Average number of times homeless 1.5 |
| Schaffer[33] | Observational study of Veterans in the criminal justice system who received VA outreach services | 399 Veterans who received VA outreach services in criminal justice settings | 74% were homeless once; 50% were homeless more than once |

(continued)

*Table 6.2* **Continued**

| Authors | Study Design | Sample Size | Prevalence of Homelessness |
|---|---|---|---|
| Stainbrook et al.[34] | Observational study of Veterans in a multisite jail diversion evaluation from January 2009–April 2014 | 1,274 Veterans in jail diversion program | 15% of Veterans were homeless at baseline |
| Stainbrook et al.[35] | Observational study of Veterans in a multisite jail diversion evaluation from January 2009–April 2014 | 1,025 Veterans in jail diversion program | 17% homeless in past 30 days |
| Stovall et al.[36] | Observational study of Veterans in jail who received outreach services | 62 male Veterans in jail with mental illness | 26% were homeless at arrest; 75% had a prior episode of homelessness |
| Tsai et al.[37] | Observational study of incarcerated Veterans who received VA outreach services in prison from October 2007–April 2011 | 30,348 incarcerated Veterans | 30% had a homeless history<br><br>8% were transiently homeless = homeless at the time of incarceration for less than one month or homeless only once in the past three years<br><br>11% were episodically homeless = homeless at the time of incarceration for one month or more and less than one year and/or homeless three times or less in the past three years<br><br>11% were chronically homeless = homeless at the time of incarceration for one year or more or homeless more than 3 times in the past three years |

| Tsai et al.[38] | Observational study of criminal justice–involved Veterans who received VA outreach services in jail or court from July 2010 to Nov 2015 | 22,708 Veterans who received VJO outreach services: 8,083 in Veterans Treatment Courts 680 in other treatment courts 13,945 not in treatment courts | 12% of Veterans in Veterans Treatment Court participants, 15% of Veterans in other treatment courts, and 18% of Veterans not in treatment courts were chronically homeless |
| Williams et al.[39] | Observational study of people incarcerated in prison who were within two years of release in 2004 | 142 Veterans age 55 years or older who were exiting prison | 10% had a history of homelessness, including being homeless at the time of arrest (2.5%) or in the year before arrest (8.7%) or being marginally housed at the time of arrest (3.5%) |

lowest rate of chronic homelessness (12%) compared with Veterans in other treatment courts (15%) and Veterans not in treatment courts (18%).[38] Among Veterans in Veterans Treatment Courts, not having minor children was associated with a higher prevalence of homelessness than having minor children (18% vs. 14%).[24] Homeless Veterans with minor children are a priority group for VA supportive housing, which may explain the differences between the groups. Two studies examining Veterans entering VA supportive housing programs found that Veterans with criminal justice or incarceration histories did not have delays in obtaining housing through the program compared with other Veterans with no criminal justice history.[13,14]

History of homelessness was examined among Veterans who received VA outreach services while incarcerated. Among a sample of 1,676 Veterans who were contacted by VA homeless outreach staff while in jail, 21% had experienced homelessness for 6 months or more.[29] Another study of 91 incarcerated women Veterans who received VHA homeless outreach services found that 60% had a history of homelessness.[31]

A few studies examined recent homelessness among Veterans in jail or jail diversion programs. Among 62 male Veterans in jail with mental illness, 26% were homeless at arrest.[36] Homelessness in the past 30 days was observed among 17% of Veterans in a jail diversion program.[34]

A small number of studies examined homelessness after criminal justice involvement. National samples of Veterans who received VA outreach services while in jail or court indicate roughly one-fourth are homeless during the year after their first contact with outreach staff[25]; however, gender differences were observed, with 19% of women Veterans and 24% of men Veterans homeless in the year after contact with outreach staff.[26] Among Veterans who received VA outreach services while in prison, 5% were homeless the day of their first face-to-face visit at a VHA facility.[27] Among 29 women Veterans who were homeless, 47% were on probation or parole and explained that they were restricted from leaving the county in which they were paroled or on probation, which prevented them from using housing options with family members who lived elsewhere.[28]

Although difficult to generalize because of variations in the samples, roughly one-fourth to three-fourths of criminal justice–involved Veterans experience homelessness, both before and after their criminal justice involvement. The majority of these studies were conducted with Veterans who received VA outreach services, so we are unable to determine whether these results generalize to the larger population of criminal justice–involved Veterans who do not receive VA outreach services or who do not use VA care. A few studies examined women Veterans separately from men Veterans, and one study examined transgender Veterans; however, these results were limited to prevalence rates. In addition, there is a dearth of information on the intersection of criminal justice involvement and homelessness among Veterans by socio-demographic factors such as race or ethnicity, rural or urban residence, disability status, or period of service. We also know very little about the scope of treatment needs among Veterans who are both homeless and criminal justice involved, treatment interventions that would help break the cyclical relationship of homelessness and criminal justice involvement, and the appropriate timing of interventions because Veterans who become incarcerated cannot receive VHA services while serving their sentence—a policy that interrupts their continuity of care and limits treatment options to those provided by the custodial agency.

Notably, most studies focused on lifetime criminal justice histories of Veterans. However, the current VA programs focus on outreach services for Veterans who are actively involved in the justice system. In the context of homelessness, recent criminal justice convictions—rather than arrests—are important because Veterans may lose their housing or employment while incarcerated or may have difficulty finding housing or employment after being released from jail or prison. Convictions that are more than seven years old are generally less problematic for Veterans when seeking employment, except in the case of Veterans who have sexual offense convictions. Individuals who are required to register on lifetime sex offender registries have persistent difficulties obtaining housing and employment and an elevated risk for homelessness.[41-43] Veterans on lifetime registries are prohibited by HUD from using the HUD-VASH program, a major national program that provides Housing Choice vouchers, formerly Section 8 vouchers, to Veterans.[44]

## RISK FACTORS

A few studies have examined criminal justice involvement as a risk factor for homelessness among Veterans. A study of VHA patients with bipolar disorder examined links between lifetime and recent incarceration and homelessness.[45] Veterans with a lifetime history of incarceration had four times higher odds of lifetime homelessness than Veterans with no incarceration history. Veterans with a recent incarceration (past four weeks) had 26 times higher odds of recent homelessness (past four weeks) than Veterans with no recent incarceration. Another study with 1,060 male Veterans in VA supportive housing found that a history of incarceration, either before entering supportive housing or during the time of the program, was linked to 50% higher odds of returning to homelessness within 600 days of leaving the program.[46] Transitional or supportive housing provided by the VA may help attenuate the risk for homelessness among some Veterans exiting incarceration. However, in a study of Veterans in VA supportive housing in Los Angeles, 51 Veterans who exited the program before locating permanent housing ("exiters") were compared with a matched sample of Veterans who were housed ("stayers") before the program end; comparisons were on Veterans' characteristics at the time of program entry.[9] More exiters were on probation or parole at the time of program entry compared with stayers (29% vs. 14%). This suggests that Veterans with a criminal justice history may have more difficulty staying in housing than other Veterans. After exiting the program, 24% of exiters were incarcerated and 31% became homeless. No studies that we know of examined additional factors that may explain the link between criminal justice involvement and homelessness among Veterans.

## The VA's Role in Addressing Criminal Justice Involvement to Prevent Homelessness

Historically, spikes in crime among returning military Veterans in the United States have been observed after every major conflict starting with the Civil War.[47,48] Following World War II and the Korean War, a comprehensive movement to offer treatment to incarcerated Veterans emerged. State departments of corrections and the then-emerging Veteran Service Organizations became prominent in both providing direct services and serving an advocacy role to highlight the issues among Veterans who were incarcerated. After the Vietnam War, there was a shift away from federal and state governments providing services to incarcerated Veterans, with advocacy organizations instead providing these services. During the 1980s and 1990s, there was some provision of services from the VA to incarcerated Veterans. However, the extent to which homelessness was a major issue among incarcerated Veterans and whether the provision of homeless services was the focus of these programs are unknown.

In 1999, federal regulations were issued that barred incarcerated Veterans from receiving VA health care while incarcerated,[49] which effectively ended systematic VA programming. In response to congressional inquiry, the VA created a workgroup on incarcerated Veterans that embraced partnerships with Department of Justice Bureau of Prisons and Veterans Service Organizations, expansion of outreach for Veterans exiting incarceration, and establishment of a best practice network in the VA. The modern delivery of VA services for incarcerated Veterans relied on the 2001 workgroup and was expanded based on opportunities created by H.R. 1593, the Second Chance Act of 2007, and a philosophical shift in the United States during the 2000s from a dramatic expansion of incarceration to a focus on critical needs during re-entry. President George W. Bush's signature quote (2004), "America is the land of the second chance, and when the gates of the prison open, the path ahead should lead to a better life," was a precursor to programming and re-engagement with services to Veterans who were incarcerated.

## HEALTH CARE FOR RE-ENTRY VETERANS

The VA began the modern interventions for Veterans who are criminal justice involved with an explicit understanding of the intertwined nature of homelessness and incarceration.[50] Aligned with the Sequential Intercept Model,[51] the first focus of intervention was at intercept 4 (i.e., community re-entry from jail or prison), to address the re-entry needs of Veterans incarcerated in state and federal prisons. Started in 2007, the HCRV program hired staff at the VA's regional levels to partner with state and federal prisons.[2] HCRV staff come primarily from social work and counseling backgrounds and are responsible for contacting Veterans while they are incarcerated and developing an individualized re-entry plan that works to address a full complement of psychosocial needs, including housing, as well as medical and mental health care. Program staff also provide short-term case management after Veterans are released to ensure Veterans engage with needed clinical services that support healthy re-entry.

The HCRV program works to overcome a number of complications in its efforts to serve incarcerated Veterans. First, state and federal prison facilities, which have oversight of Veterans while they are incarcerated, have no mandate that requires them to create or allow special programming for Veterans or to allow access to facilities for staff members of other agencies such as the VA. HCRV staff work to cross boundaries, developing partnerships with federal and state agencies to allow them to have access to controlled facilities.

Second, identifying Veterans among the incarcerated population is difficult. Military service is not among the demographic indicators that all prison facilities collect, and Veterans are not required to disclose their military history or status. Initially, HCRV staff members held open information sessions announcing their presence onsite at a prison and requesting attendance by Veterans. Subsequently, some prison facilities have added an intake question requesting that incarcerated people self-disclose their history of military service. Most recently, the VA has developed an online tool called the Veterans Re-entry Search Service that allows a criminal justice entity (such as a state department of corrections) to upload their entire list of incarcerated persons, which is matched against U.S. Department of Defense records to determine who among the entire inmate population has a history of U.S. military service. VA outreach staff and correctional staff are then provided with a list of Veterans identified in the prison or jail. Before development of this tool, roughly 2% to 3% of incarcerated persons were identified as Veterans. In locations where it is used, 8% to 9% of incarcerated persons are often identified as Veterans. The improvement in identification of Veterans who are incarcerated has allowed more direct outreach to individual Veterans by the VA and better opportunities for HCRV to serve Veterans who do not self-identify.

Finally, HCRV makes efforts to overcome the barrier that state and federal prison facilities are often located in communities that are a far distance from where an individual committed a crime and is required to be released. As a result, HCRV is often challenged with traveling long distances to provide onsite outreach to prisons and with coordinating re-entry services for Veterans who are incarcerated hundreds of miles from the communities where they will release. HCRV relies on the national network of VA medical centers and colleagues across the country who assist in coordinating a package of housing, medical, mental health, substance use, and employment interventions in the community closest to where each Veteran will release.

## VETERANS JUSTICE OUTREACH PROGRAM

In 2009, building on the experience gained in HCRV, the VA developed a second intervention, the Veterans Justice Outreach (VJO) program. VJO focuses on Veterans who encounter law enforcement (intercept 1 in the Sequential Intercept Model), are incarcerated in local jails (intercepts 2 and 3), or are involved in oversight through specialty courts, including Veterans Treatment Courts (intercepts 3 and 4).[2] Staff from this program also address the re-entry and/or probation needs of Veterans exiting jail (intercepts 4 and 5). Like HCRV staff, VJO staff are primarily drawn from social work and counseling backgrounds and share similar responsibilities. The VJO program focuses on intervening at earlier points in the criminal justice system in order to divert Veterans away from incarceration and into treatment before they are sentenced and incarcerated in state and federal prison facilities.

VJO staff share the same challenge as HCRV staff of gaining access to secure facilities and identifying Veterans who are incarcerated. In addition, the short-term incarceration of Veterans in jail creates the challenge of having high-volume, quick-turnover caseloads; over one million Veterans may be arrested over the course of a year.[52] Strategies used by VJO staff when working with Veterans who are incarcerated in local jails are similar to those employed by HCRV; they become experts at partnering with local criminal justice agencies to develop access to secure jail facilities, assist in developing self-report or data matching protocols to identify Veterans who are incarcerated, and then meet with Veterans to develop individualized plans that address housing, medical, mental health, and employment needs.

# Future Directions for Researchers

As the HCRV and VJO programs continue to grow, research can help inform resource allocation and programming to serve Veterans who are homeless and/or criminal justice involved. However, the current body of literature is limited for a number of reasons. First, the extant studies are limited to Veterans who seek treatment or housing at the VA, and most national studies are limited to Veterans in housing or justice programs. Veterans who do not have contact with the VA or who are not in the homeless or justice programs were not captured in these studies; thus, we have no information on what support they may need to attenuate their risks for homelessness or criminal justice involvement. Using more comprehensive data sources that include Veterans who do not use the VA, as well as other sources for criminal justice involvement such as arrest records, will provide a clearer picture of this population. Second, we know very little about demographic groups such as women, people of color, rural Veterans, Veterans with disabilities, and Veterans from different periods of service. Research is needed to examine the extent to which these Veterans differ from white male Veterans who live in urban areas and what unique programmatic needs they may have. Third, the cyclical nature of homelessness and criminal justice involvement and the mechanisms that explain the link between these two life experiences are largely unexplored. Homeless Veterans may become criminal justice involved because they are arrested for things related to homelessness such as panhandling or vagrancy. They may also engage in stealing or other illegal acts in order to survive on the streets. Criminal justice–involved Veterans may become homeless because they lost their housing while incarcerated or are unable to find a job after exiting incarceration so cannot afford housing. Mental health and substance use disorders are common among both homeless Veterans[17,53] and criminal justice–involved Veterans[25,27] and, unaddressed by treatment, may contribute to chronic homelessness and criminal justice involvement. Without critical research in these areas, outreach and intervention programs will be limited in their ability to provide targeted programmatic efforts to homeless and criminal justice–involved Veterans.

# Future Directions for Providers of Housing, Legal, Health, and Social Services to Homeless and Criminal Justice–Involved Veterans

While research continues on the link between homelessness and criminal justice involvement in the Veteran population, current literature provides few suggestions for providers who work with homeless, criminal justice–involved Veterans. First, many homeless Veterans in VA mental health and substance use disorder treatment programs had criminal justice involvement. Efforts by these programs to connect Veterans with legal services in their area may help reduce their risk for continued criminal justice involvement. For example, Veterans who need to resolve minor charges or bench warrants may benefit from short-term legal services that clear up their criminal justice involvement and allow them to refocus on their treatment. The VA currently hosts more than 160 free legal clinics in its medical centers and other facilities. Although most of these clinics focus on Veterans' civil legal issues, some can assist Veterans facing criminal charges, and approximately 40% of the clinics can help Veterans seek to expunge old charges or convictions from their records. Expanding the availability of these services in VA settings may increase their accessibility to Veterans, particularly those with limited resources.

Second, Veterans with criminal justice involvement are particularly vulnerable to homelessness in the period after release from incarceration. Ensuring that they have housing immediately on release, a difficult task given changes in release dates and availability of beds, may help reduce this risk period. Veterans exiting prison incarceration are also at high risk for overdose and have mental health and substance use disorder treatment needs that may be exacerbated by homelessness. Furthermore, 44% of Veterans who received VA outreach while in prison do not enter VA treatment in the year following their outreach visit, and those who do enter VA treatment often leave mental health or substance use disorder treatment quickly.[27] Following Veterans as they leave prison and ensuring they receive needed treatment, either at the VA or in a community treatment setting, may help limit the risk for homelessness and other health problems experienced by this population.

Finally, employment training may be a critical treatment service to help reduce Veterans' risk for homelessness or criminal justice involvement. In a national study of Veterans in VA supportive housing, homeless Veterans with a criminal history were less skilled and held jobs for shorter time periods than their counterparts without criminal justice involvement.[16] Difficulty maintaining employment and low wages associated with unskilled work may have contributed to homelessness or criminal involvement among this population. Offering employment training in VA supportive housing programs may ensure that the population that most needs this training receives it. Other programs geared toward criminal justice–involved Veterans, such as Moral Reconation Therapy, which addresses criminogenic thinking, could also be offered in housing program settings through homeless programs staff.

# Conclusion

The apparent link between homelessness and criminal justice involvement among Veterans is recognized, but the extant literature reveals that much is still to be learned. For homeless Veterans, identifying and understanding their recent criminal justice involvement and how such involvement shapes their risk for return to or continued homelessness will inform homeless programs, both inside and outside the VA. For criminal justice–involved Veterans, delivery of homeless and other support services immediately on release from incarceration will help limit their risk for homelessness. The VA's HCRV and VJO programs, as well as homeless programs more broadly, address some of the needs of this population. However, more focused research on the mechanisms explaining homelessness and criminal justice involvement, attention to different socio-demographic groups, and more comprehensive data from a variety of sources are needed to inform and guide future efforts to serve homeless and criminal justice–involved Veterans.

# References

1. Metraux S, Roman CG, Cho R. Incarceration and homelessness. Paper presented at the National Symposium on Homelessness Research; 2007, March; Washington, DC.
2. Blue-Howells JH, Clark SC, van den Berk-Clark C, McGuire JF. The U.S. Department of Veterans Affairs Veterans Justice Programs and the sequential intercept model: Case examples in national dissemination of intervention for justice-involved veterans. *Psychol Serv.* 2013;10(1):48–53.
3. Greenberg GA, Rosenheck RA. Jail incarceration, homelessness, and mental health: A national study. *Psych Serv.* 2008;59(2):170–177.
4. Benda BB, Rodell DE, Rodell L. Crime among homeless military veterans who abuse substances. *Psychiatr Rehabil J.* 2003;26(4):332–345.
5. Benda BB, Rodell DE, Rodell L. Differentiating nuisance from felony offenses among homeless substance abusers in a V.A. medical center. *J Offender Rehabil.* 2003;37(1):41–65.
6. Buchholz JR, Malte CA, Calsyn DA, et al. Associations of housing status with substance abuse treatment and service use outcomes among veterans. *Psychiatr Serv.* 2010;61(7):698–706.
7. Cheung RC, Hanson AK, Maganti K, Keeffe EB, Matsui SM. Viral hepatitis and other infectious diseases in a homeless population. *J Clin Gastroenterol.* 2002;34(4):476–480.
8. Douyon R, Guzman P, Romain G, et al. Subtle neurological deficits and psychopathological findings in substance-abusing homeless and non-homeless veterans. *J Neuropsychiatry Clin Neurosci.* 1998;10(2):210–215.
9. Gabrielian S, Burns AV, Nanda N, Hellemann G, Kane V, Young AS. Factors associated with premature exits from supported housing. *Psychiatr Serv.* 2016;67(1):86–93.
10. Kashner TM, Rosenheck R, Campinell AB, et al. Impact of work therapy on health status among homeless, substance-dependent veterans: A randomized controlled trial. *Arch Gen Psychiatry.* 2002;59(10):938–944.
11. Schaffer BJ. Homeless military veterans and the intersection of partner violence. *J Hum Behav Soc Environ.* 2012;22(8):1003–1013.

12. Seidner AL, Burling TA, Fisher LM, Blair TR. Characteristics of telephone applicants to a residential rehabilitation program for homeless veterans. *J Consult Clin Psychol.* 1990;58(6):825–831.

13. Tejani N, Rosenheck R, Tsai J, Kasprow W, McGuire JF. Incarceration histories of homeless veterans and progression through a national supported housing program. *Community Ment Health J.* 2014;50(5):514–519.

14. Tsai J, O'Connell M, Kasprow WJ, Rosenheck RA. Factors related to rapidity of housing placement in Housing and Urban Development–Department of Veterans Affairs Supportive Housing program of 1990s. *J Rehabil Res Dev.* 2011;48(7):755–762.

15. Tsai J, Rosenheck RA. Homeless veterans in supported housing: Exploring the impact of criminal history. *Psychol Serv.* 2013b;10(4):452–458.

16. Tsai J, Rosenheck RA. Psychosis, lack of job skills, and criminal history: Associations with employment in two samples of homeless men. *Psychiatr Serv.* 2016;67(6):671–675.

17. Tsai J, Rosenheck RA, Kane V. Homeless female U.S. veterans in a national supported housing program: Comparison of individual characteristics and outcomes with male veterans. *Psychol Serv.* 2014;11(3):309–316.

18. Wenzel SL, Bakhtiar L, Caskey NH, et al. Dually diagnosed homeless veterans in residential treatment: Service needs and service use. *J Nerv Ment Dis.* 1996;184(7):441–444.

19. Wenzel SL, Gelberg L, Bakhtiar L, et al. Indicators of chronic homelessness among veterans. *Hosp Community Psychiatry.* 1993;44(12):1172–1176.

20. Westermeyer J, Lee K. Residential placement for veterans with addiction: American Society of Addiction Medicine criteria vs. a veterans homeless program. *J Nerv Ment Dis.* 2013;201(7):567–571.

21. McLellan AT, Luborsky L, O'Brien CP, Woody GE. An improved diagnostic instrument for substance abuse patients: The Addiction Severity Index. *J Nerv Ment Dis.* 1980;168:26–33.

22. Tsai J, Rosenheck RA. Childhood antecedents of incarceration and criminal justice involvement among homeless veterans. *Am J Orthopsychiatry.* 2013;83(4):545–549.

23. Brown GR, Jones KT. Health correlates of criminal justice involvement in 4,793 transgender veterans. *LGBT Health.* 2015;2(4):297–305.

24. Clark S, Blue-Howells J, McGuire J. What can family courts learn from the Veterans Treatment Courts? *Fam Ct Rev.* 2014;52(3):417–424.

25. Finlay AK, Smelson D, Sawh L, et al. U.S. Department of Veterans Affairs Veterans Justice Outreach program: Connecting justice-involved veterans with mental health and substance use disorder treatment. *Crim Justice Policy Rev.* 2016;27(2):203–222.

26. Finlay AK, Binswanger IA, Smelson D, et al. Sex differences in mental health and substance use disorders and treatment entry among justice-involved veterans in the Veterans Health Administration. *Med Care.* 2015;53(Suppl 1):S105-S111.

27. Finlay AK, Stimmel M, Blue-Howells J, et al. Use of Veterans Health Administration mental health and substance use disorder treatment after exiting prison: The Health Care for Reentry Veterans program. *Adm Policy Ment Health.* 2017;44(2):177–187.

28. Hamilton AB, Poza I, Washington DL. "Homelessness and trauma go hand-in-hand": Pathways to homelessness among women Veterans. *Womens Health Issues.* 2011;21(4 Suppl):S203–209.

29. McGuire J, Rosenheck RA, Kasprow WJ. Health status, service use, and costs among veterans receiving outreach services in jail or community settings. *Psychiatr Serv.* 2003;54(2):201–207.

30. Schaffer B. Veteran sex offenders and reentry problems. *J Correct Health Care.* 2011;17(3):266–270.

31. Schaffer BJ. Female military veterans: Crime and psychosocial problems. *J Hum Behav Soc Environ.* 2014;24(8):996–1003.

32. Schaffer BJ. Military veterans in the criminal justice system: Partner violence and the impact of relationships with fathers. *J Evid Inf Soc Work.* 2016;13(4):394–400.

33. Schaffer BJ. Incarcerated Veterans Outreach Program. *J Evid Inf Soc Work.* 2016;13(3):293–304.

34. Stainbrook K, Penney D, Elwyn L. The opportunities and challenges of multi-site evaluations: Lessons from the jail diversion and trauma recovery national cross-site evaluation. *Eval Program Plann.* 2015;50:26–35.

35. Stainbrook K, Hartwell S, James A. Female veterans in jail diversion programs: Differences from and similarities to their male peers. *Psychiatr Serv.* 2015;67(1):133–136.

36. Stovall JG, Cloninger L, Appleby L. Identifying homeless mentally ill veterans in jail: A preliminary report. *J Am Acad Psychiatry Law.* 1997;25(3):311–315.

37. Tsai J, Rosenheck RA, Kasprow WJ, McGuire JF. Homelessness in a national sample of incarcerated veterans in state and federal prisons. *Adm Policy Ment Health.* 2014b;41(3):360–367.

38. Tsai J, Flatley B, Kasprow WJ, Clark S, Finlay A. Diversion of veterans with criminal justice involvement to treatment courts: Participant characteristics and outcomes. *Psychiatr Serv.* 2017;68(4):375–383.

39. Williams BA, McGuire J, Lindsay RG, et al. Coming home: Health status and homelessness risk of older pre-release prisoners. *J Gen Intern Med.* 2010;25(10):1038–1044.

40. Tsai J, Rosenheck RA, Kasprow WJ, McGuire JF. Homelessness in a national sample of incarcerated veterans in state and federal prisons. *Adm Policy Ment Health.* 2014;41(3):360–367.

41. Levenson JS, D'Amora DA, Hern AL. Megan's Law and its impact on community re-entry for sex offenders. *Behav Sci Law.* 2007;25(4):587–602.

42. Mercado CC, Alvarez S, Levenson J. The impact of specialized sex offender legislation on community reentry. *Sex Abuse.* 2008;20(2):188–205.

43. Socia KM, Levenson JS, Ackerman AR, Harris AJ. "Brothers under the bridge": Factors influencing the transience of registered sex offenders in Florida. *Sex Abuse.* 2015;27(6):559–586.

44. VA National Center on Homelessness Among Veterans. HUD-VASH resource guide for permanent housing and clinical care. Washington, DC: US Department of Veterans Affairs; 2004.

45. Copeland LA, Miller AL, Welsh DE, McCarthy JF, Zeber JE, Kilbourne AM. Clinical and demographic factors associated with homelessness and incarceration among VA patients with bipolar disorder. *Am J Public Health.* 2009;99(5):871–877.

46. Cusack M, Montgomery AE. Examining the bidirectional association between veteran homelessness and incarceration within the context of permanent supportive housing. *Psychol Serv.* 2017;14(2):250–256.

47. Hunter BD. Echoes of war: The combat veteran in criminal court. Vet Court Con: Veterans Treatment Court Conference; 2013; Washington DC.

48. Seamone ER. A historical touchstone for Nebraska in the mission to divert criminally-involved veterans from confinement. *Nebraska Lawyer.* 2013;16(6):7–15.

49. Principi A. *Letter to The Honorable Bart Gordon, U.S. House of Representatives concerning the exclusion of incarcerated veterans from Department of Veterans Affairs (VA) health care benefits.* Washington, D.C.: The Secretary of Veterans Affairs; 2001.

50. McGuire J. Closing a front door to homelessness among veterans. *J Prim Prev.* 2007;28(3):389–400.

51. Munetz MR, Griffin PA. Use of the sequential intercept model as an approach to decriminalization of people with serious mental illness. *Psychiatr Serv.* 2006;57:544–549.

52. Mumola CJ, Noonan ME. Justice-involved veterans: National estimates and research resources. VHA National Veterans Justice Outreach Planning Conference; December 2, 2008; Baltimore, MD.

53. Tsai J, Kasprow WJ, Rosenheck RA. Alcohol and drug use disorders among homeless veterans: Prevalence and association with supported housing outcomes. *Addict Behav.* 2014;39(2):455–460.

# 7

# Homelessness and Money Management in Military Veterans

ERIC B. ELBOGEN

> Too many veterans carrying the burdens of PTSD or
> TBI, compounded by limited financial literacy and
> atypical behaviors, begin a downward spiral towards
> isolation, depression, substance abuse, joblessness,
> failed relationships, homelessness—and sometimes
> suicide. It usually doesn't happen overnight—it's a long,
> slow slide. But it begins somewhere, and it would be
> shortsighted for any of us to presume that these
> conditions only ensue after the uniform comes off.
> Former Secretary of Veterans Affairs Eric Shinseki

Explaining the historically disproportionate number of Veterans in the homeless population is a challenge that has stymied policymakers (Institute of Medicine, 2010). Researchers have identified links between Veteran homelessness and posttraumatic stress disorder (PTSD) (Metraux, Cusack, Byrne, Hunt-Johnson, & True, 2017), depression (Institute of Medicine, 2010; Rosenheck & Fontana, 1994), bipolar disorder (Copeland et al., 2009), military sexual trauma (Washington et al., 2010; Brignone et al., 2016), alcohol and drug abuse (Edens, Mares, Tsai, & Rosenheck, 2011; Institute of Medicine, 2010; Rosenheck & Fontana, 1994; Tsai, Hoff, & Harpaz-Rotem, 2017), and traumatic brain injury (TBI) (Metraux, Clegg, Daigh, Culhane, & Kane, 2013; Russell et al., 2013). Studies demonstrate that criminal justice involvement and postemployment arrests (Copeland et al., 2009; Institute of Medicine, 2010) and military misconduct (Gundlapalli et al., 2015) are potential correlates of Veteran homelessness. Sociodemographic variables have also been investigated, with research showing that lower education and being unmarried increase the odds of homelessness among Veterans (Copeland et al., 2009; Montgomery, Dichter, Thomasson, Fu, & Roberts, 2015; Tsai et al., 2017; Washington et al., 2010).

An additional, though often overlooked, contributor to homelessness is difficulty achieving financial stability (Elbogen et al., 2013; Steen & MacKenzie, 2013). On Veterans Day 2010, National Public Radio (NPR) reported this story: "Over the past decade, the number of female veterans who have become homeless has nearly doubled to roughly 6,500, according to the Department of Veterans Affairs. Most of them are younger than 35. One of them is Cherish Cornish. Since June, the 29-year-old has lived on the fifth floor of a temporary housing facility run by Father Bill's & Main Spring, a private nonprofit group in Brockton, Massachusetts. Cornish lives in one of five rooms reserved for homeless female veterans. She's struggling to make a life for herself after the military. 'When I joined the Army, I was barely 20 years old,' Cornish says with a Southern accent, a legacy of years growing up in Texas. 'I come out, and I'm 23, and so I just kind of came of age in the military. I wind up on my own again in an apartment. It's the first time I've had to pay rent since I was a teenager. It's the first time I had to pay a light bill— pretty much ever—and all these responsibilities and budgeting and stuff that I'd really never had to deal with in the military'"(Kaplan, 2010).

Ms. Cornish was clear about how she became homeless after separating from the military: she had little to no experience managing her own finances before transitioning to civilian life. Military Veterans can face an array of barriers in the financial domain, so is money management another risk factor that should be considered when assessing risk for Veteran homelessness? Or when implementing policy to reduce Veteran homelessness? If so, what money management problems do Veterans experience? How are financial problems linked to mental and behavioral health problems? What approaches lead to improved money management in Veterans? How can these be configured to optimize effectiveness? What programs are available during and after military service?

This chapter reviews the link between money management and homelessness in military Veterans. First, money management challenges and issues faced by Veterans are outlined, emphasizing some of the unique characteristics of military service and Veteran status that may play a role. Second, the link between mental health problems—one of the most consistent predictors of homelessness—and money management in Veterans is examined. Third, the role of money management in Veteran homelessness is examined, while noting that successful homelessness programs typically include at least informal money management. Fourth, research on how to effectively improve money management and financial literacy in Veterans, as well as in the civilian population, is summarized. Fifth, both U.S. Department of Veterans Affairs (VA) and military programs aimed at improving financial literacy are reviewed, and suggestions for extending money management interventions are offered. In the end, recognizing the role of money management in Veterans' lives is seen as an important component of efforts to combat, and ultimately eliminate, Veteran homelessness.

## Money Management in Military Veterans

Many Veterans who return home from combat cope with injuries related to their war experiences, including PTSD, TBI, and major depressive disorder (MDD) (Hoge et al., 2004; Seal et al., 2009; Tanielian & Jaycox, 2008). On top of these mental health issues, however, Veterans also often need to overcome financial barriers, which themselves are associated with symptoms of mental and physical disorders (Richardson, Elliott, & Roberts, 2013).

Reports show that military experience can uniquely affect financial well-being (Department of Labor, 2012; Elbogen, Johnson, Wagner, Newton, & Beckham, 2012; FINRA, 2010; Institute of Medicine, 2010). First, psychological and physical war injuries can reduce a Veteran's employability, and many military personnel also require retraining to learn skills and education (Tinoco, 2014) to transfer skills from the military to civilian work (Horton et al., 2013), found to be a significant problem among women Veterans (Greer, 2017). Second, when service members live on a military base, their basic needs are met; therefore, many recently discharged Veterans might find themselves financially independent for the first time in their mid to late 20s or even 30s, a decade after most civilians do. Third, service members' sense of financial security may be adversely affected by multiple deployments that disrupt family stability or lead to job loss.

Fourth, although mental illnesses such as bipolar disorder and PTSD could involve impulsive behavior that leads to unwise spending, recent data indicate that predatory lenders target military and Veterans; in addition, the largest concentration of payday lending businesses in the country are in zip codes near military bases, and active-duty service members are three times more likely than civilians to take out payday loans (Institutes of Medicine, 2010). However, recent empirical studies question whether this has an actual impact on military service members, finding few adverse effects of payday loan access (Carter & Skimmyhorn, 2017). As of October 3, 2016, lenders to active-duty service members and their dependents have to comply with the Military Lending Act (which expanded the Talent-Nelson Military Lending Act, 10 U.S.C. § 987, enacted in 2006) for most types of consumer loans, including payday loans, deposit advance products, vehicle title loans, overdraft lines of credit but not traditional overdraft services, and installment loans.

Data from National Financial Capability Study (Financial Industry Regulatory Authority, 2010), conducted in collaboration with the Department of Treasury and the President's Advisory Counsel on Financial Literacy, show that military service members are the same as civilians in terms of saving money and opening up bank accounts, are less likely than civilians to meet their basic needs, and are more likely than civilians to have significant credit card debt. Credit card misman-agement was also a noted problem for Veterans in particular, leading to heavy debt, fees, and interest accumulation. Military families were found to display financial capability in the following ways: keeping up with monthly expenses, calculating how much they need to save for retirement, contributing regularly to retirement accounts, shopping around and comparing financial products, checking their credit score and credit report, and demonstrating higher levels of financial literacy. Those who had been enlisted personnel and junior noncom-missioned officers while serving in the military also exhibited greater problems in planning for financial emergencies. Recent empirical analyses examining data from the 2009 and 2012 National Financial Capability Studies find that compared with civilian households, military households have more types of sav-ings accounts, more problematic credit card behaviors, and equivalent use of alternative financial services (Skimmyhorn, 2016).

Recently, researchers examined food insecurity, defined as lack of access to sufficient food for a healthful lifestyle, among Veterans of the wars in Iraq and Afghanistan (Widome, Jensen, Bangerter, & Fu, 2015). Specifically, in this study, food security was measured using the U.S. Household Food Security Module, which includes items such as: "The food that (I/we) bought just didn't last, and (I/we) didn't have money to get more" and "(I/we) couldn't afford to eat balanced meals." The authors found that more than one in four Veterans reported past-year food insecurity, with 12% reporting very low food security. Correlates of food insecurity among Veterans included being younger, not being married or having a partner, living in households with more children, earning lower incomes, having a lower final military pay grade, being more likely to use tobacco, engaging in more frequent binge drinking, and sleeping less.

Another study (Miller, Larson, Byrne, & DeVoe, 2016) using data from the 2005–2013 waves of the Current Population Survey—Food Security Supplement to identify rates of food insecurity in Veteran and non-Veteran households concluded: "Though adjusting eliminated many differences between veteran and non-veteran households, veterans who served from 1975 and onwards may be at higher risk for [food insecurity] and should be the recipients of targeted outreach to improve nutritional outcomes." For this reason, a subset of Veterans may benefit from the Supplemental Nutrition Assistance Program (SNAP), which offers nutrition assistance to low-income individuals and families (www.fns.usda.gov/snap).

Both Veteran- and non-Veteran–specific factors contribute to financial in-security as well. Poor money management, bad financial decisions, and lack of knowledge of how to at least establish a baseline level of financial well-being can result in, or perpetuate, Veteran homelessness. Some Veterans might accrue severe debt by covering minimum payments on credit cards; they may not understand that interest rates are charged on outstanding credit card balances. Others may spend freely and regularly on tobacco products or lottery tickets, without awareness of how this could affect their monthly budget. Veterans may be unaware of vocational programs available through the VA or that many companies and stores provide military/Veterans savings discounts. They mistakenly may believe they will lose disability benefits if they work, which researchers have noted would be a disincentive for seeking steady employment (Rosenheck, Frisman, & Sindelar, 1995). Veterans receiving disability may be vulnerable to financial exploitation by predatory lenders or even family members. Veterans may lack knowledge of financial benefits, such as not knowing that many companies and stores provide military/Veterans savings discounts.

Despite the numerous factors playing a role in Veterans' financial well-being, there has been relatively little research published regarding how Veterans manage their money, but what we do know indicates that Veterans struggle with debt (Heisler, Wagner, & Piette, 2005), unemployment (Rosenheck et al., 1995), and money *mis*management (Black et al., 2008). Studies of consumer behavior have documented that "vulnerable" populations, such as Veterans with psychiatric disabilities, may be at higher risk for being taken advantage of by predatory lenders (Hill & Kozup, 2007). Rosenheck and colleagues found reduced significantly lower employment among Veterans with psychiatric disabilities receiving benefits compared with those who were not (Rosenheck, Dausey, Frisman, & Kasprow, 2000). As indicated early, work disincentive following receipt of disability for Veterans has been demonstrated using national data sets (Rosenheck et al., 1995).

Veterans with psychiatric disabilities can garner more than $4,000 per month in disability benefits combined from the VA and U.S. Social Security Administration (SSA), whereas non-Veterans with psychiatric disabilities may receive less than $1,000 from the SSA alone. Further, Veterans first obtaining disability often get retroactive checks that can amount to tens of thousands of dollars. Still, it is important to recognize that these increased benefits to Veterans with psychiatric disabilities may paradoxically (1) increase available funds to purchase alcohol or drugs; (2) increase risk for severe debt because of increased capacity to obtain credit cards and other unsecured loans; (3) decrease incentive to work as policies at the VA and SSA are distinct, ever-changing, and often difficult to navigate; and (4) increase vulnerability to financial exploitation and victimization by family, friends, and strangers as a result of greater income than non-Veterans with psychiatric disabilities.

A recent study provides some empirical support that Veterans, even when homeless, use at least a portion of their funds for substance abuse. Tsai and Rosenheck (2015) analyzed data from 1,160 Veterans from nearly 20 sites on entry into the U.S. Housing and Urban Development–Veterans Affairs Supportive Housing (HUD-VASH) program (Tsai & Rosenheck, 2015). They specifically examined the amount of money homeless Veterans spent on alcohol and drugs and the interrelationships between public support income, including VA disability compensation, and expenditures on alcohol and drugs. Although the investigators found that one-third of Veterans reported spending money on alcohol and 22% reported spending money on drugs in the past month, no significant association was found between public support income, VA disability compensation, and money spent on alcohol and drugs. The authors concluded that while a substantial proportion of homeless Veterans spend some income on alcohol and drugs, disability income, including VA compensation, is unrelated to substance use or money spent on addictive substances.

## Money Management and Mental Health in Veterans

Money management is a cornerstone of psychosocial rehabilitation for Veterans (Elbogen, Tiegreen, Vaughan, & Bradford, 2011; Klee, Armstrong, & Harkness, 2016; Rowe, Serowik, Ablondi, Wilber, & Rosen, 2013). Because it affects daily independent living, money management can be seen as an essential component of psychiatric rehabilitation and recovery. People with psychiatric disabilities consistently rank better financial management and improving money skills as among their most important personal goals (Barbato, Monzani, & Schiavi, 2004; Borras et al., 2007; Eklund, 2009; Evans, Wright, Svanum, & Bond, 2004; Foldemo, Ek, & Bogren, 2004; Perron, Ilgen, Hasche, & Howard, 2008). A common "unmet" need reported by people with psychiatric disabilities is having enough money to cover food, clothes, and shelter (Gater et al., 1997; Hanrahan et al., 2002; Perese, 1997; Stansfeld, Orrell, Mason, Nicholls, & D'Ath, 1998). Improving money management is thus seen as enhancing self-determination (Elbogen & Tomkins, 1999, 2000; Shaner, Tucker, Roberts, & Eckman, 1999). Scholars support the need to broaden the focus of reintegration of Veterans to include the financial domain of functioning (Sherman, Larsen, & Borden, 2015).

Research has accumulated strong evidence for the effectiveness of a psychiatric rehabilitation framework guided by the following principles: (1) the goal of treatment is to minimize disability and maximize self-determination and independent functioning (Cook, Russell, Grey, & Jonikas, 2008; Liberman, 1992); (2) consumers must be empowered to play an active role in making decisions about their treatment and, ultimately, their lives (Lecomte, Wallace, Perreault, & Caron, 2005); (3) clinical assessment must include articulation of the functional nature of the disabilities, such as how cognitive deficits influence capacity for independent living (Spaulding et al., 1999); (4) treatment must address as many of the skill deficits and disabilities of the disorder as possible (Liberman, Kopelowicz, & Young, 1994; Spaulding, Sullivan, & Poland, 2003); and (5) outcomes must be judged on the balance of symptom control, neutralization of disability, improved independent living skills, subjective well-being, empowerment and autonomy, and objective quality of life (Spaulding, Poland, Elbogen, & Ritchie, 2000).

A recovery orientation therefore postulates that a person with mental illness can achieve better functioning in specific domains, including living, work, and social environments (Anthony, 1998; Menditto et al., 1999). Money management skills intersect with each of these (Klee et al., 2016). In the living environment, a person creates a budget, pays bills and utilities, buys groceries, opens a bank account and saves money, and ensures that rent, food, and clothing are paid for. In the work environment, basic money management skills are needed to understand wages, taxes, and earnings and how these relate to one's labor input (Dunn, Wewiorski, & Rogers, 2008). In the social environment, going out to a restaurant on a date, joining a social club, going to a movie, and buying a cup of coffee rely on basic money management skills. Affording transportation in any of these environments, or getting to a mental health center, also depends on a person with mental illness having a certain level of basic money management skills. Independent functioning implicitly relies on a person being able to handle finances adequately.

Financial difficulties are strongly linked to mental health problems (Dohrenwend & et al., 1992; Eaton, Bovasso, & Smith, 2001; Luo & Waite, 2005; Marmot, 2001; Pomerantz, 2003; Weich, Lewis, & Jenkins, 2001), one of the most often cited set of factors that increase risk for homelessness in Veterans (Copeland et al., 2009; Institute of Medicine, 2010; Rosenheck & Fontana, 1994). Broadly, empirical research shows that individuals with greater debt are significantly more likely to suffer from physical and mental health problems (Richardson et al., 2013) as well as mental disorders (Jenkins et al., 2008; Muntaner, Eaton, Miech, & O'Campo, 2004; Reading & Reynolds, 2001), a finding replicated internationally (Patel & Kleinman, 2003; Weich & Lewis, 1998). Research demonstrates significantly elevated risk for completed suicide (Chan et al., 2009) and self-harm behaviors (Hatcher, 1994) among those with unemployment and unmanageable debt. Finances rank among the biggest stressors in families (Ochoa et al., 2008).

Among people with severe mental illness such as schizophrenia, bipolar disorder, and MDD, better financial status is associated with higher quality of life, greater self-efficacy, and fewer psychiatric symptoms (Barbato et al., 2004; Dufort, Dallaire, & Lavoie, 1997; Heider et al., 2007; Laliberte-Rudman, Yu, Scott, & Pajouhandeh, 2000; Olusina & Ohaeri, 2003). Indeed, finances have been shown in some studies to be a stronger predictor of consumer quality of life than clinical symptoms (Kovess-Masfaty et al., 2006). Conversely, financial instability has been consistently linked to increased risk for relapse (Mattsson, Topor, Cullberg, & Forsell, 2008), increased family burden and strain (Gutierrez-Maldonado, Caqueo-Urizar, & Kavanagh, 2005; Lowyck et al., 2004; Ochoa et al., 2008; Shibre et al., 2003), increased stress in the environment (de Souza & Coutinho, 2006), increased substance abuse (Black et al., 2008; Dixon, 1999), and increased homelessness (Wolf, Burnam, Koegel, Sullivan, & Morton, 2001). Such findings have been replicated across countries and cultures (Gaite et al., 2002). Consumers who mismanage funds (Rosen et al., 2003) or who have financial troubles (Koppel & McGuffin, 1999) have been found to use greater number of inpatient hospital days. Psychiatric treatment costs were found to be twice as high for consumers earning no money (Warner & Polak, 1995). Among people with severe mental illness, financial issues also predict family arguments, conflict, and even violence (Elbogen, Swanson, Swartz, & Van Dorn, 2005).

A VA chart review of Veterans of the Iraq and Afghanistan conflicts indicates that finances were an area of psychosocial concern for 42% of the sample, which included difficulty paying bills, child support, a mortgage, tuition, or loans; facing foreclosure; or difficulty obtaining benefits of the GI Bill or disability claims (Strong et al., 2014). Research shows that military Veterans' experiences with suicidal ideation are associated with postdeployment situational stressors such as financial stability and not having money (Denneson et al., 2015). Researchers examined the impact of financial resources on soldiers' well-being in data from a large Army installation in the Midwest (Bell et al., 2014), finding that (1) soldiers with higher credit card debt and lower perceived net worth had lower levels of subjective well-being; (2) soldiers with greater perceived financial knowledge and larger emergency savings accounts had higher levels of subjective well-being; and (3) automobile loan debt may play a small role in the subjective well-being of soldiers.

The National Post-Deployment Adjustment Survey (NPDAS), comprised of 1,388 Operation Enduring Freedom and Operation Iraqi Freedom (OEF/OIF) Veterans from all 50 states representing all branches of the military, found the following regarding financial well-being and mental health (Elbogen et al., 2012):

- Forty-two percent of OEF/OIF Veterans in this national sample reported not having enough money to pay for basic needs like food, shelter, or transportation.
- Analyses show relevance of financial strain on all OEF/OIF Veterans and that both disabled and nondisabled OEF/OIF Veterans appear to have money management difficulties, though the former group is at higher risk.

- Veterans with probable PTSD, MDD, or TBI were substantially less likely to have money to cover expenses for clothing and social activities than other Veterans and more than twice as likely to have been referred to a collection agency.
- Participants screening positive for PTSD, MDD, or TBI had lower income and more debt and were significantly less satisfied with their financial status.
- Compared with Veterans meeting basic needs, Veterans without enough money to cover basic needs were significantly more likely to be criminally arrested (5% vs. 15%), become homeless (1% vs. 9%), misuse alcohol (24% vs. 36%) or drugs (4% vs. 12%), endorse suicidal ideation/behavior (9% vs. 27%), and report violence/aggression (23% vs. 45%).
- On these variables, Veterans with higher income (>$50,000 annual) but poor money management generally fared about the same as those with lower income (<$50,000 annual) and good money management.
- Multivariable analyses revealed not only that these problems were related to diagnosis or income but also that money mismanagement (e.g., being turned over to a collection agency, going over credit limit, being scammed) predicted the aforementioned adverse outcomes among OEF/OIF Veterans.

Although financial variables were related to adverse outcomes, the data underscored that merely increasing income may not be enough to eliminate behavioral problems. Specifically, efforts may need to target money *mismanagement* as well. Indeed, we also found that money mismanagement in the past year—defined as bouncing/forging a check, going over one's credit limit, being turned over to a collection agency, or falling victim to a money scam—was reported by 30% of the national random sample of OEF/OIF Veterans (Elbogen, Sullivan, Wolfe, Wagner, & Beckham, 2013).

Importantly, these money mismanagement variables still predicted poor outcomes such as suicidal ideation and violent behavior when modeled with individual demographics, military characteristics, and clinical diagnosis. Finally, it was also noteworthy that Veterans with mental health disorders had concurrent financial problems. Money mismanagement and the use of funds to purchase alcohol and drugs occurred more frequently among Veterans with disabilities, who typically have the fewest financial resources. Veterans with psychiatric disabilities were also at highest risk for financial exploitation, and they were more likely to have been laid off or fired, which mirrors research findings in civilian populations (Elbogen, Tiegreen, Vaughan, & Bradford, 2011; Hill & Kozup, 2007).

# Money Management and Veteran Homelessness

Over the past decade, there has been significant progress in interventions to reduce homelessness. Housing First is premised on the belief that housing is a basic right and involves placing homeless individuals immediately into residences without requiring mental health or substance abuse treatment (Tsemberis, Gulcur, & Nakae, 2004). There have been many recent studies showing that this approach not only is cost-effective but also improves living stability (Larimer et al., 2009; Sadowski, Kee, VanderWeele, & Buchanan, 2009; Tsemberis et al., 2004). Most Housing First programs mandate that participants use approximately one-third of their income to pay rent for housing (Edens et al., 2011; Larimer et al., 2009; Sadowski et al., 2009; Tsemberis et al., 2004). In this way, such programs create a spending plan for participants that is so rudimentary one might argue it is not a spending plan at all. But for many individuals, this is the first budget they have ever had made for them and the first budget they have ever been asked to stick with. Indeed, Housing First programs provide exactly the type of basic structure for money management that many participants may have previously lacked (Kertesz & Weiner, 2009). In other words, difficulty making good financial decisions (either dependent or independent of mental health problems) may have led at least some people to become homeless.

There are many VA homeless programs that at the very least offer informal money management assistance. The Homeless Providers Grant and Per Diem Program provides grants and per diem payments (as funding is available) to help public and nonprofit organizations establish and operate supportive housing and service centers for homeless Veterans. HUD-VASH is a joint effort between HUD and the VA. HUD allocated nearly 38,000 Housing Choice Section 8 vouchers across the country. These vouchers allow Veterans and their families to live in market rate rental units while the VA provides case management services. A housing subsidy is paid to the landlord on behalf of the participating Veteran. The Veteran then pays the difference between the actual rent charged by the landlord and the amount subsidized by the program. The Acquired Property Sales for Homeless Providers Program makes all VA foreclosed properties available for sale to homeless provider organizations—at a 20% to 90% discount—to shelter homeless Veterans.

The Supportive Services for Veteran Families (SSVF) program provides grants and technical assistance to community-based, nonprofit organizations to help Veterans and their families stay in their homes. The VA's Health Care for Homeless Veterans (HCHV) program offers outreach, exams, treatment, referrals, and case management to Veterans who are homeless and dealing with mental health issues, including substance use. At HCHV sites, trained, caring VA specialists provide tools and support necessary for Veterans to get their lives on a better track. Project CHALENG (Community Homelessness Assessment, Local Education and Networking Groups) brings together providers, advocates, and other concerned citizens to identify the needs of homeless Veterans and work to meet those needs through planning and cooperative action. This process has helped build thousands of relationships between VA and community agencies so that together they can better serve homeless Veterans.

Elbogen et al. (2013) examined the link between money mismanagement and subsequent homelessness in Iraq and Afghanistan Veterans using longitudinal data from the national survey described previously, which included a random sample of OEF/OIF Veterans. This sample of 1,090 Veterans, from 50 states and all military branches, completed two waves of data collection one year apart. At the first wave, money mismanagement in the past year was reported by 30% of the national random sample of OEF/OIF Veterans. Multivariable analysis revealed that money mismanagement at wave 1—defined as bouncing/forging a check, going over one's credit limit, being turned over to a collection agency, or falling victim to a money scam—was associated with quadruple the rate of homelessness in the next year (odds ratio [OR] = 4.09, 95% confidence interval [CI] = 1.87, 8.94), along with arrest history (OR = 2.65, 95% CI = 1.33, 5.29), mental health diagnosis (OR = 2.59, 95% CI = 1.26, 5.33), and income (OR = 0.30, 95% CI = 0.13, 0.71). In the end, financial management was as important a factor as personal income when it came to predicting future homelessness among Veterans and was even a more robust indicator than PTSD or TBI.

Just as important was the interaction found between money mismanagement, income, and Veteran homelessness. Not surprisingly, when annual income was dichotomized as high (at least median $50,000) versus low (less than median $50,000), the highest rates of homelessness were found among those with low income (15%) and those who reported money mismanagement; conversely, the lowest rates were found among those with high income and no money mismanagement (<1%). What was surprising was that the group of Veterans with high income and money mismanagement experienced approximately the same level of homelessness in the next year (6%) compared with Veterans with low income and no money mismanagement (4%).

The findings have implications for policymakers and clinicians, suggesting that financial education programs may eventually be targeted to effectively address Veteran homelessness. There is some empirical research to support this notion. Specifically, researchers in Australia examined the effects of the HOME Advice Program, which used a strengths-based case management practice framework to address financial issues and provide support and assistance to 2,190 families at risk for homelessness; support included teaching Veterans how to budget, making referrals to financial counseling and advice services, assisting with a current financial crisis, and resolving government benefit issues (Steen & MacKenzie, 2013). These investigators found that:

- Ten percent of clients left the program with no debt (i.e., debt reduced to zero).
- A little more than one-half of clients (55%) reduced their debts while in the program.
- For about one-third of clients (33%) debt remained about the same, and for 2% of clients, debt actually increased.
- About one-fourth of families had no information recorded against debt before and after support; however, they had other issues that placed them at risk for homelessness.
- There were a small number of families who had mortgages and were more likely to report no change in their debt position, but none said their debt had worsened.

The authors concluded that "evidence that suggests that case management and support which incorporates financial counselling and financial literacy can assist in moderating the impact of financial stress and help those at risk of homelessness" (Steen & MacKenzie, 2013).

## Improving Money Management in Veterans

Can Veterans' financial well-being be improved and their risk for homelessness reduced by enhancing financial literacy and money management? Fundamentally, "financial literacy is the ability to make informed judgments and to take effective decisions regarding the use and management of money" (Beal & Delpachitra, 2003; Huston, 2010). Scholars indicate that financial literacy encompasses both knowledge and application of knowledge (Huston, 2010). With respect to the application dimension, scholars have used the social-cognitive framework of goal-setting theory to guide programs to improve money management behavior (Hollenbeck & Klein, 1987; Mandell & Klein, 2007). Goal-setting theory posits that conscious goals and intentions drive results and therefore assumes that to change behavior, an individual must be committed to a goal, must get continuous feedback, and must demonstrate repeated ability to perform the task (Hollenbeck & Klein, 1987; Locke & Latham, 1990; Mandell & Klein, 2007). Based on goal-setting theory, financial literacy programs are more effective when individuals are motivated by perceptions and concerns about financial well-being (Mandell & Klein, 2007).

Reviews of empirical research demonstrate that such financial literacy programs can increase savings, reduce debt, and lower delinquency in mortgage payments by encouraging increased budgeting and reduced impulsive spending (Braunslein & Welch, 2002; Fox, Bartholomae, & Lee, 2005; Lusardi & Mitchell, 2007). However, a meta-analysis of the relationship of financial literacy and of financial education to financial behaviors in 168 papers covering 201 prior studies found that interventions to improve financial literacy explain very little of the variance in financial behaviors studied, with weaker effects in low-income samples, and that financial education decays over time (Fernandes, Lynch, & Netemeyer, 2014). Still, researchers have identified several principles associated with improved money management interventions.

First, *"Financial illiteracy will not be 'cured' by a one-time benefit fair or a single seminar on financial economics. This is not because financial education is ineffective, but because the cure is inadequate for the disease"*(Lusardi & Mitchell, 2007). Specifically, research indicates that when it comes to changing spending habits, a one-time educational session is not sufficient to lead to actual adjustment of behavior because motivation (Mandell & Klein, 2007) and self-regulation (Howlett, Kees, & Kemp, 2008) are needed to permanently change spending habits and financial decisions. Generally, this is consistent with literature on interventions to change a variety of behaviors: while a single session of any intervention (e.g., to quit smoking, lose weight, or reduce impulse buys) might help a fraction of people, multiple sessions are needed to optimally improve outcomes among participants (e.g., to substantially alter motivation and self-regulation in smoking, overeating, or impulsive spending habits). For example, meta-analyses of smoking cessation efforts indicate that longer and more intensive interventions are most efficacious; indeed, the U.S. Department of Health and Human Services clinical practice guidelines indicate that to change behavior, "intensive interventions are more effective than less intensive interventions and should be used whenever possible" (Fiore, Bailey, & Cohen, 2000). Correspondingly, reviews of financial literacy programs show that more intensive interventions (i.e., more than one session) lead to greater improvement (Braunslein & Welch, 2002; Fox et al., 2005; Lusardi & Mitchell, 2007).

Second, *"The finding that people have difficulty following through on planned actions suggests that education alone may not be sufficient. Rather, it is important to give consumers the tools to change their behaviors, rather than simply delivering financial education"* (Lusardi & Mitchell, 2007). Thus, financial literacy cannot involve didactics imparting financial knowledge only. Rather, it must also teach and reteach trainees how to create a budget, avoid financial scams, open a bank account, balance a checkbook, obtain a credit report, borrow money knowledgeably, avoid financial exploitation, use a calendar to pay bills on time, and learn daily strategies to save money.

Third, *"Education programs will be most effective if they are targeted to particular population subgroups, so as to address differences in savings needs and in preferences"* (Lusardi & Mitchell, 2007). As noted previously, military Veterans face unique challenges in maintaining stable employment and financial security. As illustrated by the National Financial Capability Study (FINRA, 2010) conducted in collaboration with the U.S. Department of Treasury and the President's Advisory

Council on Financial Literacy, Veterans were less likely than civilians to meet their basic needs and more likely to have significant credit card debt.

Broadly, money management has been an important component of several evidence-based practices and treatments for severe mental illness. Supported employment is optimal when people know how to use the money they earn from their jobs (Becker, Drake, & Naughton, 2005; Bond et al., 2001; Browne, 1999; Ellison, Russinova, Lyass, & Rogers, 2008; Mueser et al., 1997; Peckham & Muller, 1999) and when programs consider careers that allow consumers to experience some potential for future economic progress (Baron & Salzer, 2000). Assertive Community Treatment client teams frequently engage and help consumers learn to manage money (McCarthy et al., 2009; Neale & Rosenheck, 2000). Dual diagnosis treatment has frequently incorporated money management given funds required to purchase alcohol and drugs (Rosen, Carroll, Stefanovics, & Rosenheck, 2009). Given that finances are one of the biggest stressors reported by families of consumers with psychiatric disabilities (Elbogen, Wilder, Swartz, & Swanson, 2008), family psychoeducational interventions also likely address issues of money management. A skill-based rehabilitation intervention showed increases in money management skills using a psychiatric rehabilitation skills module among people with schizophrenia (Liberman et al., 1998).

There have been several projects aimed at improving money management among Veterans. A randomized trial of a contingency management showed reduced substance abuse among dually diagnosed Veterans (Rosen et al., 2009). Assigning representative payees to manage Veterans' disability benefits (Conrad et al., 2006) led to increased quality of life and reduced substance abuse. The Adviser-Teller Money Manager program targets Veterans with substance use and/or psychiatric problems and offers weekly meetings with money managers who monitor access to funds, train Veterans to budget, and link spending to treatment goals (Rowe et al., 2013). More recently, the efficacy of a psychoeducational intervention called $teps for Achieving Financial Empowerment ($AFE) was examined in a clinical trial of Veterans with psychiatric disabilities (Elbogen, Hamer, Swanson, & Swartz, 2016). The $AFE intervention:

1. Outlines specific strategies for military Veterans to save money (e.g., providing information about Veteran discounts for goods and services).
2. Teaches Veterans how to create a viable budget by first distinguishing between expense needs and expense wants and then listing their own income and expenses.
3. Calculates how much Veterans could earn without losing disability SSA benefits and reviews different VA vocational rehabilitation programs available to Veterans.

4. Summarizes strategies for avoiding various forms of financial exploitation.
5. Provides local and national mental health, vocational, and Veterans' resources.

Veterans who reported using the $AFE budget showed significantly higher "responsible spending" behaviors at six-months follow-up compared with control participants, while Veterans who used more $AFE skills were significantly less likely than participants in the control condition to engage in "impulsive spending" at six months. Veterans who specifically reported using $AFE information to look for work were significantly more likely than control participants at six months to be engaged in any vocational activity and to have increased number of hours worked. Veterans who reported use of $AFE skills had significantly greater improvement in money knowledge than participants in the control group. The data from the $AFE randomized clinical trial suggest that efforts are needed to increase actual use of money skills, tailored to the Veteran's individualized money management needs.

Overall, interventions of Veterans with psychiatric disabilities should include components facilitating continued interactions (Rosen et al., 2002) to better ensure effective money management, as do some of the aforementioned interventions (Conrad et al., 2006; Rosen et al., 2009). Current findings imply that future approaches to implementation would be improved by increasing number of sessions and enhancing motivation to use financial skills to address a Veteran's individualized financial needs. The data indicate that for money management interventions to be more effective for Veterans, they must both teach Veterans the necessary skills and facilitate ongoing and increased use of these critical life skills to provide benefit across different domains of psychosocial functioning.

## Money Management Programs for Veteran Populations

The U.S. military provides financial training when soldiers are first enlisted and when they are discharged from services. Personal Financial Management Training (PFMT) is a one-day course mandated by the U.S. Department of the Army for all first term Soldiers. This training consists of Principles of Personal Finance, Planning and Budgeting, Banking and Checking Accounts, Using Credit Wisely, Insurance, Savings and Investing, Making Large Purchases, Consumer Scams, and getting help. Other PFMT dates are scheduled at Brigade level throughout the year. Finally, before separation, soldiers complete a one-week Transition Assistance Program implemented by the U.S. Departments of Defense,

Labor, Veteran Affairs, and Transportation, one hour of which involves a soldier creating a budget.

Military bases also offer Financial Readiness Programs (FRPs) that include educational classes for the military community, keeping families financially aware and prepared. FRP staff are available by appointment for one-on-one financial counseling. This program focuses on improving soldiers' personal financial status and their ability to perform as informed consumers. Assistance is provided to unit commanders and leaders on training soldiers and family members in personal financial readiness. There is a basic preventive education program for soldiers and family members in personal financial readiness/soldier money management and consumer affairs. Classes are given to units to fulfill their training requirements and to other organizations as requested. Also, bases offer emergency relief as reactive assistance when soldiers and family members require emergency financial assistance. However, there is no requirement that soldiers enroll in the myriad of classes offered through the FRP.

Some VA centers offer money management classes to Veterans in the context of psychosocial rehabilitation and recovery centers (PRRCs). The VA Fiduciary Program assigns third parties to manage disability funds for Veterans determined to be incompetent to manage their financial affairs, though it should be noted that assigning a fiduciary is not intended to address immediate homelessness and involves a process arguably more rigorous (and thereby potentially lengthier) than used for assigning a representative payee in the SSA (Wilder, Elbogen, & Moser, 2015). As mentioned previously, VA homeless programs— HUD-VASH, SSVF, and HCHV— provide informal money management through case managers. Veteran Justice Outreach provides eligible, justice-involved Veterans with timely access to the VA's mental health and substance use services when clinically indicated and to other VA services and benefits as appropriate. The VA's Substance Use Disorder Treatment Enhancement Initiative provides substance use services in the community to aid homeless Veterans' recovery. The Health Care for Re-entry Veterans program helps incarcerated Veterans successfully rejoin the community through supports, including those addressing mental health and substance use problems. The Readjustment Counseling Service's Vet Center Programs feature community-based locations and outreach activities that help to identify homeless Veterans and match homeless Veterans with necessary services.

Veterans could benefit by additional financial literacy training before and after separation. This could be modeled on the earlier PFMT and be offered as a refresher course. VA homelessness programs that assist Veterans in finding stable residences could add formal money management training focused on teaching Veterans the financial skills necessary to maintain a home over time. Contact with Veterans during disability screening may also present another opportunity to assess current money management skills or plan for needed training and to encourage financial health screenings at medical and psychiatric appointments. Financial education, even on simple issues such as how to create a budget, avoid financial scams, open a bank account, balance a checkbook, obtain a credit report, apply for and manage loans, use a calendar to pay bills on time, and daily strategies to save money, could readily and inexpensively be added to work with Veterans before and after separation from military service.

## Conclusion

To date, there has been little research examining whether improving financial literacy reduces homelessness in Veteran populations. Still, financial strain has been shown to be associated with suicidal ideation, violence, criminal arrest, and substance abuse in Veterans. Further, money mismanagement was found to markedly increase risk for Veteran homelessness. What we do know has clinical implications for case management services of homeless Veterans, which more typically involves less formal money management assistance than some of the interventions and programs described previously.

Military personnel and Veterans could benefit by completing more financial literacy training before separation, perhaps a refresher course of PFMT. VA homelessness programs could assist Veterans in finding stable residences as well as adding formal training to teach Veterans financial skills to maintain their home in the future. Financial education on how to create a budget, avoid financial scams, open a bank account, balance a checkbook, obtain a credit report, borrow money knowledgeably, use a calendar to pay bills on time, and learn daily strategies to save money can readily (and inexpensively) be added before separation from service or after return home. One context in which additional financial literacy training would be especially important is when a Veteran first receives disability benefits, which sometimes includes a large sum payment that, if mismanaged, could lead to significant long-term debt or other financial problems for the Veteran in the future.

Former Secretary of the VA Eric Shinseki underscored potential links between money management and other poor outcomes, including homelessness: "Too many veterans carrying the burdens of PTSD or TBI, compounded by *limited financial literacy* and atypical behaviors, begin a downward spiral towards isolation, depression, substance abuse, joblessness, failed relationships, homelessness—and sometimes suicide. It usually doesn't happen overnight— it's a long, slow slide. But it begins somewhere, and it would be shortsighted for any of us to presume that these conditions only ensue after the uniform comes off" (Shinseki, 2011). In the end, efforts to house Veterans at risk for homelessness could be usefully complemented by teaching Veterans skills for maintaining housing and thereby reduce risk for future homelessness.

Empirical research on Veterans and civilian populations indicate that improvement in savings and reduction in debt are possible after taking financial literacy and money management courses, especially if repeated to adjust to constantly changing budgets and financial situations. Certainly, VA facilities and military bases are aware of the importance of financial well-being and offer service members opportunities to teach this set of basic skills to succeed economically when returning to civilian life. To the extent that they are actively encouraged, or even required, to take advantage of such services, Veterans will be gaining needed abilities and strengths to avoid the path toward homelessness and instead to move toward living a life of success in the community, fitting for those who have defended our country so honorably.

# References

Anthony, W. A. (1998). Psychiatric rehabilitation technology: Operationalizing the "black box" of the psychiatric rehabilitation process. In P. W. Corrigan & D. F. Giffort (Eds.), *Building teams and programs for effective psychiatric rehabilitation* (pp. 79–87). San Francisco, CA: Jossey-Bass.

Barbato, A., Monzani, E., & Schiavi, T. (2004). Life satisfaction in a sample of outpatients with severe mental disorders: A survey in northern Italy. *Quality of Life Research: An International Journal of Quality of Life Aspects of Treatment, Care & Rehabilitation, 13*(5), 969–973.

Baron, R. C., & Salzer, M. S. (2000). The career patterns of persons with serious mental illness: Generating a new vision of lifetime careers for those in recovery. *Psychiatric Rehabilitation Skills, 4*(1), 136–156.

Beal, D. J., & Delpachitra, S. B. (2003). Financial literacy among Australian university students. *Economic Papers, 22*(1), 65–78.

Becker, D. R., Drake, R. E., & Naughton, W. J., Jr. (2005). Supported employment for people with co-occurring disorders. *Psychiatric Rehabilitation Journal, 28*(4), 332–338.

Bell, M. M., Nelson, J. S., Spann, S. M., Molloy, C. J., Britt, S. L., & Goff, B. N. (2014). The impact of financial resources on soldiers' well-being. *Journal of Financial Counseling and Planning, 25*, 41–52.

Black, R. A., Rounsaville, B. J., Rosenheck, R. A., Conrad, K. J., Ball, S. A., & Rosen, M. I. (2008). Measuring money mismanagement among dually diagnosed clients. *Journal of Nervous and Mental Disease, 196*(7), 576–579.

Bond, G. R., Resnick, S. G., Drake, R. E., Xie, H., McHugo, G. J., & Bebout, R. R. (2001). Does competitive employment improve nonvocational outcomes for people with severe mental illness? *Journal of Consulting and Clinical Psychology, 69*(3), 489–501.

Borras, L., Mohr, S., Boucherie, M., Dupont-Willemin, S., Ferrero, F., & Huguelet, P. (2007). Patients with schizophrenia and their finances: How they spend their money. *Social Psychiatry and Psychiatric Epidemiology, 42*(12), 977–983.

Braunslein, S., & Welch, C. (2002). Financial literacy: An overview of practice, research, and policy. *Federal Reserve Bulletin, 88*(Nov.), 445–458.

Brignone, E., Gundlapalli, A. V., Blais, R. K., Carter, M. E., Suo, Y., Samore, M. H., . . . Fargo, J. D. (2016). Differential risk for homelessness among US male and female veterans with a positive screen for military sexual trauma. *JAMA Psychiatry*, 73(6), 582–589. doi:10.1001/jamapsychiatry.2016.0101

Browne, S. (1999). Rehabilitation programmes and quality of life in severe mental illness. *International Journal of Social Psychiatry*, 45(4), 302–309.

Carter, S. P., & Skimmyhorn, W. (2017). Much ado about nothing? New evidence on the effects of payday lending on military members. *Review of Economics and Statistics*, 99(4), 606–621. doi: 10.1162/REST_a_00647

Chan, S. S. M., Chiu, H. F. K., Chen, E. Y. H., Chan, W. S. C., Wong, P. W. C., Chan, C. L. W., . . . Yip, P. S. F. (2009). Population-attributable risk of suicide conferred by Axis I psychiatric diagnosis in a Hong Kong Chinese population. *Psychiatric Services*, 60(8), 1135–1138.

Conrad, K. J., Lutz, G., Matters, M. D., Donner, L., Clark, E., & Lynch, P. (2006). Randomized trial of psychiatric care with representative payeeship for persons with serious mental illness. *Psychiatric Services*, 57(2), 197–204.

Cook, J. A., Russell, C., Grey, D. D., & Jonikas, J. A. (2008). A self-directed care model for mental health recovery. *Psychiatric Services*, 59(6), 600–602.

Copeland, L. A., Miller, A. L., Welsh, D. E., McCarthy, J. F., Zeber, J. E., & Kilbourne, A. M. (2009). Clinical and demographic factors associated with homelessness and incarceration among VA patients with bipolar disorder. *American Journal of Public Health*, 99(5), 871–877. doi:10.2105/ajph.2008.149989

de Souza, L. A. J., & Coutinho, E. S. F. (2006). The quality of life of people with schizophrenia living in community in Rio de Janeiro, Brazil. *Social Psychiatry and Psychiatric Epidemiology*, 41(5), 347–356.

Denneson, L. M., Teo, A. R., Ganzini, L., Helmer, D. A., Bair, M. J., & Dobscha, S. K. (2015). Military Veterans' experiences with suicidal ideation: Implications for intervention and prevention. *Suicide and Life-Threatening Behavior*, 45(4), 399–414. doi:10.1111/sltb.12136

Dixon, L. (1999). Dual diagnosis of substance abuse in schizophrenia: Prevalence and impact on outcomes. *Schizophrenia Research*, 35, s93–ss100.

Dohrenwend, B. P., Levav, I., Shrout, P. E., et al. (1992). Socioeconomic status and psychiatric disorders: The causation-selection issue. *Science*, 255(5047), 946–952.

Dufort, F., Dallaire, L., & Lavoie, F. (1997). Factors contributing to the perceived quality of life of people with mental disorders. *Social Work and Social Sciences Review*, 7(2), 89–100.

Dunn, E. C., Wewiorski, N. J., & Rogers, E. S. (2008). The meaning and importance of employment to people in recovery from serious mental illness: Results of a qualitative study. *Psychiatric Rehabilitation Journal*, 32(1), 59–62.

Eaton, W. W., Bovasso, G., & Smith, C. (2001). Socioeconomic status and depression. *Journal of Health and Social Behavior*, 42, 277–293.

Edens, E. L., Mares, A. S., Tsai, J., & Rosenheck, R. A. (2011). Does active substance use at housing entry impair outcomes in supported housing for chronically homeless persons? *Psychiatric Services*, 62(2), 171–178. doi:10.1176/appi.ps.62.2.171

Eklund, M. (2009). Work status, daily activities and quality of life among people with severe mental illness. *Quality of Life Research: An International Journal of Quality of Life Aspects of Treatment, Care & Rehabilitation*, 18(2), 163–170.

Elbogen, E. B., Hamer, R. M., Swanson, J. W., & Swartz, M. S. (2016). A randomized clinical trial of a money management intervention for Veterans with psychiatric disabilities. *Psychiatric Services*, 67(10), 1142–1145. doi:10.1176/appi.ps.201500203

Elbogen, E. B., Johnson, S. C., Wagner, H. R., Newton, V. M., & Beckham, J. C. (2012). Financial well-being and postdeployment adjustment among Iraq and Afghanistan war Veterans. *Military Medicine*, 177(6), 669–675.

Elbogen, E. B., Sullivan, C. P., Wolfe, J., Wagner, H. R., & Beckham, J. C. (2013). Homelessness and money mismanagement in Iraq and Afghanistan Veterans. *American Journal of Public Health*, 103(S2), S248–S254.

Elbogen, E. B., Swanson, J. W., Swartz, M. S., & Van Dorn, R. (2005). Family representative payeeship and violence risk in severe mental illness. *Law and Human Behavior*, 29(5), 563–574.

Elbogen, E. B., Tiegreen, J., Vaughan, C., & Bradford, D. (2011). Money management, mental health, and psychiatric disability: A recovery-oriented model for improving financial skills. *Psychiatric Rehabilitation Journal*, *34*, 223–231.

Elbogen, E. B., & Tomkins, A. J. (1999). The psychiatric hospital and therapeutic jurisprudence: Applying the law to promote mental health. In W. Spaulding (Ed), *The role of the state hospital in the twenty-first century: New directions for mental health services* (pp. 71–84). San Francisco, CA: Jossey-Bass.

Elbogen, E. B., & Tomkins, A. J. (2000). From the psychiatric hospital to the community: Integrating conditional release and contingency management. *Behavioral Sciences & the Law*, *18*(4), 427–444.

Elbogen, E. B., Wagner, H. R., Fuller, S. R., Calhoun, P. S., Kinneer, P. M., & Beckham, J. C. Correlates of anger and hostility in Iraq and Afghanistan war Veterans. *American Journal of Psychiatry*, *167*(9), 1051–1058.

Elbogen, E. B., Wilder, C., Swartz, M. S., & Swanson, J. W. (2008). Caregivers as money managers for adults with severe mental illness: How treatment providers can help. *Academic Psychiatry*, *32*(2), 104–110.

Ellison, M. L., Russinova, Z., Lyass, A., & Rogers, E. S. (2008). Professionals and managers with severe mental illnesses: Findings from a national survey. *Journal of Nervous and Mental Disease*, *196*(3), 179–189.

Evans, J. D., Wright, D. E., Svanum, S., & Bond, G. R. (2004). Psychiatric disorder and unmet service needs among welfare clients in a representative payee program. *Community Mental Health Journal*, *40*(6), 539–548.

Fernandes, D., Lynch J. G., Jr., & Netemeyer, R. G. (2014). Financial literacy, financial education, and downstream financial behaviors. *Management Science*, *60*(8), 1861–1883.

Financial Industry Regulatory Authority. (2010). Financial capability among military personnel: Initial report of research findings from the 2009 Military Survey. Retrieved from http://www.usfinancialcapability.org/downloads/NFCS_2009_Mil_Full_Report.pdf

Fiore, M. C., Bailey, W. C., & Cohen, S. J. (2000). Treating tobacco use and dependence: Clinical practice guideline. Retrieved from https://www.aarc.org/wp-content/uploads/2014/08/sc_guidelines.pdf

Foldemo, A., Ek, A. C., & Bogren, L. (2004). Needs in outpatients with schizophrenia, assessed by the patients themselves and their parents and staff. *Social Psychiatry and Psychiatric Epidemiology*, *39*, 381–385.

Fox, J., Bartholomae, S., & Lee, J. (2005). Building the case for financial education. *Journal of Consumer Affairs*, *39*(1), 195–214.

Gaite, L., Vázquez-Barquero, J. L., Borra, C., Ballesteros, J., Schene, A., Welcher, B., . . . Herránthe, A. (2002). Quality of life in patients with schizophrenia in five European countries: The EPSILON study. *Acta Psychiatrica Scandinavica*, *105*(4), 283–292.

Gater, R., Goldberg, D., Jackson, G., Jennett, N., Lowson, K., Ratcliffe, J., . . . Warner, R. (1997). The care of patients with chronic schizophrenia: A comparison between two services. *Psychological Medicine*, *27*(6), 1325–1336.

Greer, T. W. (2017). Career development for women veterans. *Advances in Developing Human Resources*, *19*(1), 54–65. doi:doi:10.1177/1523422316682737

Gundlapalli, A. V., Fargo, J. D., Metraux, S., Carter, M. E., Samore, M. H., Kane, V., & Culhane, D. P. (2015). Military misconduct and Homelessness Among US Veterans separated from active duty, 2001–2012. *JAMA*, *314*(8), 832–834. doi:10.1001/jama.2015.8207

Gutierrez-Maldonado, J., Caqueo-Urizar, A., & Kavanagh, D. J. (2005). Burden of care and general health in families of patient with schizophrenia. *Social Psychiatry and Psychiatric Epidemiology*, *40*, 899–904.

Hanrahan, P., Luchins, D. J., Savage, C., Patrick, G., Roberts, D., & Conrad, K. J. (2002). Representative payee programs for persons with mental illness in Illinois. *Psychiatric Services*, *53*(2), 190–194.

Hatcher, S. (1994). Debt and deliberate self-poisoning. *British Journal of Psychiatry*, *164*, 111–114.

Heider, D., Angermeyer, M. C., Winkler, I., Schomerus, G., Bebbington, P. E., Brugha, T., . . . Toumi, M. (2007). A prospective study of quality of life in schizophrenia in three European countries. *Schizophrenia Research, 93*(1), 194–202.

Heisler, M., Wagner, T. H., & Piette, J. D. (2005). Patient strategies to cope with high prescription medication costs: Who is cutting back on necessities, increasing debt, or underusing medications? *Journal of Behavioral Medicine, 28*(1), 43–51.

Hill, R. P., & Kozup, J. C. (2007). Consumer experiences with predatory lending practices. *Journal of Consumer Affairs, 41*(1), 29–46.

Hoge, C. W., Castro, C., Messer, S., McGurk, D., Cotting, D., & Koffman, R. (2004). Combat duty in Iraq and Afghanistan: Mental health problems and barriers to care. *New England Journal of Medicine, 351*(1), 13–22.

Hollenbeck, J. R., & Klein, H. J. (1987). Goal commitment and the goal-setting process: Problems, prospects, and proposals for future research. *Journal of Applied Psychology, 72*, 212–220.

Horton, J. L., Jacobson, I. G., Wong, C. A., Wells, T. S., Boyko, E. J., Smith, B., . . . Smith, T. C. (2013). The impact of prior deployment experience on civilian employment after military service. *Occup Environ Med, 70*(6), 408–417.

Howlett, E., Kees, J., & Kemp, E. (2008). The role of self-regulation, future orientation, and financial knowledge in long-term financial decisions. *Journal of Consumer Affairs, 42*(2), 223–242.

Huston, S. J. (2010). Measuring financial literacy. *Journal of Consumer Affairs, 44*(2), 296–315.

Institute of Medicine. (2010). *Returning home from Iraq and Afghanistan: Preliminary assessment of readjustment needs of Veterans, service members, and their families.* Washington, DC: National Academies Press.

Jenkins, R., Bhugra, D., Bebbington, P., Brugha, T., Farrell, M., Coid, J., . . . Meltzer, H. (2008). Debt, income and mental disorder in the general population. *Psychological Medicine, 38*(10), 1485–1493.

Kaplan, S. (2010). No place to call home for many female Veterans. Retrieved from http://www.npr.org/2010/11/11/131192165/no-place-to-call-home-for-many-female-Veterans

Kertesz, S. G., & Weiner, S. J. (2009). Housing the chronically homeless: High hopes, complex realities. *JAMA: Journal of the American Medical Association, 301*(17), 1822–1824.

Klee, A., Armstrong, M., & Harkness, L. (2016). Money management for returning service members and Veterans. In N. D. Ainspan, C. J. Bryan, W. E. Penk, N. D. Ainspan, C. J. Bryan, & W. E. Penk (Eds.), *Handbook of psychosocial interventions for Veterans and service members: A guide for the non-military mental health clinician* (pp. 211–222). New York, NY: Oxford University Press.

Koppel, S., & McGuffin, P. (1999). Socio-economic factors that predict psychiatric admission at a local level. *Psychological Medicine, 29*, 1235–1241.

Kovess-Masfaty, V., Xavier, M., Kustner, B. M., Suchocka, A., Sevilla-Dedieu, C., Dubuis, J., . . . Walsh, D. (2006). Schizophrenia and quality of life: A one-year follow-up in four EU countries. *BMC Psychiatry, 6.*

Laliberte-Rudman, D., Yu, B., Scott, E., & Pajouhandeh, P. (2000). Exploration of the perspectives of persons with schizophrenia regarding quality of life. *American Journal of Occupational Therapy, 54*(2), 137–147.

Larimer, M. E., Malone, D. K., Garner, M. D., Atkins, D. C., Burlingham, B., Lonczak, H. S., . . . Marlatt, G. A. (2009). Health care and public service use and costs before and after provision of housing for chronically homeless persons with severe alcohol problems. *JAMA, 301*, 1349–1357.

Lecomte, T., Wallace, C. J., Perreault, M., & Caron, J. (2005). Consumers' goals in psychiatric rehabilitation and their concordance with existing services. *Psychiatric Services, 56*(2), 209–211.

Liberman, R. P. (1992). *Effective psychiatric rehabilitation.* San Francisco, CA: Jossey-Bass.

Liberman, R. P., Kopelowicz, A., & Young, A. S. (1994). Biobehavioral treatment and rehabilitation of schizophrenia. *Behavior Therapy, 25*(1), 89–107.

Liberman, R. P., Wallace, C. J., Blackwell, G., Kopelowicz, A., Vaccaro, J. V., & Mintz, J. (1998). Skills training versus psychosocial occupational therapy for persons with persistent schizophrenia. *American Journal of Psychiatry, 155*(8), 1087–1091.

Locke, E. A., & Latham, G. P. (1990). *A theory of goal setting and task performance.* Englewood Cliffs, NJ: Prentice-Hall.

Lowyck, B., De Hert, M., Peeters, E., Wampers, M., Gilis, P., & Peuskens, J. (2004). A study of the family burden of 150 family members of schizophrenic patients. *European Psychiatry, 19*(7), 395–401.

Luo, Y., & Waite, L. J. (2005). The impact of childhood and adult SES on physical, mental, and cognitive well-being in later life. *Journals of Gerontology: Series B: Psychological Sciences and Social Sciences, 60*(2), S93–SS101.

Lusardi, A., & Mitchell, O. (2007). Financial literacy and retirement preparedness: Evidence and implications for financial education. *Business Economics, 42* (1), 35–44.

Mandell, L., & Klein, L. S. (2007). Motivation and financial literacy. *Financial Services Review, 16*, 105–116.

Marmot, M. G. (2001). Inequalities in health. *N Engl J Med, 345*, 134–136.

Mattsson, M., Topor, A., Cullberg, J., & Forsell, Y. (2008). Association between financial strain, social network and five-year recovery from first episode psychosis. *Social Psychiatry and Psychiatric Epidemiology, 43*(12), 947–952.

McCarthy, J. F., Valenstein, M., Dixon, L., Visnic, S., Blow, F. C., & Slade, E. (2009). Initiation of assertive community treatment among Veterans with serious mental illness: Client and program factors. *Psychiatric Services, 60*(2), 196–201.

Menditto, A. A., Wallace, C. J., Liberman, R. P., Vander Wal, J., Jones, N. T., & Stuve, P. (1999). Functional assessment of independent living skills. *Psychiatric Rehabilitation Skills, 3*(2), 200–219.

Metraux, S., Clegg, L. X., Daigh, J. D., Culhane, D. P., & Kane, V. (2013). Risk factors for becoming homeless among a cohort of Veterans who served in the era of the Iraq and Afghanistan conflicts. *Am J Public Health, 103*(Suppl 2), S255–261. doi:10.2105/ajph.2013.301432

Metraux, S., Cusack, M., Byrne, T. H., Hunt-Johnson, N., & True, G. (2017). Pathways into homelessness among post-9/11-era Veterans. *Psychological Services, 14*(2), 229–237. doi:10.1037/ser0000136

Miller, D. P., Larson, M. J., Byrne, T., & DeVoe, E. (2016). Food insecurity in Veteran households: Findings from nationally representative data. *Public Health Nutrition, 19*(10), 1731–1740.

Montgomery, A. E., Dichter, M. E., Thomasson, A. M., Fu, X., & Roberts, C. B. (2015). Demographic characteristics associated with homelessness and risk among female and male Veterans accessing VHA outpatient care. *Women's Health Issues, 25*(1), 42–48. doi:10.1016/j.whi.2014.10.003

Mueser, K. T., Becker, D. R., Torrey, et al. (1997). Work and nonvocational domains of functioning in persons with severe mental illness: A longitudinal analysis. *Journal of Nervous and Mental Disease, 185*(7), 419–426.

Muntaner, C., Eaton, W. W., Miech, R., & O'Campo, P. (2004). Socioeconomic position and major mental disorders. *Epidemiologic Reviews, 26*, 53–62.

Neale, M. S., & Rosenheck, R. A. (2000). Therapeutic limit setting in an assertive community treatment program. *Psychiatric Services, 51*(4), 499–505.

Ochoa, S., Vilaplana, M., Haro, J. M., Villalta-Gil, V., Martínez, F., Negredo, M. C., . . . Autonell, J. (2008). Do needs, symptoms or disability of outpatients with schizophrenia influence family burden? *Social Psychiatry and Psychiatric Epidemiology, 43*(8), 612–618.

Olusina, A. K., & Ohaeri, J. U. (2003). Subjective quality of life of recently discharged Nigerian psychiatric patients. *Social Psychiatry and Psychiatric Epidemiology, 38*(12), 707–714.

Patel, V., & Kleinman, A. (2003). Poverty and common mental disorders in developing countries. *WHO Bulletin, 81*, 609–615.

Peckham, J., & Muller, J. (1999). Employment and schizophrenia: Recommendations to improve employability for individuals with schizophrenia. *Psychiatric Rehabilitation Journal, 22*(4), 399–402.

Perese, E. F. (1997). Unmet needs of persons with chronic mental illnesses: Relationship to their adaptation to community living. *Issues in Mental Health Nursing, 18*(1), 19–34.

Perron, B. E., Ilgen, M. A., Hasche, L., & Howard, M. O. (2008). Service needs of clients in outpatient substance-use disorder treatment: A latent class analysis. *Journal of Studies on Alcohol and Drugs, 69*(3), 449–453.

Pomerantz, J. M. (2003). The relationship between psychosis and poverty. *Drug Benefit Trends, 15*(3), 31–32.

Reading, R., & Reynolds, S. (2001). Debt, social disadvantage and maternal depression. *Social Science and Medicine, 53,* 441–453.

Remarks by Secretary Eric K. Shinseki. (2011). Retrieved from http://www.va.gov/opa/speeches/2011/11_07_2011.asp

Richardson, T., Elliott, P., & Roberts, R. (2013). The relationship between personal unsecured debt and mental and physical health: A systematic review and meta-analysis. *Clinical Psychology Review, 33*(8), 1148–1162. doi:10.1016/j.cpr.2013.08.009

Rosen, M. I., Carroll, K. M., Stefanovics, E., & Rosenheck, R. A. (2009). A randomized controlled trial of a money management based substance use intervention. *Psychiatric Services, 60*(4), 498–504.

Rosen, M. I., Rosenheck, R. A., Shaner, A., Eckman, T., Gamache, G., & Krebs, C. (2002). Veterans who may need a payee to prevent misuse of funds for drugs. *Psychiatric Services, 53*(8), 995–1000. doi:10.1176/appi.ps.53.8.995

Rosen, M. I., Rosenheck, R., Shaner, A., Eckman, T., Gamache, G., & Krebs, C. (2003). Do patients who mismanage their funds use more health services? *Administration and Policy in Mental Health, 31*(2), 131–140.

Rosenheck, R. A., Dausey, D. J., Frisman, L., & Kasprow, W. (2000). Outcomes after initial receipt of social security benefits among homeless Veterans with mental illness. *Psychiatric Services, 51*(12), 1549–1554. doi:10.1176/appi.ps.51.12.1549

Rosenheck, R., & Fontana, A. (1994). A model of homelessness among male Veterans of the Vietnam War generation. *American Journal of Psychiatry, 151*(3), 421–427.

Rosenheck, R., Frisman, L., & Sindelar, J. (1995). Disability compensation and work among Veterans with psychiatric and nonpsychiatric impairments. *Psychiatric Services, 46*(4), 359–365.

Rowe, M., Serowik, K. L., Ablondi, K., Wilber, C., & Rosen, M. I. (2013). Recovery and money management. *Psychiatric Rehabilitation Journal, 36*(2), 116.

Russell, L. M., Devore, M. D., Barnes, S. M., Forster, J. E., Hostetter, T. A., Montgomery, A. E., . . . Brenner, L. A. (2013). Challenges associated with screening for traumatic brain injury among US Veterans seeking homeless services. *Am J Public Health, 103*(Suppl 2), S211–212. doi:10.2105/ajph.2013.301485

Sadowski, L. S., Kee, R. A., VanderWeele, T. J., & Buchanan, D. (2009). Effect of a housing and case management program on emergency department visits and hospitalizations among chronically ill homeless adults: A randomized trial. *Journal of the American Medical Association, 301*(17), 1771–1778.

Seal, K., Metzler, T., Gima, K., Bertenthal, D., Maguen, S., & Marmar, C. (2009). Trends and risk factors for mental health diagnoses among Iraq and Afghanistan Veterans using Department of Veterans Affairs health care, 2002–2008. *American Journal of Public Health, 99,* 1651–1658.

Shaner, A., Tucker, D. E., Roberts, L. J., & Eckman, T. A. (1999). Disability income, cocaine use, and contingency management among patients with cocaine dependence and schizophrenia. In: S. T. Higgins & K. Silverman (Eds.), *Motivating behavior change among illicit-drug abusers: Research on contingency management interventions* (pp. 95–121). Washington, DC: American Psychological Association.

Sherman, M. D., Larsen, J., & Borden, L. M. (2015). Broadening the focus in supporting reintegrating Iraq and Afghanistan Veterans: Six key domains of functioning. *Professional Psychology: Research and Practice, 46*(5), 355.

Shibre, T., Kebede, D., Alem, A., Negash, A., Deyassa, N., Fekadu, A., . . . Kullgren, G. (2003). Schizophrenia: Illness impact on family members in a traditional society—Rural Ethiopia. *Social Psychiatry & Psychiatric Epidemiology, 38*(1), 27–34.

Skimmyhorn, W. L. (2016). Comparing military and civilian household finances: Descriptive evidence from recent surveys. *Journal of Consumer Affairs, 50*(2), 471–483.

Spaulding, W. D., Fleming, S. K., Reed, D., Sullivan, M., Storzbach, D., & Lam, M. (1999). Cognitive functioning in schizophrenia: Implications for psychiatric rehabilitation. *Schizophrenia Bulletin, 25*(2), 275–289.

Spaulding, W. D., Poland, J., Elbogen, E., & Ritchie, A. J. (2000). Applications of therapeutic jurisprudence in rehabilitation for people with severe and disabling mental illness. *Cooley Law Review., 17*(1), 135–170.

Spaulding, W. D., Sullivan, M. E., & Poland, J. S. (2003). *Treatment and rehabilitation of severe mental illness.* New York, NY: Guilford Press.

Stansfeld, S., Orrell, M., Mason, R., Nicholls, D., & D'Ath, P. (1998). A pilot study of needs assessment in acute psychiatric inpatients. *Social Psychiatry and Psychiatric Epidemiology, 33*(3), 136–139.

Steen, A., & MacKenzie, D. (2013). Financial stress, financial literacy, counselling and the risk of homelessness. *Australasian Accounting Business & Finance Journal, 7*(3), 31.

Strong, J., Ray, K., Findley, P. A., Torres, R., Pickett, L., & Byrne, R. J. (2014). Psychosocial concerns of Veterans of Operation Enduring Freedom/Operation Iraqi Freedom. *Health & Social Work, 39*(1), 17–24. doi:10.1093/hsw/hlu002

Tanielian, T., & Jaycox, L. (2008). *Invisible wounds of war: Psychological and cognitive injuries, their consequences, and services to assist recovery.* Retrieved from https://www.rand.org/content/dam/rand/pubs/monographs/2008/RAND_MG720.pdf

Tinoco, E. M. (2014). Student Veterans in higher education: A transitional challenge. *Community Investments, 26*(3), 28–44.

Tsai, J., Hoff, R. A., & Harpaz-Rotem, I. (2017). One-year incidence and predictors of homelessness among 300,000 U.S. Veterans seen in specialty mental health care. *Psychological Services, 14*(2), 203–207. doi:10.1037/ser0000083

Tsai, J., & Rosenheck, R. A. (2015). VA disability compensation and money spent on substance use among homeless Veterans: A controversial association. *Psychiatric Services, 66*(6), 641–644. doi:10.1176/appi.ps.201400245

Tsemberis, S., Gulcur, L., & Nakae, M. (2004). Housing first, consumer choice, and harm reduction for homeless individuals with a dual diagnosis. *Am. J. Public Health, 94*, 651–656.

US Department of Labor. (2012). *Employment situation of Veterans.* Retrieved from http://www.bls.gov/news.release/vet.nr0.htm

Warner, R., & Polak, P. (1995). The economic advancement of the mentally ill in the community: II. Economic choices and disincentives. *Community Mental Health Journal, 31*(5), 477–492.

Washington, D. L., Yano, E. M., McGuire, J., Hines, V., Lee, M., & Gelberg, L. (2010). Risk factors for homelessness among women Veterans. *Journal of Health Care for the Poor and Underserved, 21*(1), 81–91.

Weich, S., & Lewis, G. (1998). Poverty, unemployment and common mental disorders. *British Medical Journal, 317*, 115–119.

Weich, S., Lewis, G., & Jenkins, S. P. (2001). Income inequality and the prevalence of common mental disorders in Britain. *British Journal of Psychiatry, 178*, 222–227.

Widome, R., Jensen, A., Bangerter, A., & Fu, S. S. (2015). Food insecurity among Veterans of the US wars in Iraq and Afghanistan. *Public Health Nutrition, 18*(5), 844–849.

Wilder, C. W., Elbogen, E.B., & Moser, L. (2015). Fiduciary services for veterans with psychiatric disabilities. *Federal Practitioner, 32*, 12–19.

Wolf, J., Burnam, A., Koegel, P., Sullivan, G., & Morton, S. (2001). Changes in subjective quality of life among homeless adults who obtain housing: A prospective examination. *Social Psychiatry and Psychiatric Epidemiology, 36*(8), 391–398.

# 8

## Unique Considerations for Homeless Female Veterans

ANN ELIZABETH MONTGOMERY, THOMAS H. BYRNE, AND MELISSA E. DICHTER

> When you're a woman alone, security is very important.
> I have experienced abuse. I'm apprehensive about being put
> in a living situation where I'm going to be put in a position
> where I could be abused.
> —Female Veteran

With expansions in service roles over the past several decades, the number of women in the United States who join the armed services has grown substantially, increasing the size of the female Veteran population overall as well as the number of women Veterans who may experience housing instability. While women Veterans' pathways into and experiences with homelessness parallel, to an extent, those of women non-Veterans and male Veterans, they are a distinct population with unique experiences that characterize their housing instability.

In this chapter, we describe the importance of understanding homelessness among women Veterans as a discrete problem that, while overlapping with the broader problem of homelessness among Veterans, merits a specific response calibrated to their particular needs and experiences. We first provide an overview of the epidemiology of homelessness among women Veterans to contextualize what is known about the scope and nature of this problem and its likely future trajectory, focusing on key qualitative differences between women Veterans and their male counterparts. Identifying the ways in which women Veterans and their experiences of homelessness may differ from their male counterparts is especially important given that women have served—and are now being served as Veterans—in largely male-dominated systems, including the U.S. Departments of Defense (DoD) and Veterans Affairs (VA), and responses may need to be tailored to address their specific needs. We describe the risk factors for homelessness and the lived experiences of unstably housed women Veterans—with a particular focus on gender-specific experiences (i.e., trauma, social roles)—and how they may contribute to women Veterans' pathways into homelessness. We then discuss the unique challenges that women may face while reintegrating into their communities after military deployment or discharge, a time when they may be particularly vulnerable and that may be a potentially crucial window during which to intervene to mitigate risk for homelessness. Finally, we conclude by taking stock of the available responses to the problem of homelessness among women Veterans and offer thoughts on potential future responses and recommendations for future research.

# Epidemiology of Homelessness Among Women Veterans

To begin to understand the problem of homelessness among women Veterans, it is important to first address questions about the extent of the problem and the characteristics of those affected by it. Epidemiological questions such as these have been the primary focus of much of the empirical research on homelessness among women Veterans conducted to date. Before summarizing key findings from these studies, we must take a step back and consider broader trends in the number of women among both the active-duty military and Veteran populations, which helps to illustrate the increasing salience of homelessness among female Veterans as a distinct issue and why it is likely to require ongoing attention.

## WOMEN SERVICE MEMBERS AND VETERANS

Both the DoD and VA have historically employed or served a largely male population: the vast majority of military recruits, service members, and Veterans are male. However, during the recent decades, and especially during the most recent military conflicts, the presence of women in the military has rapidly increased and continues to rise. Over the past 40 years, there has been a roughly five-fold increase overall in the proportion of women as a share of the active-duty population. In 1975, women represented roughly 4.6% of the armed forces[1]; during 2015, 15.5% ($n$ = 201,403) of active-duty service members and 19% ($n$ = 157,052) of the Selective Reserve force were women.[2]

Along with the increase in women service members, there has been a corresponding increase in the number of women Veterans; as shown in Figure 8.1, as of 2015, there were approximately 2 million women Veterans, making up 10% of all living Veterans; by 2035, women Veterans are expected to represent 15% of all Veterans.[3] This trend has obvious implications for the VA in terms of both the volume and type of services that it will be tasked with providing to female

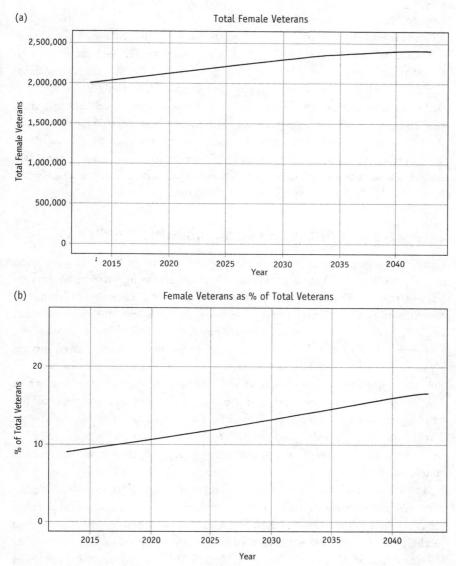

*Figure 8.1* Projection of female Veteran population and female Veterans as share of total Veteran population. From US Department of Veterans Affairs, Veteran Population Projection Model 2014 (VetPop2014), Table 1L.

Veterans. Indeed, the VA is already affected by the growth in the population of women Veterans: the number of women Veterans accessing Veterans Health Administration (VHA) care increased by 80% between FY 2003 and FY 2012.[4]

Data collected by the U.S. Census Bureau through the American Community Survey point to significant differences between men and women Veterans. On average, women Veterans are about 15 years younger than men (median age of 50 years compared with 65 for men) and are more racially and ethnically diverse (65.9% identify as White/non-Hispanic compared with 78.8% of men). Women Veterans also have a higher level of education (78.8% have at least some college compared with 63.1% of men) and are less likely to be married (49.4% are married compared with 64.7% of men). Despite having higher levels of education, women Veterans appear to experience higher levels of economic hardship than their male counterparts: they have incomes that are, on average, 7% lower and are more likely to be living in poverty (10.3% compared with 6.5% of men) and receiving means-based entitlements such as Supplemental Nutrition Assistance Program (SNAP) (13% compared with 6.3% of men).[5]

## ESTIMATES OF HOMELESSNESS AMONG WOMEN VETERANS

Early estimates found an underrepresentation of women Veterans within the larger population of Veterans experiencing and accessing services to address homelessness: 1.6% of Veterans served by the VA's Homeless Chronically Mentally Ill (HCMI) Veterans program between 1988 and 1991 were women, while 3.6% of all Veterans in the general population at that time were women.[6] However, more recent data indicate an *overrepresentation* of women among Veterans experiencing homelessness: national estimates of the number of Veterans experiencing homelessness and accessing shelter over the course of a year have revealed that, over time, female Veterans have become overrepresented in the population of homeless Veterans (if not equally representative, as in 2014).[7] Further, it is estimated that 1% to 2% of all women Veterans and 13% to 15% of women Veterans living in poverty experience homelessness over the course of a year.[8,9]

There are particular considerations that present a challenge to obtaining accurate estimates of the homeless female Veteran population. Given the historical focus on male military service members and Veterans, women who have served in the military may not identify themselves—or be identified by others—as Veterans. Indeed, there is evidence that female Veterans are almost three times as likely as their male counterparts to be incorrectly identified as not being a Veteran in records maintained by community-based shelter systems.[10] Also, because of needs related to caregiving or personal safety that are more prominent among women than men, women may be more likely to double up with family or friends rather than access emergency shelter or stay in an unsheltered location.[11] Based on how enumeration of the homeless population is typically conducted, women Veterans may be less likely to be counted as homeless despite lacking safe and stable housing of their own.[12]

Estimates of homelessness are based on a number of methodologies— including point-in-time (PIT) counts of homeless services users and people staying in unsheltered situations as well as analysis of administrative data, each of which have advantages and disadvantages. Each of these estimates relies on different yet overlapping populations; for example, not all women Veterans are engaged with VA care, so any estimates using VA administrative data are limited to the minority (41%) of women Veterans who access VA health care (through the VHA) or other VA benefits such as service-connected disability compensation.[13] In addition, studies have shown that Veterans may use services provided by community-based (non-VA) homeless services system only, VA Homeless Programs only, or both, meaning that counts of Veterans using either system do not include all Veterans experiencing homelessness.[14,15] Therefore, it is important to note that each estimate of female Veteran homelessness is likely an underestimate and that, given the populations from which they are drawn, each estimate should be considered both separately and collectively.

### Point-in-Time Count Administered by the U.S. Department of Housing and Urban Development

Each January, communities across the country conduct a one-night census to estimate the number of people experiencing unsheltered or sheltered (i.e., staying in emergency shelters or transitional housing) homelessness. These PIT counts assess the number of the total homeless population as well as certain subpopulations—based on self-report—such as families with children, youth, adults experiencing chronic homelessness, and Veterans. The most recent estimate provided by the U.S. Department of Housing and Urban Development (HUD) used data collected during January 2017, which identified 3,571 women Veterans who were experiencing homelessness on a single night, representing 8.9% of the Veteran homeless population identified by this method. Among these women Veterans, roughly 60% were staying in sheltered situations, while the remaining 40% were living in unsheltered situations or places not intended for human habitation.[16] As mentioned previously, there is concern that this method represents a significant undercount of women Veterans experiencing homelessness because of the nature of their homelessness (e.g., being doubled up) and the potentially higher rate at which they may be classified incorrectly as non-Veterans in data collected by the community-based emergency shelter system.[10]

### Estimates from Veterans Health Administration Medical Records

Administrative records provide an alternative means to estimate the number of women Veterans experiencing homelessness. VHA medical records include at least three data elements that may identify Veterans experiencing housing instability: (1) use of a VHA Homeless Program, (2) indications of homelessness documented by diagnostic information codes (e.g., International Classification of Diseases [ICD]-9 V codes and ICD-10 Z codes indicating unstable housing), and (3) positive responses to VHA's universal screen for homelessness and risk. Each of these are described further here.

Note that, while the VHA is in an enviable position to have access to a great deal of information about Veterans' health, health care use, and social determinants of health through its electronic medical record system, these data are limited both to the population of Veterans who engage with VHA care and to the information that is documented within their electronic medical records in a standardized way. Among the more than 2 million women Veterans in the United States, 22.4% access VA health care (through the VHA), which means that a significant proportion of women Veterans are not represented in these data.[13] Women Veterans may forego or leave VHA care due to access to private care outside of the VA system or because of negative experiences with or perceptions of, or lack of knowledge about, VA care.[17] Others may be ineligible for VA care because of inadequate active service or nonqualifying discharge from military service and may be among the Veterans most vulnerable to housing instability.

### Veterans Health Administration Homeless Programs

In addition to health care, VHA offers Veterans services to address important social determinants of health, such as housing and homelessness through VHA Homeless Programs that range from outreach and drop-in services to transitional housing and permanent supportive housing (PSH). Between 2010 and 2015, the number of women Veterans accessing VHA Homeless Programs or otherwise identified as homeless by VHA through diagnostic information codes or self-report increased from 11,016 to 36,443, or 231%, due in part to massive increases in funding for services to address housing instability among Veterans as well as a growing female Veteran population. Additional analysis that draws on projections in the likely growth of the number of women separating from the military suggests that the number of women Veterans who may access VHA Homeless Programs is likely to increase by an additional 9% by 2025.[18]

### Diagnostic Information Codes

VHA health care providers can flag certain social conditions, including a patient's experience of homelessness, using the ICD-9 V-60 codes indicating lack of or inadequate housing and ICD-10 Z-59 codes indicating homelessness or inadequate housing. Although these codes maybe be inconsistently or not uniformly applied—and may or may not be removed when a Veteran achieves housing stability—they can be used to identify patients experiencing homelessness who may not be identified through other data points in the medical record (e.g., not formally enrolled in a VHA Homeless Program).

*Universal Screening for Homelessness and Risk*

The VHA administers a universal screen for housing instability to all Veterans who access VHA outpatient care and who are not already engaged with VHA homelessness services. This screen asks Veterans if they have been living in stable housing for the past two months (a "no" answer indicates homelessness) or if they are worried or concerned that they will not have stable housing in the next two months (a "yes" answer indicates imminent risk for homelessness). During FY 2016, 2,872,092 Veterans responded to these questions and 1.31% indicated that they were experiencing housing instability (i.e., either current homelessness or imminent risk); this accounts for 35,467 Veterans, 3,898 of whom were women. The rate of positive screens among women was 1.78%, approximately 30% greater than the rate among men (1.27%).[20]

Among a cohort of 8,427 women Veterans receiving VHA care between 2014 and 2016, between 1.6% and 6.7% had evidence of accessing a VHA Homeless Program, 6% had a homelessness-related diagnosis code documented in their VHA medical record, and 2.2% had a positive screen for housing instability based on the VHA's universal screen for homelessness and risk. Combined, 11.3% of women Veterans had any indicator of housing instability[20] (Table 8.1 and Figure 8.2).

## CHARACTERISTICS OF WOMEN VETERANS EXPERIENCING HOMELESSNESS

Much of the existing research assessing the characteristics of women Veterans experiencing homelessness has compared them with their male counterparts. Findings from these studies indicate that female and male Veterans experiencing homelessness differ on a number of key dimensions, many of which have implications for tailoring interventions specifically to the needs of women Veterans. For example, prior studies show that, compared with their male counterparts, women Veterans *experiencing homelessness* are younger[21-23] and more likely to have minor children in their care.[21,24] They are less likely to have a history of incarceration[21,22] as well as current employment.[23] They are more likely than their male counterparts to have served during Operations Enduring Freedom, Iraqi Freedom, and New Dawn (OEF/OIF/OND),[21,22] reflective of the age difference of men and women participating in military service; further, they are less likely to have a disability but more likely to be *receiving compensation for* a service-connected disability.[21] A number of studies have found that while women Veterans experiencing homelessness are more likely to have a diagnosis of a mental health condition[6,21,23]—including affective, post-traumatic stress, and anxiety disorders[21]—they are less likely to have a diagnosis of a substance use disorder compared with male Veterans experiencing homelessness.[6,21-23]

*Table 8.1* **Indicators of Housing Instability**

|  | Total | |
| --- | --- | --- |
|  | N | % |
| **Diagnoses and Services Use** | | |
| V60 or Z59 Code | 509 | 6.0 |
| HCHV | 567 | 6.7 |
| GPD | 135 | 1.6 |
| HUD-VASH | 451 | 5.4 |
| Other VHA Homeless Program | 169 | 2.0 |
| Any diagnosis or service use | 844 | 10.0 |
| **Response to HSCR** | | |
| Homeless | 99 | 1.2 |
| At risk | 84 | 1.0 |
| Homeless or at risk | 183 | 2.2 |
| Any indicator of housing instability | 950 | 11.3 |

GPD, Grant and Per Diem; HCHV, Health Care for Homeless Veterans; HUD-VASH; U.S. Department of Housing and Urban Development–VA Supported Housing; VHA, Veterans Health Administration.

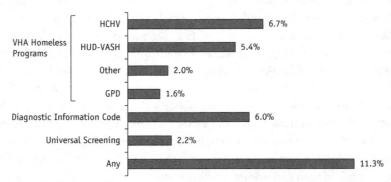

*Figure 8.2* Indicators of housing instability among women Veterans. GPD, Grant and Per Diem; HCHV, Health Care for Homeless Veterans; HUD-VASH; U.S. Department of Housing and Urban Development–VA Supported Housing; VHA, Veterans Health Administration. From Montgomery AE, Sorrentino AE, Cusack MC, Bellamy SL, Medvedeva E, Roberts CB, Dichter ME. Recent intimate partner violence and housing instability among women Veterans. *American Journal of Preventive Medicine.* 2018;54(4):584–590. doi:10.1016/j.amepre.2018.01.020

In addition to differences in sociodemographic and clinical characteristics between male and female Veterans experiencing homelessness, *how* they experience homelessness looks different. Women are less likely than their male counterparts to be literally homeless,[21] chronically homeless,[21–23,25] or staying in an unsheltered situation (again, making it more difficult to enumerate the population).[26] In addition, male and female Veterans vary on the types of services that they receive from VHA Homeless Programs: while women are more likely to access PSH through the HUD–VA Supportive Housing (HUD-VASH) program—which provides a deep permanent subsidy in a setting that is not gender specific and can accommodate children—men are more likely to access transitional housing through VA's Grant and Per Diem (GPD) program, which often has gender-specific housing and is intended for Veterans only (i.e., other family members cannot receive services through GPD).[21,22]

It is also important to note that, in addition to characteristic differences between male and female Veterans experiencing homelessness, research suggests that there is meaningful heterogeneity *within* the population of women Veterans experiencing homelessness. Specifically, an analysis of 19,684 women Veterans who accessed a VHA Homeless Program in 2014 identified six distinct subgroups of this population (in descending order from largest to smallest subgroup):

(1) Middle-aged women with limited VHA health care service use;
(2) Older women (i.e., >50 years) who make limited use of VHA health care services;
(3) OEF/OIF/OND Veterans who are younger women;
(4) Women Veterans with moderate rates of behavioral health diagnoses and relatively high rates of chronic medical conditions;
(5) Women older than 40 years who have high rates of substance use disorders, serious mental illness, and chronic health conditions and who make heavy use of VHA health care services; and
(6) Women Veterans younger than 29 years who appear to have only limited contact with the VHA health care system.[18]

The heterogeneity in the characteristics and needs of these subgroups of women Veterans experiencing homelessness suggests that there is meaningful variation within this population with respect to their housing and other service needs; that is, there is not one "type" of female Veteran who is homeless, requiring a sophisticated set of responses to the problem. The range of needs among this population is highly variable because there are young women Veterans who have recently returned from the wars in Afghanistan and Iraq, older women Veterans with high needs and related services use, and women Veterans who infrequently access VHA care, presenting a need for varied interventions.

## RISK FACTORS FOR HOMELESSNESS AMONG WOMEN VETERANS

While evidence suggests that women Veterans experience homelessness at higher rates than their male Veteran and female non-Veteran counterparts, there is limited understanding about the origins of this differential risk. In the following section, we summarize findings from studies that have identified both sociodemographic and clinical characteristics that may be associated with risk for homelessness among women Veterans. In a subsequent section, we describe a theoretical model for risk for homelessness among women Veterans that helps to illustrate potential pathways into homelessness, based heavily on their experience of trauma over the life course.

### Comparative Risk for Homelessness: Non-Veteran Women and Male Veterans

Generally, and specifically for Veterans, the research exploring homelessness from the perspective of gender is fairly limited. In addition, it is often difficult to conduct research comparing Veterans with non-Veterans because there are not many samples based on administrative data, requiring more time- and resource-intensive primary data collection. However, a number of studies have identified differential risk for homelessness among women Veterans compared with non-Veteran women and Veteran men. A study using data from community-based emergency shelters in several communities across the country found that women Veterans were more than twice as likely as their female non-Veteran counterparts to experience homelessness; when looking specifically at the population living in poverty, women Veterans were more than three times as likely as their female non-Veteran counterparts to spend at least one night in a homeless shelter.[8]

Although *differences* in the risk for men and women VHA patients accessing VHA Homeless Programs have not been identified,[27] the rates at which women have a positive screen for homelessness or risk on the VHA's universal screen for housing instability are disproportionately high, as discussed previously.[19] However, one study of OEF/OIF Veterans did not find a significant relationship between gender and homelessness risk.[28]

### Sociodemographic Characteristics

Several sociodemographic characteristics appear to increase risk for homelessness among women Veterans. Recent studies have identified younger age as a risk factor for homelessness among women Veterans, although a study using data from the mid-1990s identified women ages 45 to 54 years to be at greatest risk.[29] Among Veterans who served in the recent conflicts in Iraq and Afghanistan, women were as likely as men to use a VHA Homeless Program, but those aged 26 to 35 years were significantly (approximately 20%) more likely to do so compared with women in other age groups.[26] Data from community-based homeless shelters found that women Veterans aged 18 to 29 years were at increased risk for homelessness relative to other age groups.[8] Among women in VHA care, being 55 years or older was protective against screening positive for homelessness; women aged 65 years and older were significantly less likely than younger women to screen positive for imminent risk for homelessness, but those aged 35 to 54 years were more likely than their younger counterparts to screen positive for homelessness risk.[30] While these findings generally indicate that younger women who are either of childbearing age or likely to have young children appear to be at elevated risk and older women Veterans are more likely to have stable housing, it is difficult to compare studies that were conducted during different time periods and using different sources of data. Age clearly is a factor in homelessness risk, but the research to date is fairly inconclusive regarding which age groups may have the greatest risk.

Other characteristics associated with housing instability among women Veterans include having a disability,[31] identifying as Black,[8,30] and living in the Northeast region of the United States.[27] Women Veterans who receive a service-connected disability rating by the VA (i.e., have been certified by the VA to have a disability incurred during military service and are likely receiving compensation for that disability) may have increased risk for housing instability owing to the presence of a disability; however, receipt of compensation related to the disability may be protective against homelessness because of income and benefits, including housing supports that they may receive as a consequence of their service-connected disability.[30] While women Veterans are more likely than their non-Veteran counterparts to be recently employed and married,[29] unmarried status[30,31] and unemployment[31] are both associated with an increased risk for homelessness among women Veterans.

*Clinical Characteristics*
A number of studies have found an increased risk for homelessness among women Veterans with mental health issues or substance use disorders,[32] but there is limited evidence that physical health conditions are important predictors of homelessness. A study assessing disparities in self-reported housing status associated with Veterans' diagnosed medical, cognitive, and behavioral health conditions found that chronic medical conditions were not associated with an increased likelihood of Veterans reporting current or imminent housing instability; however, women Veterans who had a diagnosis of traumatic brain injury (TBI), post-traumatic stress disorder (PTSD), depression, schizophrenia and other psychoses, alcohol abuse, drug abuse, or a previous suicide attempt or intentional self-inflicted injury were at increased risk for reporting recent or expected housing instability. Each of these conditions independently, with the exception of TBI, increased the odds that a woman Veteran would report

housing instability; having a substance use disorder or a history of suicide or self-inflicted injury was associated with the greatest odds of women Veterans reporting housing instability.[33] Another study found that, among a cohort of women Veterans, those with a diagnosis of anxiety disorder were more than four times as likely to be homeless as those without such a diagnosis.[31]

PTSD is a significant issue for women Veterans generally, and it appears to pose particular risk for homelessness among women Veterans. Homeless women Veterans' exposure to traumatic events and experience of PTSD is high: in one study, 98% of a sample of women Veterans reported exposure to a high-magnitude stressor and 81% reported experiencing persistent post-traumatic distress, rates that are significantly higher than those found among a non-Veteran sample.[34] In addition, studies have found that PTSD is a significant predictor of a number of indicators of housing instability, including using a VHA Homeless Program[27] or reporting current or imminent homelessness,[33] and may increase the likelihood of homelessness among women Veterans by a factor of five.[31] Symptoms of PTSD emerge as a result of experience of trauma and adversity and pose challenges to the stability of relationships, employment, mental and physical health, and housing.[35-37] The role of trauma is explored in the next section.

# Pathways into Homelessness Among Women Veterans and the Role of Trauma

Studies focusing on individual risk factors, such as those described earlier, are not entirely sufficient for understanding the complex dynamics of risk for homelessness generally and among women Veterans specifically. Homelessness is likely a result of a little-understood and complex mechanism by which individual and structural factors—as well as life experiences and related responses—come together to increase vulnerability or risk. This recognition has led to more in-depth work to begin to understand pathways into homelessness among women Veterans.

A team of VHA researchers conducted a series of focus groups with women Veterans experiencing homelessness to examine how individual risk factors may accrue over time and interact with one another, leading to complex pathways into homelessness. This study identified a "web of vulnerability" that included five "roots" of Veteran women's "downward spiral" into homelessness, often exacerbated by both personal and structural factors: childhood adversity; trauma or substance abuse during military service; abuse, adversity, and relationship termination as well as mental health, substance abuse, and medical problems during the period following discharge from the military; and unemployment. A common theme among these roots of homelessness is the experience of trauma before, during, and after military service.[32] These pathways are represented in Figure 8.3.

Another study that characterized types of trauma experienced by homeless women Veterans identified six common categories of trauma: having been robbed, subjected to accidents or disasters, subjected to illness or death of others, engaged in combat, experienced sexual assault, and experiences physical assault. This study found that almost all of the women in the study had been exposed to multiple potential traumas and that a previous experience of sexual trauma was specifically associated with an increase in the number of days the women spent homeless.[38] Women Veterans frequently report experience of a variety of types of trauma both in civilian and military contexts as well as over the course of their life. In addition, PTSD is prevalent among women Veterans and may have a particularly important link with homelessness among this population.

What emerges from these studies is a theoretical model of pathways into homelessness among women that focuses on pre-military, military, and post-military experiences, consistent with a model of pathways into homelessness that has been proposed and tested for the male Veteran population.[39] However, what distinguishes the model specifically for women Veterans is the central role that trauma appears to play—and gender-specific experiences of trauma such as sexual assault—at each time period. What follows is a summary of the evidence that is relevant to understanding how pre-military, military, and post-military factors, and particularly experience of trauma during these periods, influence pathways into homelessness.

## BEFORE MILITARY SERVICE

Studies indicate that, as a group, women Veterans report higher rates of childhood maltreatment, including physical, emotional, and sexual abuse, compared with women who have not served in the military.[40] In fact, about one-third of enlisted women enter the military with a history of childhood sexual abuse[41,42]; some women Veterans have reported that they joined the military to escape violent or other unhealthy family dynamics.[32,42–44] In a qualitative study, *homeless* women Veterans discussed ways in which experiences of pre-military adversity, including child abuse and intimate partner violence, contributed to their decisions to enter the military and to their cumulative experiences of trauma that contributed to their housing instability.[32]

## DURING MILITARY SERVICE

Primary sources of trauma during military service for women include exposure to combat and sexual harassment or assault, both of which may be exacerbated

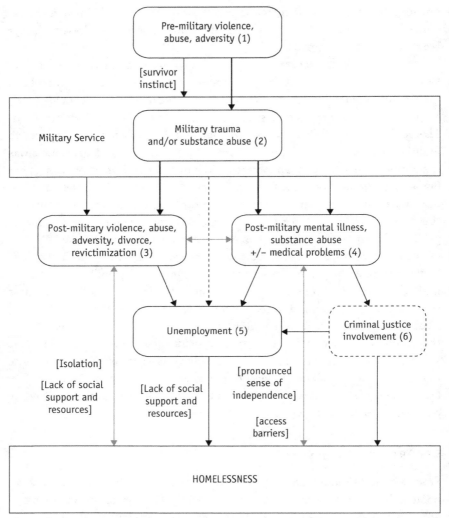

*Figure 8.3* Web of vulnerability illustrating interrelated pathways into homelessness for women Veterans. 1–5: Roots of homelessness. namely, initiators or precipitating factors for the path toward homelessness. 6: Subsidiary factor. *Arrows* indicate links, or pathways, from roots toward homelessness, and the weight of the arrow conveys the strength of the link. Contextual factors are individual characteristics or structural factors that, when present, promote the pathway. A pronounced sense of independence inhibits care-seeking, and access barriers (mental health, social service) lead to unmet need. *Note:* Not all roots, links (pathways), or contextual factors are present in all individuals, (e.g., military trauma without an adverse pre-military history could initiate the pathway). From Hamilton AB, Poza I, Washington DL. Homelessness and trauma go hand-in-hand: Pathways to homelessness among women Veterans. *Women's Health Issues.* 2011;21(4):S203–S209.

by the social and hierarchical male-dominated nature of the military setting.[45] Military sexual trauma (MST)—defined as "experiences of sexual assault or repeated, threatening sexual harassment that a Veteran experienced during his or her military service"[46]—receives the most attention in the literature related to trauma experienced by women during military service. VHA conducts a one-time, universal screen for MST among all Veterans who present for care. This screen has found that about one of every five women Veterans served by VHA reports that she experienced threatening sexual harassment or assault during military service.[47] Survey research has identified that as many as 25% to 40% of women Veterans experienced sexual assault,[41,42,48] 74% experienced sexual harassment,[49] and 50% to 54% experienced nonsexual assault[48,49] while serving in the military.

The nature of women's roles in combat (i.e., often experiencing the aftermath of combat rather than participating in active combat) has received less attention.[50] Women may experience both MST and combat-related trauma; in fact, deployment to areas with combat-like experiences—characterized as male-dominated and high stress, leading to less accountability for perpetrators—is associated with increased risk for MST.[51]

Women face substantial barriers to reporting MST during military service: stigma, concerns about confidentiality,[52] secondary victimization,[52,53] worries about poor job performance or risking one's job,[52,54] disruption of the cohesion of one's unit and greater importance placed on the unit than the individual,[52,53] and being actively discouraged not to report.[53] Further, as a numerical minority, some women in the military may face limited opportunities to establish strong social networks with other women service members, contributing to experience of isolation, especially in situations of gender-based violence.

Women's "gendered experience as women entering and existing in a male-dominated institution" generally, and MST experience specifically, lead to particular vulnerabilities,[44] including mental health conditions,[47,55] especially PTSD[47,55-57]; substance abuse[41]; poorer health, quality of life, and emotional and psychological functioning[54]; premature discharge from the military[44,58,59] and difficulties with reintegration[60,61]; and ongoing victimization and trauma,[42,56] all of which also increase risk for housing instability. Having experienced MST is common among women Veterans experiencing homelessness[62] and increases the odds of an experience of homelessness by more than a factor of four.[31] Studies of women Veterans experiencing homelessness have found that as many as four of five have been traumatized by a colleague or superior while serving in the military,[31] and two of five screen positive on the VHA MST screen.[55]

## AFTER MILITARY SERVICE

Trauma experience before and during a woman's military career may be compounded by further ongoing trauma after military service.[56] One significant source of ongoing trauma is intimate partner violence (IPV). Experience of IPV has been found to increase the odds of homelessness among women by a factor of four[63] and is a significant pathway to homelessness among women Veterans.[12,31] The rate of lifetime IPV experience is significantly higher among women who have served in the military compared with those who have not[64]; as many as one in five women Veterans report experiencing IPV in the past year.[65] IPV is associated with a host of negative outcomes, including substance use,[66,67] mental health issues,[66,68] and economic hardship, including housing instability.[12,19,63,65,69]

### Women Veterans' Experience of Post-traumatic Stress Disorder

Women *entering* the military are at high risk for PTSD as indicated by high prevalence of early abuse, increased risk for assault while in the military, and a high likelihood of post-traumatic stress related to MST among this population.[56] Among women Veterans, PTSD is associated with early trauma experienced before military service, exposure to war-zone traumas, and post-war factors such as stressful life events and the presence or absence of social support.[70] Other significant contributors to PTSD include experience of IPV and MST, both of which may confer greater risk for PTSD than other traumas[68,71,72]; specifically, sexual trauma has been found to be more influential than war trauma in the development of PTSD among women Veterans.[73]

### Reintegration After Deployment or Military Discharge

Reintegration into civilian life after military service is a crucial time period during which women Veterans may need to navigate new realities with respect to familial and other interpersonal relationships, child care, employment, housing, health care, and role identity. While there is scant evidence specifically about whether and to what extent difficulties navigating this terrain may lead to homelessness, the challenges of reintegration for the minority population of women Veterans in particular may contribute, either directly or indirectly, to an increased risk for homelessness in a number of ways, including through the potential loss of reintegration supports because of premature discharge from the military and lack of social support.

As described earlier, women's experiences in the military may have exposed them to a number of stressors, including combat and MST[50] or long-term separation from their families, which is characteristic of the more frequent and longer deployments of the recent conflicts.[74] Women may even leave the military early because of some of these experiences, which can result in their lack of access to potential benefits that would ultimately assist them in achieving economic stability during their post-deployment or post-military reintegration.[58,75] This may have a considerable impact on women Veterans' transition to civilian life, including difficulty obtaining stable housing and, particularly, employment, which women Veterans report among the most important post-reintegration stressors.[76]

Many women enter military service at the age of 18 years, moving directly from the home of their family of origin to the regimented world of military life that provides employment, income, services, and, often, housing. On discharge from military service, Veterans may need to find their own housing for the first time in their life; a first stop following discharge from the armed services may be a return to their parents' home or to a home they have established with a spouse or partner. However, women Veterans who have entered military service in part (or wholly) to escape adversity in their families of origin may not have the option of safely returning to that home; among those who do have that option, this living arrangement may lead to conflict and ultimate housing instability.[77]

While in the military, active service members are more likely than civilian counterparts to be married—although women service members are less likely than their male peers to be married—and have access to many resources that are family-friendly, including health insurance for the family, family housing, and child care. However, after they leave military service, they are three times as likely to divorce than those who have not served and, while many of the benefits received during military service may be protective for marriage and generally pro-family, they are not available after one becomes a Veteran.[78] The potential loss of social support—including both instrumental and emotional support from a spouse or partner—combined with the loss of supportive resources provided in the military environment may pose significant difficulties for women Veterans during their reintegration period.

Another complicating factor is that service members cannot fully control where they are stationed, and it may be at a distance from family or other sources of support; after leaving military service, most Veteran families remain, at least for a time, in the location of their last station, which may lead to an additional lack of social support during the period of reintegration to civilian life when such support may be particularly important in helping obtain employment, child care, and housing.[78] Further, as a minority population, women Veterans may have more difficulty than male Veterans identifying and establishing or integrating into social networks of other Veterans in the civilian world and may also have trouble connecting with other women and community members who do not share or understand their military-related experiences.[35]

# Implications for Policy and Practice

The existing literature related to women Veterans generally and homelessness among women Veterans specifically points very clearly to several implications for policy and practice as well as directions for future research. These include assessing for and addressing trauma among women Veterans; building on the strengths of women Veterans experiencing homelessness; addressing the needs of younger women Veterans and those with dependent children; ensuring appropriate gender-responsive resources for women Veterans who are transitioning into permanent housing; and addressing the needs of women Veterans as they reintegrate after deployment or military discharge.

## ASSESS FOR AND ADDRESS TRAUMA

Trauma experienced before, during, and after military service must be addressed among women Veterans.[21,32,38,55,79,80] A trauma-informed approach to care recognizes the impact of trauma on the individual and requires a basic understanding of trauma, providing services in an environment that feels safe, and using a strengths-based approach,[81,82] recognizing that "major or repeated trauma such as partner violence can impact all aspects of a woman's life including her sense of self, behavior, coping, ability to respond to treatment, and intimate relationships."[71 (p. 109)]

VHA has offered a number of responses to trauma among women Veterans, including routine screening for MST and IPV and response programs including resources such as sexual trauma treatment programs that work with Veterans with complex histories of trauma and life stressors (e.g., homelessness, substance use disorder).[83] Given the overlap between women Veterans who have experienced trauma and those who have experienced homelessness, it is important for VHA Homeless Programs to continue to engage in best practices with respect to trauma-informed care, including recognizing the potential impacts of trauma in individuals' lives and behaviors, responding to impacts of trauma, and working to avoid revictimization. Both VA and non-VA providers that serve women Veterans should be trained to identify and recognize the military experience of women Veterans, engage principles of trauma-informed care, and recognize and understand the potentially unique characteristics and experiences of Veteran consumers.

## ADDRESS NEEDS OF YOUNGER WOMEN AND THOSE WITH CHILDREN

As the age and gender distribution of the Veteran population continues to shift,[4] it is particularly important to consider the unique needs of younger women Veterans and those with dependent children. This is particularly true given that VHA Homeless Programs have traditionally been oriented toward serving a population of older, single, male adults; are often ill-equipped to meet the needs of younger women Veterans; and, in many cases, cannot accommodate women Veterans and their children. A specific policy response that should be implemented immediately is increasing young women Veterans' (both those with and without children) access to transitional housing with individually focused services.[84] It is important that policymakers and practitioners tailor interventions to the emerging population of women Veterans and recognize that interventions developed for older women Veterans may not be appropriate for this younger cohort.[85]

Beyond realigning VHA Homeless Programs to meet the needs of a new and growing generation of women Veterans, the VA may consider other supports oriented toward economic and housing stability, either as adjuncts to existing VHA Homeless Programs or as separate programs entirely. One need that should receive priority moving forward is child care,[21,27] given that approximately one-third of women Veterans experiencing homelessness do so with children.[24] Because women Veterans experiencing homelessness are younger and less disabled than their male counterparts, they are also likely to be more active participants in the labor market. Thus, providing child care may be a critical support for helping women Veterans obtain and maintain employment and could be linked with other forms of support that are geared toward promoting economic (and housing) stability.

The characteristics of women Veterans that are dissimilar as a group from male Veterans—for example, younger age, more recent discharge from military service, less extensive homelessness or incarceration histories, less unhealthy substance use—may also place them at an advantage in terms of accessing housing and employment.[22] Policies and programs should embrace a strengths-based and empowerment-oriented approach to services provision.[43]

## ENSURE APPROPRIATE RESOURCES FOR WOMEN VETERANS TRANSITIONING INTO PERMANENT HOUSING

Findings related to differential utilization of VHA Homeless Programs, as described previously, suggest that while women may be less in need of the intensive, longer-term transitional housing provided by GPD, they may nonetheless need more time-limited housing as they leverage the homelessness prevention or rapid rehousing assistance provided by the Supportive Services for Veteran Families (SSVF) program or other resources to obtain permanent housing or as they navigate the process of leasing an apartment through HUD-VASH. Moving forward, it is especially important to fill this niche and ensure that appropriate resources, such as shelters and transitional housing, are available specifically for the purpose of temporarily accommodating women Veterans who are actively engaged in the process of transitioning into permanent housing.[21] Appropriate resources would also be responsive to women Veterans' preferences, which may include providing women-only programs or adapting mixed-gender programs to address particular needs or concerns of women Veterans such as safety and the use of peer support in the deployment of interventions.[43] There is also a need to work with Veterans who are homeless but are not engaged in VHA Homeless Programs and may need assistance to access preventive care.[15]

## ADDRESS REINTEGRATION NEEDS OF WOMEN VETERANS

As noted earlier, periods of reintegration from deployment or after discharge from the military represent crucial windows during which increased attention to housing, vocational, and interpersonal issues is warranted and could meaningfully reduce the risk for homelessness and promote positive outcomes in a number of other domains. Some research has found peer support to be effective in promoting successful transitions, but more is needed.[86] Additional efforts should adapt existing interventions that have proved to be effective in similar contexts to the specific needs of women Veterans reintegrating after a deployment or after discharge from the military. One such intervention that could prove highly effective in this regard is Critical Time Intervention (CTI), which is a time-limited intervention explicitly geared toward helping individuals successfully navigate challenging transitions. Initially developed for persons with serious mental illness exiting emergency shelters and psychiatric settings, the intervention is, by design, flexible and has been implemented with other populations, including persons exiting incarceration and families experiencing homelessness. Adapting CTI to the unique needs of women who are either in the process of reintegrating after a long deployment or transitioning out of the military to civilian life could prove highly effective in disrupting pathways to homelessness.[87,88]

# Future Research

Existing research exploring homelessness among women Veterans has been instrumental in uncovering the magnitude of the problem, pathways into homelessness among this population, and potential responses to prevent or mitigate this outcome. However, there is much more to be learned to understand the nature of the problem and how to address it, especially among particular populations of women Veterans.

A better understanding of homelessness among both younger and older women Veterans would inform the development of interventions to address housing instability among these unique populations. Work exploring the particular risk factors for homelessness among younger women Veterans—with a focus on children and family issues as well as reintegration after military service—is especially important for intervening among this new and growing Veteran population. In addition, given that women Veterans are also aging, it is important to better understand their unique needs related to housing, including the extent of the need and appropriate responses, such as aging in place. It is important for research to consider how these two populations are different and how services should be specifically tailored for their needs.

Another specific subpopulation to consider would be women Veterans living in rural areas. Given the unique nature of housing instability in these areas and the potential challenges that the characteristics of rural areas may confer on the reintegration process, it is important to better understand the characteristics and needs of women Veterans who may be experiencing housing instability in rural areas. Little research has been conducted about rural Veteran homelessness, and none has focused specifically on women Veterans. Issues of particular concern would be access to adequate and affordable housing; the availability of supportive services, including child care; and employment opportunities. Other subpopulations of interest include women Veterans who are involved in the criminal legal system and the relationship with experience of and homelessness as well as the unique vulnerabilities of sexual and gender minority (e.g., lesbian, gay, bisexual, and transgender) Veterans, who may be at increased risk for housing instability.

More generally, there is a need for research on housing instability more broadly among women, especially those who are homeless with children. While women may be less likely to experience literal homelessness, that does not necessarily mean that they are not experiencing chronic housing insecurity. Again, a significant need among women Veterans experiencing housing instability, particularly younger women Veterans, is not only housing but also employment. Work related to the development and evaluation of interventions should consider options that pair housing assistance with employment resources, such as supported employment.

# References

1. US Department of Defense. Population representation in the military services, appendix table D13. 2014. https://www.cna.org/pop-rep/2014/appendixd/d_13.html. Accessed March 10, 2016.
2. US Department of Defense, Office of the Deputy Assistant Secretary of Defense for Military Community and Family Policy. 2015 Demographics profile of the military community. http://download.militaryonesource.mil/12038/MOS/Reports/2015-Demographics-Report.pdf. Accessed March 13, 2017.

3. US Department of Veterans Affairs, National Center for Veterans Analysis and Statistics. Veteran population project. http://www.va.gov/Vetdata/Veteran_population.asp. Accessed April 26, 2016.

4. Frayne SM, Mattocks KM. Sourcebook: Women Veterans in the Veterans Health Administration. Volume 2: Sociodemographics and use of VHA and non-VA care (fee). 2012. https://www.womenshealth.va.gov/WOMENSHEALTH/docs/SourcebookVol2_508c_FINAL.pdf. Accessed April 24, 2017.

5. US Department of Veterans Affairs, National Center for Veterans Analysis and Statistics. (2016, December). Profile of women Veterans: 2015. Data from the American Community Survey. https://www.va.gov/Vetdata/docs/SpecialReports/Women_Veterans_Profile_12_22_2016.pdf. Accessed April 24, 2017.

6. Leda C, Rosenheck R, Gallup P. Mental illness among homeless female Veterans. *Hosp Commun Psychol*. 1992;43(10):1026–1028.

7. US Department of Housing and Urban Development. The 2014 Annual Homeless Assessment Report to Congress. Part 2: Estimates of homelessness in the United States. Washington, DC: Author.    https://www.hudexchange.info/onecpd/assets/File/2014-AHAR-Part-2.pdf. Accessed May 30, 2017.

8. Fargo JD, Metraux SM, Byrne TH, Munley E, Montgomery AE, Jones H, Sheldon G, Kane VR, Culhane DP. Prevalence and risk of Homelessness Among US Veterans. *Prev Chron Dis*. 2012;9:110–112.

9. US Department of Housing and Urban Development. Veteran homelessness: A supplemental report to the 2010 annual homeless assessment report to Congress. Washington, DC: Author.    https://www.va.gov/HOMELESS/docs/2010AHARVeteransReport.pdf.    Accessed May 30, 2017.

10. Metraux S, Stino M, Culhane DP. Validation of self-reported Veteran status among two sheltered homeless populations. *Publ Health Rep*. 2014;129(1):73–77.

11. Yu B, Montgomery AE, True JG, Cusack MC, Butler A, Chhabra M, Dichter ME. The intersection of interpersonal violence and housing instability: Perspectives from women Veterans. Unpublished data.

12. Casura, L. Down for the count: Women Veterans likely underestimated in federal homelessness figures. *Huffington Post*. April 13, 2017. http://www.huffingtonpost.com/entry/down-for-the-count-women-Veterans-likely-underestimated_us_58e9216ee4b06f8c18beec64.

13. US Department of Veterans Affairs, National Center for Veterans Analysis and Statistics. (2016). Unique Veteran users profile, FY 2015. https://www.va.gov/Vetdata/docs/SpecialReports/Profile_of_Unique_Veteran_Users_2015.pdf. Accessed June 11, 2017.

14. Byrne TH, Montgomery AE, Treglia D, Roberts CB, Culhane DP. Health services use among Veterans using VA and mainstream homeless services. *World Med Health Pol*. 2013;5(4):347–361.

15. Montgomery AE, Byrne TH. Services utilization among recently homeless Veterans: A gender-based comparison. *Mil Med*. 2014;179(3):236–239.

16. US Department of Housing and Urban Development. The 2017 annual homeless assessment report to Congress. Part 1: Point-in-time estimates of homelessness. Washington, DC: Author.    https://www.hudexchange.info/resources/documents/2017-AHAR-Part-1.pdf. Accessed February 26, 2018.

17. Hamilton AB, Frayne SM, Cordasco KM, Washington DL. Factors related to attrition from VA healthcare use: Findings from the National Survey of Women Veterans. *J Gen Intern Med*. 2013 Jul;28(suppl 2):S510–516.

18. Byrne TH. *Emerging populations: Female, OEF/OIF/OND, and older veterans*. Philadelphia, PA: National Center on Homelessness Among Veterans; 2016.

19. Montgomery AE. *Universal screening for homelessness and risk in the VHA: Fiscal year 2016 annual report*. Philadelphia, PA: National Center on Homelessness Among Veterans; 2017.

20. Montgomery AE, Sorrentino AE, Cusack MC, Bellamy SL, Medvedeva E, Roberts CB, Dichter ME. Recent intimate partner violence and housing instability among women Veterans. *Am J Prev Med*. 2018;54(4):584–590. doi:10.1016/j.amepre.2018.01.020

21. Tsai J, Kasprow WJ, Kane V, Rosenheck RA. National comparison of literally homeless male and female VA service users: Entry characteristics, clinical needs, and service patterns. *Womens Health Issues.* 2014;24(1):e29–e35.

22. Tsai J, Rosenheck RA, Kane VR. Homeless female US Veterans in a national supported housing program: Comparisons of individual characteristics and outcomes with male Veterans. *Psychol Serv.* 2014;11(3):309–316.

23. Tsai J, Rosenheck RA, McGuire JF. Comparison of outcomes of homeless female and male Veterans in transitional housing. *Commun Ment Health J.* 2012;48:705–710.

24. Tsai J, Rosenheck RA, Kasprow WJ, Kane V. Characteristics and use of services among literally homeless and unstably housed US Veterans with custody of minor children. *Psychol Serv.* 2015;66(10):1083–1090.

25. Montgomery AE, Byrne TH, Treglia D, Culhane DP. Characteristics and likelihood of ongoing homelessness among unsheltered Veterans. *J Health Care Poor Underserved.* 2016;27:911–922.

26. Byrne TH, Montgomery AE, Fargo JD. Unsheltered homelessness among Veterans: Correlates and profiles. *Commun Mental Health J.* 2016;52(2):148–157.

27. Blackstock OJ, Haskell SG, Brandt CA, Desai RA. Gender and the use of Veterans Health Administration homeless services programs among Iraq/Afghanistan Veterans. *Med Care.* 2012;50(4):347–352.

28. Metraux S, Clegg LX, Daigh JD, Culhane DP, Kane V. Risk factors for becoming homeless among a cohort of Veterans who served in the era of the Iraq and Afghanistan conflicts. *AJPH.* 2013;103(S2):S255–S261.

29. Gamache G, Rosenheck R, Tessler R. Overrepresentation of women Veterans among homeless women. *AJPH.* 2003;93(7):1132–1136.

30. Montgomery AE, Dichter ME, Thomasson AM, Fu X, Roberts CB. Demographic characteristics associated with homelessness and risk among female and male Veterans accessing VHA outpatient care. *Womens Health Issues.* 2015;25(1):42–48.

31. Washington DL, Yano EM, McGuire J, Hines V, Lee M, Gelberg L. Risk factors for homelessness among women Veterans. *J Health Care Poor Underserved.* 2010;21:81–91.

32. Hamilton AB, Poza I, Washington DL. Homelessness and trauma go hand-in-hand: Pathways to homelessness among women Veterans. *Womens Health Issues.* 2011;21(4):S203–S209.

33. Montgomery AE, Dichter ME, Thomasson AM, Roberts CB, Byrne TH. Disparities in housing status among Veterans with general medical, cognitive, and behavioral health conditions. *Psychol Serv.* 2015;66(3):317–320.

34. Carlson EB, Garvert DW, Macia KS, Ruzek JI, Burling TA. Traumatic stressor exposure and post-traumatic symptoms in homeless Veterans. *Mil Med.* 2013;178(9):970–973.

35. Mattocks KM, Haskell SG, Krebs EE, Justice AC, Yano EM. Women at war: Understanding how women Veterans cope with combat and military sexual trauma. *Soc Sci Med.* 2012;74:537–545.

36. Schnurr PP, Lunney CA, Bovin MJ, Marx BP. Posttraumatic stress disorder and quality of life: extension of findings to Veterans of the wars in Iraq and Afghanistan. *Clin Psychol Rev.* 2009;29(8):727–735.

37. Tsai J, Harpaz-Rotem I, Pietrzak RH, Southwick SM. The role of coping, resilience, and social support in mediating the relation between PTSD and social functioning in Veterans returning from Iraq and Afghanistan. *Psychiatry.* 2012;75(2):135–149.

38. Tsai J, Rosenheck RA, Decker SE, Desai RA, Harpaz-Rotem I. Trauma experience among homeless female Veterans: Correlates and impact on housing, clinical, and psychosocial outcomes. *J Trauma Stress.* 2012;25:624–632.

39. Rosenbeck R, Fontana A. A model of homelessness among male Veterans of the Vietnam War generation. *Am J Psychol.* 1994;151:421.

40. Blosnich JR, Dichter ME, Cerulli C, Batten SV, Bossarte RM. Disparities in adverse childhood experiences among individuals with a history of military service. *JAMA Psychiatry.* 2014;71(9):1041–1048.

41. Booth BM, Mengeling M, Torner J, Sadler AG. Rape, sex partnership, and substance use consequences in women Veterans. *J Trauma Stress.* 2011;24(3):287–294.

42. Sadler AG, Booth BM, Mengeling MA, Doebbeling BN. Life span and repeated violence against women during military service: Effects on health status and outpatient utilization. *J Womens Health*. 2004;13(7):799–811.

43. Hamilton AB, Poza I, Hines V, Washington DL. Barriers to psychosocial services among homeless women Veterans. *J Social Work Pract Addict*. 2012;12(1):52–68.

44. Hamilton AB, Washington DL, Zuchowski JL. Gendered social roots of homelessness among women Veterans. *Ann Anthropol Pract*. 2014;37(2):92–107.

45. Sadler AG, Booth BM, Cook BL, Doebbeling BN. Factors associated with women's risk of rape in the military environment. *Am J Industrial Med*. 2003;43:262–273.

46. US Department of Veterans Affairs, National Center for PTSD. Military sexual trauma. (2015). https://www.ptsd.va.gov/public/types/violence/military-sexual-trauma-general.asp. Accessed June 11, 2017.

47. Kimerling R, Gima K, Smith MW, Street A, Frayne S. The Veterans Health Administration and military sexual trauma. *AJPH*. 2007;97(12):2160–2166.

48. Street AE, Gradus JL, Giasson HL, Vogt D, Resick PA. Gender differences among Veterans deployed in support of the wars in Afghanistan and Iraq. *JGIM*. 2013;28(suppl 2):S556–S562.

49. Gibson CJ, Gray KE, Katon JG, Simpson TL, Lehavot K. Sexual assault, sexual harassment, and physical victimization during military service across age cohorts of women Veterans. *Womens Health Issues*. 2015;26(2):225–231.

50. Street AE, Vogt D, Dutra L. A new generation of women Veterans: Stressors faced by women deployed to Iraq and Afghanistan. *Clin Psychol Rev*. 2009;29:685–694.

51. LeardMann CA, Pietrucha A, Magruder KM, Smith B, Murdoch M, Jacobson IG, Ryan MAK, Gackstetter G, Smith TC. Combat deployment is associated with sexual harassment or sexual assault in a large, female military cohort. *Womens Health Issues*. 2013;23(4):e215–e223.

52. Burns B, Grindlay K, Holt K, Manski R, Grossman D. Military sexual trauma among U.S. servicewomen during deployment: A qualitative study. *AJPH*. 2014;104(2):345–349.

53. Campbell R, Raja S. The sexual assault and secondary victimization of female Veterans: Help-seeking experiences with military and civilian social systems. *Psychol Women Q*. 2005;29:97–106.

54. Pavao J, Turchik JA, Hyun JK, Karpenko J, Saweikis M, McCutcheon S, Kane VR, Kimerling R. Military sexual trauma among homeless Veterans. *JGIM*. 2013;28(suppl 2):S536–S541.

55. Suris A, Lind L, Kashner TM, Borman PD. Mental health, quality of life, and health functioning in women Veterans: Differential outcomes associated with military and civilian sexual assault. *J Interpers Violence*. 2007;22:179–197.

56. Himmelfarb N, Yaeger D, Mintz J. Posttraumatic stress disorder in female Veterans with military and civilian sexual trauma. *J Trauma Stress*. 2006;19(6):837–846.

57. Kimerling R, Street AE, Pavao J, Smith MW, Cronkite C, Holmes TH, Frayne SM. Military-related sexual trauma among Veterans Health Administration patients returning from Afghanistan and Iraq. *AJPH*. 2000;100(8):1409–1412.

58. Dichter ME, True JG. "This is the story of why my military career ended before it should have": Premature separation from military service among U.S. women Veterans. *J Women Social Work*. 2015;30(2):187–199.

59. Dichter ME, Wagner C, True G. Women Veterans' experience of intimate partner violence and non-partner sexual assault in the context of military service: Implications for women's health and well-being. *J Interpers Violence*. 2016. doi:10.1177/0886260516669166.

60. Brignone E, Gundlapalli AV, Blais RK, Carter ME, Suo Y, Samore MH, Kimerling R, Fargo JD. Differential risk for homelessness among US male and female Veterans with a positive screen for military sexual trauma. *JAMA Psychiatry*. 2016;73(6):582–589.

61. Katz LS, Bloor LE, Cojucar G, Draper T. Women who served in Iraq seeking mental health services: Relationships between military sexual trauma, symptoms, and readjustment. *Psychol Serv*. 2007;4(4):239–249.

62. Decker SE, Rosenheck RA, Tsai J, Hoff R, Harpaz-Rotem I. Military sexual assault and homeless women Veterans: Clinical correlates and treatment preferences. *Womens Health Issues*. 2013;23(6):e373–e380.

63. Pavao J, Alvarez J, Baumrind N, Induni M, Kimerling R. Intimate partner violence and housing instability. *Am J Prev Med*. 2007;32(2):143–146.

64. Dichter ME, Cerulli C, Bossarte RM. Intimate partner violence victimization among women Veterans and associated heart health risks. *Womens Health Issues.* 2011;21:S190–94.
65. Kimerling R, Iverson KM, Dichter ME, Rodriguez AL, Wong A, Pavao J. Prevalence of intimate partner violence among women Veterans who utilize Veterans Health Administration primary care. *JGIM.* 2016;31(8):888–894.
66. Bonomi AE, Anderson ML, Reid RJ, Rivara FP, Carrell D, Thompson RS. Medical and psychosocial diagnoses in women with a history of intimate partner violence. *Arch Intern Med.* 2009;169(18):1692–1697.
67. Gobin RL, Green KE, Iverson KM. Alcohol misuse among female Veterans: Exploring associations with interpersonal violence and mental health. *Substance Use Misuse.* 2015;50(14):1765–1777.
68. Lagdon S, Armour C, Stringer M. Adult experience of mental health outcomes as a result of intimate partner violence victimisation: A systematic review. *Eur J Psychotraumatol.* 2014;5:1–12.
69. Dichter ME, Wagner C, Borrero S, Broyles L, Montgomery AE. Intimate partner violence, unhealthy alcohol use, and housing instability among women Veterans in the Veterans Health Administration. *Psychol Serv.* 2017;14(2):246.
70. King DW, King LA, Foy DW, Keane TM, Fairbank JA. Posttraumatic stress disorder in a national sample of female and male Vietnam Veterans: Risk factors, war-zone stressors, and resilience-recovery variables. *J Abnorm Psychol.* 1999;108(1):164–170.
71. O'Campo P, Woods A, Jones S, Dienemann J, Campbell J. Depression, PTSD, and comorbidity related to intimate partner violence in civilian and military women. *Brief Treatm Crisis Intervent.* 2006;6(2):99–110.
72. Yaeger D, Himmelfarb N, Cammack A, Mintz J. DSM-IV diagnosed posttraumatic stress disorder in women Veterans with and without military sexual trauma. *JGIM.* 2006;21:S65–69.
73. Fontana A, Rosenheck R. Duty-related and sexual stress in the etiology of PTSD among women Veterans who seek treatment. *Psychol Serv.* 1998;49:658–662.
74. Carlson EB, Stromwall LK, Lietz CA. Mental health issues in recently returning women Veterans: Implications for practice. *Social Work.* 2013;58(2):105–114.
75. Kelty R, Kleykamp M, Segal DR. The military and the transition to adulthood. *Future Child.* 2010;20(1):181–207.
76. Yan GW, McAndrew L, D'Andrea EA, Lange G, Santos SL, Engel CC, Quigley KS. Self-reported stressors of National Guard women Veterans before and after deployment: The relevance of interpersonal relationships. *JGIM.* 2012;28(suppl 2):S549–S555.
77. Worthern ME, Moos M, Ahern R. Iraq and Afghanistan Veteran' experiences living with their parents after separation from the military. *Contemp Family Ther.* 2012;362–375. doi:10.1007/s10591-012-9196-4
78. Clever M, Segal DR. The demographics of military children and families. *Future Child.* 2013;23(2):13–39.
79. Atkins D, Lipson L. The role of research in a time of rapid change: Lessons from research on women Veterans' health. *Med Care.* 2015;53(4 suppl 1):S5–S7.
80. Bastian LA, Bosworth HB, Washington DL, Yano EM. Setting the stage: Research to inform interventions, practice and policy to improve women Veterans' health and healthcare. *JGIM.* 2013;28(suppl 2):S491–S494.
81. Dinnen S, Kane V, Cook JM. Trauma-informed care: A paradigm shift for services with homeless Veterans. *Prof Case Manage.* 2014;19(4):161–170.
82. Guarino KM, Beach CA, Clervil R. (2014, November). Trauma-informed care for Veterans experiencing homelessness: An organization-wide framework. American Institutes for Research. http://www.air.org/resource/trauma-informed-care-Veterans-experiencing-homelessness-organization-wide-framework. Accessed April 24, 2017.
83. Katz LS, Cojucar G, Hoff RA, Lindl C, Huffman C, Drew T. Longitudinal outcomes of women Veterans enrolled in the Renew Sexual Trauma Treatment Program. *J Contemp Psychother.* 2015;45:143–150.
84. Sturtevant L, Brennan M, Viveiros J, Handelman E. Housing and services needs of our changing Veteran population: Serving our older Veterans, female Veterans, and post-9/11 Veterans. National Housing Conference and Center for Housing Policy. 2015. http://centerforhousingpolicy.org/VeteransHousingReport_final.pdf. Accessed April 24, 2017.

85. Frayne SM, Parker VA, Christiansen CL, Loveland S, Seaver MR, Kazis LE, Skinner KM. Health status among 28,000 women Veterans: The VA Women's Health Program Evaluation Project. *JGIM*. 2006;21(S3):S40–S46.

86. Ahern J, Worthen M, Masters J, Lippman SA, Ozer EJ, Moos R. The challenges of Afghanistan and Iraq Veterans' transition from military to civilian life and approaches to reconnection. *PLoS ONE*. 2015;10(7):e0128599. doi:10.1371/journal.pone.0128599

87. Kasprow WJ, Rosenheck RA. Outcomes of critical time intervention case management of homeless Veterans after psychiatric hospitalization. *Psychol Serv*. 2007;58(7):929–935.

88. Susser E, Valencia E, Conover S, Felix A, Tsai WY, Wyatt RJ. Preventing recurrent homelessness among mentally ill men: A "critical time" intervention after discharge from a shelter. *AJPH*. 1997;87(2):256–262.

# 9

# Homeless Risk Among Post-9/11 Era Veterans

STEPHEN METRAUX AND R. TYSON SMITH

> As the Iraq war winds down and those troops return
> home . . . a new generation of Americans . . . will have to
> develop a fresh mindfulness of what these hundreds of
> thousands of men and women have been through and may be
> struggling with when they return.
> —Mike Scotti[1]

## Introduction

Homelessness among Veterans represents an uncomfortable American paradox. Over recent decades, the nation has shown support and reverence for those who have served, yet on a given night tens of thousands of Veterans of all ages are homeless and lacking basic material supports. As a result, a highly charged, moral rhetoric permeates the understanding of homelessness among Veterans. In response, the federal government, under the Obama Administration, made ending homelessness among Veterans a policy priority and, with the cooperation of Congress, greatly expanded housing and prevention services for homeless and at-risk Veterans.[2] These Obama-era assistance levels have so far continued under the Trump Administration. "We've got to keep fighting for the dignity of every veteran," Obama proclaimed at a 2016 Disabled American Veterans convention, "and that includes ending the tragedy, the travesty of veterans' homelessness."[3]

This discordance between Veteran status and homelessness is most visible among those who have served most recently. The attacks of September 11, 2001, pivotal in many respects, ushered in the recent era of military service. This post-9/11 era includes the two longest running wars in U.S. history, a military composed of people who voluntarily enlisted, and unprecedented levels of female service members. These military personnel, both during their service and subsequently as Veterans, have enjoyed a high, sustained level of public and political support.[4] Nevertheless, there has been a pervasive concern that this support has been insufficient and that, as a result, Veterans have struggled to re-establish their civilian lives.[5]

Concerns regarding homelessness—particularly among Veterans in the post-9/11–era cohort returning from Afghanistan, as part of Operation Enduring Freedom (OEF), and Iraq, as part of Operation Iraqi Freedom (OIF) or Operation New Dawn (OND)[a]—are central to a narrative of the damaged Veteran cast into an uncaring community.[6-9] The resulting perceptions of a "tsunami of homelessness"[6] among post-9/11–era Veterans have preceded more systematic, empirically based studies of the problem. This chapter examines empirical realities of post-9/11 American Veterans in light of the popular perceptions, manifested in advocacy and media accounts, that connect military service with homelessness among this most recent cohort of Veterans.

In doing so, we focus on the dimensions of homelessness that are particular to Veterans of this most recent era. This includes aspects of both their military and Veteran experiences, where military factors, insofar as they are antecedents to homelessness, interact with more general factors that occur after military service. In this manner, we take an approach consistent with Schuetz's essay "The Homecomer,"[10] in which the Veteran returns to civilian life having to face the transformations within himself or herself, as well as a civilian world that has also changed over the tenure of his or her service.[11] We do not dwell on more general, non–service-related risk factors for becoming homeless that post-9/11–era Veterans share with other Veterans and non-Veterans, such as mental illness, substance abuse, extreme poverty, and adverse childhood experiences, and that have been covered elsewhere.[12-16] Instead, we explore dimensions of military service that are particular to the post-9/11 era, the socioeconomic factors they faced on returning to civilian society, and how these military and civilian factors interact to affect the risk for homelessness.

## How Many Post-9/11 Veterans Experience Homelessness?

Tsunamis of homelessness should be quantifiable, in that numbers provide a basis for distinguishing human tidal waves from hyperbole. There have, however, not been any systematic attempts to assess the extent of homelessness

---

[a] This cohort has also been referred to as "Gulf War 2–era" Veterans. For this chapter, Gulf War 2 era and "post-9/11 era" are interchangeable, though only the latter term is used. Collectively, the subset of post-9/11–era Veterans who were deployed to Iraq and Afghanistan during this era are at times referred to by the aggregate of these acronyms, i.e., "OEF/OIF/OND veterans."

among post-9/11 Veterans. In the absence any official estimates of the homeless, post-9/11 Veteran population, the most widely disseminated unofficial estimate is that 12,700 OEF/OIF/OND Veterans experienced homelessness sometime in 2010. This estimate appears on websites of organizations as diverse the National Coalition for Homeless Veterans,[17] the American Psychological Association,[18] and the Congressional Record.[19]

None of these outlets describe who derived this estimate or how it was derived. However, it almost certainly comes from the 2010 Veteran Supplement to federal government's Annual Homelessness Assessment Report (AHAR). In this report, an estimated 12,714 Veterans aged 18 to 30 years were in shelter or transitional housing on at least one night in 2010.[20] In effect, age here became a de facto proxy for deployment.

Despite the obvious problems with using an estimate of homeless Veterans younger than 30 years to stand in for an estimate of homeless Veterans who were deployed to Iraq or Afghanistan, in 2010 this was a plausible estimate. By circumstance, the number of OEF/OIF/OND Veterans was roughly equivalent to the number of Veterans younger than 30 years, both coming in at about 1.2 million and overlapping in that a large portion of the Veterans younger than 30 years would have deployed to Iraq or Afghanistan during their service. Using either Veteran subpopulation as a denominator and the 12,700 estimate as the numerator yields an approximate annual prevalence rate of 1%. This rate roughly corresponds to annual prevalence rates found for general non-Veteran populations after adjusting for age,[21,22] suggesting that this estimate falls within a believable range.

However, this equilibrium did not hold. Between 2010 and 2015, U.S. Department of Veterans Affairs (VA) studies show that number of Veterans who deployed to Iraq and Afghanistan increased by 57%,[b] while the numbers used for the AHAR reports indicate that, over this time period, the number of all Veterans younger than 30 years increased by only 28%.[c] Moreover, the younger

---

[b] OEF/OIF/OND population increased 57%, from an estimated 1,250,000 in 2010 (based on extrapolations from 2011 to 2015 counts of OEF/OIF/OND Veterans) to 1,965,534 in 2015, as described in a series of reports by the U.S. Department of Veterans Affairs Public Health office.[24]

[c] This increase is based on numbers used for AHAR estimates. Based on numbers provided in Exhibit 3.1 (p. 7) of the 2010 AHAR Veteran Supplement,[20] there were approximately 1,164,000 Veterans younger than 30 years in 2010. The 2015 extrapolation is a bit more complex. Over the course of 2015, 132,847 Veterans used an emergency shelter or transitional housing program, which amounted to 1 in 170 Veterans experiencing sheltered homelessness during the course of that year (pp. 5–7).[23] From this (exact number is unavailable), there was a base number of approximately 22,584,000 total Veterans in 2015. Of these, the AHAR reports that 6.6% (or approximately 1,490,000) were younger than 30 years. Compared with 1,164,000 Veterans younger than 30 years in 2010, this corresponds to a 28% increase in the number of Veterans younger than 30 years since 2010.

than 30 years *homeless* Veteran estimate in the 2015 AHAR actually decreased by 5% during this period (from 12,746 in 2010[19] to 12,089[23] in 2015) so that in 2015 the annual prevalence rate dropped to 0.8%. Applying this lower prevalence rate to a 2015 estimate of almost 2 million OEF/OIF/OND[24] Veterans yields a very rough estimate of about 16,000 OEF/OIF/OND Veterans who were in shelters or transitional housing at some point in 2015. Thus, the number of homeless OEF/OIF/OND Veterans has almost certainly increased from homelessness among this group in 2010.

The numbers we calculate here are intentionally left vague because both the 2010 and our updated 2015 estimates employ decidedly back-of-the-envelope methodologies. To stretch these tenuous estimates even further, approximately half of all post-9/11 Veterans never deployed to Iraq or Afghanistan,[25] so an estimate covering the entire post-9/11 cohort would be about double what any OEF/OIF/OND estimate would be.

In place of a definitive numerical estimate, we conclude this chapter with two more general trends that should affect the extent of homelessness among the post-9/11 Veteran cohort. First, by a general consensus, overall homelessness among Veterans has declined substantially (by as much as 45% since 2009),[26] and this trend should also have affected this cohort. Second, the post-9/11 era of military service is ongoing, and as such the numbers of Veterans belonging to this era and having been deployed to Iraq and Afghanistan continues to grow. If both of these trends hold, then the past decade should have seen an increase in the number of Veterans in this cohort who became homeless (by virtue of sheer demographics), but this increase should have been limited by a corresponding decline in the rate by which these Veterans became homeless.

Taken together, "rising tide" may be a more accurate metaphor than "tsunami" for the homelessness dynamics among post-9/11 Veterans. Implicit to both metaphors is a call for increased attention and resources to the housing instability of this Veteran subpopulation, but the alarmist tsunami rhetoric appears misleading. The question of "how many" homeless post-9/11 Veterans there are is far from settled. This underscores the call made by Iraq and Afghanistan Veterans of America (IAVA) in their most recent policy agenda for the federal government to "collect data on the number of chronically homeless veterans and the number of homeless veterans by conflict-era."[27] For, in the words of former VA Secretary Eric Shinseki: "I learned a long time ago I couldn't solve a problem I can't see."[28]

## Military Factors Linked to Homelessness

Each military service era has defining features that shape Veterans' military experiences and continue to affect them in their subsequent civilian lives. Post-9/11–era Veterans have served during the time of the two longest wars in U.S.

history. The casualties of these wars have further been associated with two signature injuries: post-traumatic stress disorder (PTSD) and traumatic brain injury (TBI). Two key dynamics of this era include having women serve in unprecedented numbers and roles and conducting the first protracted modern wars without conscripted recruits. Additionally, there has been a growing number of other-than-honorable (OTH) discharges among this era's Veterans,[d] leading to concern that combat and other service-related issues are addressed in an inappropriately punitive and harmful manner. All of these issues have an impact on this Veteran cohort, as well as the perceptions and realities of homelessness among them.

## DEPLOYMENT, WARTIME EXPERIENCE, AND PTSD AND TBI

The U.S. Interagency Council on Homelessness (ICH), in its strategic plan to end and prevent homelessness, stated that: "combat and repeated deployments introduce additional factors that contribute to the risk of homelessness, including post-traumatic stress and the disruption of connections to family and community supports."[2 (p. 27)] Indeed, the most common narrative for explaining homelessness among recent Veterans underscores how wartime experiences have affected OEF/OIF/OND Veterans so that, in the extreme, they are unable to effectively reintegrate into civilian life.

Of the different ways to measure wartime exposure, deployment is perhaps the simplest. Here, deployment amounts to a largely binary measure of whether a Veteran participated in OEF, OIF, or OND. By 2015, just under 2 million Veterans were deployed to one or both of these war theaters.[24] Just spending an extended time period in a far-off, wartime environment will have lasting effects on a Veteran that may affect the risk for homelessness. Three studies assess this, but all have substantial limitations. Both Metraux and colleagues[25] and the VA's Office of the Inspector General[29] reported, based on the use of VA homeless services among 310,000 post-9/11–era Veterans, a substantially higher (albeit unadjusted) rate of homelessness among deployed Veterans compared with their nondeployed contemporaries (2.1%–1.4%). Edens and colleagues, in contrast, found OEF/OIF deployment to be associated with substantially lower risk for VA homeless services use among a large but singular group of Veterans of all ages who used VA specialty mental health services in 2009.[30] Finally, Tsai and colleagues[31] use data from the National Health and Resilience in Veterans Study[32] to look at homelessness risk among the overall Veteran population, but the small number of OEF/OIF/OND Veterans (34 total, four of whom reported

---

[d] Here we consider anyone who has served in the military, regardless of discharge status and whether they are eligible for VA benefits and services as a Veteran.

homelessness) in the survey precluded drawing any definitive conclusions about homelessness among this group.

Breaking down deployment experiences and examining the relationships of these component parts with homelessness among OEF/OIF/OND Veterans yields similarly inconclusive findings. A study by Elbogen and colleagues using the VA's National Post-Deployment Adjustment Survey found a post-military, one-year homelessness rate of 4.5% in the study group,[e] and a significant, positive bivariate association between combat experience and homelessness.[33] This association became nonsignificant, however, on introducing other covariates into a multivariate regression model. These data warrant a second look because the Elbogen's focus was on the association between money mismanagement and homelessness (see Chapter 7) and did not examine the impact of a broader set of military risk factors on homelessness beyond their role as potentially confounding factors. Other studies that examined homelessness specifically among OEF/OIF/OND Veterans do not contain any measures that even broadly differentiate aspects of Veteran deployment experiences.[25,29,34-37]

The third measure of wartime experience is PTSD. PTSD is, more precisely, a medicalized proxy for adverse wartime experience[38] that has become a means in the popular and advocacy literature for explaining negative Veteran outcomes such as homelessness. PTSD emerged following the Vietnam War as a mental health disorder based on a set of discrete psychological symptoms and reflective of the lasting behavioral responses to wartime (and other traumatic experiences) that become maladaptive in later life. The prevalence of the disorder likely ranges somewhere between 10% and 17% among combat Veterans, with lower rates when deployed noncombatants are included.[39] PTSD can impede a Veteran's ability to function in society and, in extreme manifestations, has been linked to homicide and suicide.

The empirical evidence to support the association between PTSD and homelessness has been far less robust than the popular belief in this association.[40] The most rigorous study that examined this connection looked at Vietnam Veterans and did not find a direct association between the two.[41] In the context of the Afghanistan and Iraq wars, four of the studies that examined homelessness among OEF/OIF/OND Veterans reported findings related to PTSD. Two of these studies found associations between PTSD and modestly increased risks for homelessness,[25,34] while two others[30,33] reported no significant associations after controlling for other factors.

---

[e] There is no clear explanation for why the homeless prevalence rate in the Elbogen study was higher than the comparable studies cited in this subsection, other than it used a wider ranging (and less precise) definition of homelessness.

Again, this body of evidence is an insufficient basis for drawing firm conclusions on the extent to which PTSD affects the risk for homelessness. If there is an association, it may well be an indirect one, meaning that, in addition to a PTSD diagnosis, the presence or absence of other factors will be crucial to the role that PTSD plays in becoming homeless. Other factors may include the presence of other behavioral health diagnoses because PTSD frequently co-occurs with diagnoses for depression and substance abuse disorders,[42] which both the Metraux and the Edens studies found to be associated with increased homelessness risk.[25,30] On the other hand, as suggested in the Edens study, when supports such as access to VA behavioral health care and disability benefits are available to Veterans diagnosed with PTSD, then PTSD may indirectly act as a protective factor against homelessness.[30,43]

While more research is needed to better understand the relationship between PTSD and becoming homeless, studies have found a high prevalence of PTSD among post-9/11 Veterans who experience homelessness. One study of OEF/OIF/OND Veterans who were placed into VA supportive housing called attention to the contrast between the high rates of PTSD diagnoses (67%) found in this group and the much lower rates found among older cohorts of homeless Veterans.[44] Another study, based on interviews of post-9/11 Veterans who experienced homelessness, identified PTSD as a key theme in the Veterans' accounts and showed how PTSD symptoms led to circumstances, such as difficulties maintaining employment and family relations, that directly contributed to homelessness. Furthermore, these accounts showed how PTSD and homelessness interact to exacerbate one another.[45]

There has been no evidence that links TBI, the second signature injury of the Iraq and Afghanistan wars, with increased risk for homelessness. Two studies have examined TBI among Veterans who are homeless, and although both noted a high prevalence of TBI, they found that most incidences were not military related.[46,47] Conversely, the circumstances of being homeless appear to increase the risk, regardless of Veteran status, of sustaining a TBI due to accidents, assaults, and other hazards of living on the streets.

In summary, while media reports readily link PTSD and homelessness, the research presents a less dramatic and more complicated picture. There may indeed be a higher prevalence of homelessness among this Veteran cohort that is connected to the adversities of going to war. Yet the findings to date also suggest that the wars have yet to bring on an onslaught of homelessness among post-9/11–era Veterans. Nor would homelessness disappear among this cohort in absence of any war. Yet in the midst of the uncertainty about relationships between PTSD and homelessness, addressing homelessness for an undetermined but substantial proportion of post-9/11–era Veterans involves taking into account the sequelae of their wartime experiences.

## GENDER AND FAMILY ISSUES RELATED TO MILITARY SERVICE

Recent media reports have described women as the "fastest growing demographic" among Veterans who experience homelessness.[48,49] This oft-repeated and unsupported assertion is difficult to verify, but a closer examination of it promises insights about the role of gender in homelessness among post-9/11 Veterans.

By consensus, female Veterans are at higher risk for homelessness than male Veterans.[50] Male and female Veterans differ in that, among male Veterans, the risk for experiencing homelessness increases with age up to 65 years, while among women it is the younger age groups that have the highest risk.[51] This suggests that homelessness risk among female Veterans would disproportionately fall on those in the post-9/11 cohort.

In terms of literally assessing this "fastest growing" claim, the best resource is the AHAR, referred to earlier, which provides an ongoing series of nationwide estimates of the homeless population. Based on these estimates, between 2009 and 2015 there was a net increase of 725 female Veterans, from 11,098 to 11,823. This 6.5% increase over a six-year period appears modest, although it becomes more substantial when considering that, in this same time period, the overall Veteran homeless population (as measured by annual prevalence) declined by 12.6%.[23] So while there was an increase, whether it warrants the moniker "fastest growing" will be up to the beholder and will depend on the nature of the comparison groups.

This growth in the number of female Veterans in the homeless population comes at a time of substantial growth in the number of women in the military. As a result, the female Veteran population has been increasing in size and decreasing in age, even as the overall Veteran population has been declining in size and increasing in age. While 9% of the total Veteran population are women, 17% of all post-9/11–era Veterans are women, and 40% of all female Veterans served during the post-9/11 era.[52] Among the homeless Veteran population, women also are substantially younger than men, with a higher proportion of women having served during the post-9/11 era.[53]

Studies have not found female Veterans in the post-9/11 cohort to be any more likely than their male counterparts to use VA homeless services.[34,54] However, focusing exclusively on VA services, as research on homelessness among Veterans often does, is certain to miss female Veterans who experience homelessness but do not use VA services. While no research exists on where female Veterans go when they become homeless, they are more likely than male Veterans to turn to non-VA, community-based homeless services for shelter and other assistance.[50] VA homeless services have traditionally been geared toward accommodating and serving older, single, male Veterans.[55] In such arrangements, when women seek assistance from Veteran-focused organizations, they often have to negotiate almost exclusively male environments and do not find services that meet their needs, especially when they are homeless with children. Even though the 2015 AHAR found no increase between 2009 and 2015 in the proportion of Veterans in shelters who were accompanied by children (about 3%), one study found that 57% of post-9/11–era homeless female Veterans had custody of children.[56]

The issue most frequently associated with gender with respect to Veteran homelessness is military sexual trauma (MST). An estimated 38% of female service members experienced MST compared with 4% of men,[57] with several studies finding higher rates of MST among female Veterans who experience homelessness.[58-60] One study linked MST to significantly higher risk for homelessness among both female and male OEF/OIF Veterans.[61] Furthermore, MST is associated with mental health comorbidity, including PTSD, that may contribute to a greater risk for and longer duration of homelessness.[53] Thus, MST appears to transcend gender in its association with Veteran homelessness, although because women experience MST in much higher proportions than men, MST and its sequelae are much more pervasive among women in homeless populations.

In summary, "fastest growing" in the context of homelessness among female post-9/11 Veterans reflects not only the growth in the number of women who are currently serving in the military but also the difficulties women have faced in the military and how such difficulties carry over into civilian life. Primary among these are inclusion into military and Veteran environments that remain male oriented,[62] the strain between military and family roles that manifest both in military service and Veteran services,[63] and significantly greater exposure to MST. These issues are specific to female Veterans regardless of service cohort but are particularly salient to post-9/11–era Veterans because of the increased prevalence and prominence of women in the military during this era. This has led to greater pressure on both the U.S. Department of Defense (DoD) and the VA to address these issues and provides an impetus for increasing the amount of research that currently exists on gender and Veteran homelessness.[50]

## ALL-VOLUNTEER MILITARY

The Iraq and Afghanistan wars, the longest in U.S. history, have been waged without resorting to conscription. The staffing of two wars with volunteers has created personnel challenges for the military, and these challenges may be linked to the subsequent homelessness risk among Veterans from this era.

The framework for linking recruitment to subsequent homelessness comes from the research of Rosenheck and colleagues, who ascertained that the cohort of Veterans at greatest risk for homelessness were those who served in the early years of the post-Vietnam era and during the implementation of the all-volunteer military. During this time, military service was unpopular, paid low salaries, and was forced to reduce standards in order to meet recruiting quotas. Rosenheck and colleagues argued that this brought in a higher number of recruits with factors such as behavioral health issues and criminal histories that would predispose them to a higher risk for homelessness over their post-military life course.[64] In effect, they argued that one of the most effective Veteran homeless prevention initiatives may be maintaining rigorous recruiting standards.

A similar situation may have occurred during the mid-2000s, during the early war years. As recently as 2005 the military fell substantially short of its recruiting goals, and up through 2009 the military regularly provided waivers for health and legal situations that would ordinarily bar potential recruits from enlisting.[65,66] This situation has since reversed, but these recruiting dynamics may contribute to an elevated risk for homelessness and other adverse outcomes among a subset of post-9/11–era Veterans over the life course. At this point, however, whether or not the quality of personnel recruited during the 2000s was in fact degraded is a point of contention.[67-69] And although linking of recruiting standards to homelessness risk appears compelling, in the absence of further research the evidence for such a link remains circumstantial.

Recruiting shortfalls during the course of the two wars has also led to the deployment of large numbers of National Guard and Reserve personnel and to active-duty personnel being deployed for extended periods (i.e., "stop loss"), for multiple deployments, and with less time between the multiple deployments.[70] The added stress and uncertainty of such open-ended service requirements has been linked to more difficulties with transitioning back into civilian life[71] and, conceivably, to greater vulnerability to homelessness. However, linking stop-loss to homelessness amounts to conjecture at this point, given the lack of studies that have empirically examined this relationship.

## OTHER-THAN-HONORABLE DISCHARGES

The Colorado Springs Gazette first brought public attention to an alarming increase in the number of misconduct discharges among service members leaving the military,[72] and the advocacy group Swords to Plowshares[73] subsequently provided evidence that 125,000 Veterans (6.5% of all post-9/11 Veterans) are ineligible for VA services due to OTH, bad conduct, or dishonorable discharges. The vast majority of such discharges are OTH, which are administrative discharges due to misconduct. The U.S. Government Accountability Office[74] found that 62% of service members who separated because of misconduct had PTSD or TBI diagnoses,[35,75] supporting contentions that the increase in OTH discharges were due to the military's systematically discharging personnel with medical or psychiatric conditions for punitive reasons.[72] Under these circumstances, "expedient military justice will continue to generate a hidden cost of combat."[76 (p. 1809)]

Such findings of troubled Veterans deprived of VA support have led to media headlines such as "'Bad Paper' Discharge Can Lead to Homelessness, Hopelessness."[77] This association is supported by Gundlapalli et al. (2015), who found that VA-eligible OEF/OIF Veterans with misconduct-related discharges represented 5.6% of their study group but accounted for 20.6% of those who became homeless in the subsequent five years, with a corresponding adjusted odds ratio for becoming homeless of 6.3.[37] In contrast to this study group, the large majority of post-9/11 Veterans with misconduct discharges are, by policy, ineligible for VA services, and this alone would presumably contribute to an even higher risk for homelessness. Verifying these presumptions, however, is difficult because these Veterans are invisible to the VA. They do, however, appear to be disproportionately represented among Veterans in the mainstream homeless systems, as when a 2016 survey of Minnesota's homeless population found that 11% of the Veterans (from all eras) reported negative discharges.[78] This is almost twice the rate cited earlier in the Swords to Plowshares study.

# Post-Military Factors and Homelessness

Just like there are specific features that differentiate the military service of post-9/11–era Veterans from that of their predecessors, there are also features that uniquely shape the experiences of this Veteran cohort as they subsequently seek to re-establish and resume their civilian lives. Some of these features are directly attached to their Veteran status, such as the transition process from military to civilian life, or their access to a unique set of benefits and services. Other features, such the economic vagaries of the past decade, are more general in their impact but may affect Veterans differently than they affect non-Veterans. These features have all, to some extent, been prominently linked to risk for homelessness among this cohort, either directly or in conjunction with the military factors reviewed in the previous section. Thus, they are essential to understanding the singular elements of homelessness risk specific to this cohort.

## TRANSITIONING TO CIVILIAN LIFE

A key part of the media and advocacy narrative on the vulnerability to homelessness among post-9/11–era Veterans is that homelessness occurs much sooner among this cohort, especially among Veterans returning from Iraq and Afghanistan. As Amy Fairweather, from the advocacy group Swords to Plowshares, told the San Francisco Chronicle:

> We are seeing Iraq and Afghanistan veterans, who are homeless, coming in very quickly. After Vietnam, it generally took about five to 10 years to end up on the streets. We're seeing people on the streets three months after they come home.[79]

It is unclear where Fairweather got her statistic about time to homelessness among Vietnam-era Veterans because it was more than a decade after the end of the Vietnam service era (1975) before anyone started looking at Vietnam Veterans becoming homeless.[80] In contrast, Fairweather's comments underscore how concerns about homelessness now follow the Veteran from the moment he or she starts the transition back to civilian life.

Transitioning to civilian life has received renewed attention among post-9/11 Veterans, particularly among those who were deployed to Iraq and Afghanistan. Difficulties in this process highlight the increasing incongruence between military and civilian life. The post-9/11 era has been a time of both near-constant warfare and diminishing proportions of the U.S. adults serving in the military. Attenuated connections between military personnel and the broader civilian population[4] have led to concerns about the formation of a separate "warrior caste."[81-83] Such a disconnect can make military service members feel, in the words of one Veteran, "alien."[38] Alienation, and broader issues of identity and belonging, are among the potential problems that new Veterans face during the transition period that may create increased vulnerability for homelessness.[70] In a review, Sherman, Larson, and Borden group these problems into six domains of "postdeployment impairment."[84] Three of these domains—mental health, relationship functioning and family life, and financial well-being—are closely linked to homelessness.

The extent to which homelessness occurs during the transition period is readily measurable through surveys and through linking military records and homeless services data. Two studies in particular, both based on matching DoD and VA records, have reported results on time from military discharge to onset of homeless services use for cohorts of post-9/11–era Veterans. A study by the VA's Office of Inspector General identified 5,574 Veterans as using homeless services out of the 310,685 post-9/11–era Veterans they followed over a four- to five-year period (five-year incidence rate of 3.7%). The median time period between discharge and first use of VA homeless services was three years.[29] Another study, by Blackstock and colleagues, followed 445,319 Veterans who had deployed in Afghanistan and Iraq between 2001 and 2009. For the 7,431 Veterans who were identified as using VA homeless services, the median time for their initial use of homeless services use was 1.9 years after separation from the military.[34] While the results from these two studies differ in part because of differences in the study periods they used, both indicate that relatively little homelessness occurs in the period immediately following separation from the military.

Instead of focusing on immediate onset of homelessness, qualitative research suggests that a more common trajectory involves a period of housing instability and other issues during the transition period that usually precedes literal homelessness. Here, makeshift housing arrangements, loosening social supports, and a reluctance to obtain help are common themes along a diverse range of pathways and over an extended time period.[45,62] Instead of becoming homeless in the wake of leaving the military, becoming literally homeless takes several years and, as time passes, longer. Such a perspective suggests that transition assistance could include housing and related assistance as a means for preventing homelessness in the long term.

## UNEMPLOYMENT AND HOUSING

Post-9/11–era Veterans have exited military service to fluctuating economic circumstances, depending on when their service ended. Overall, the economic outlook was relatively positive up to 2008, after which both the housing and labor markets were hit with what would be called the Great Recession. Since about 2010 the economy has been recovering, though the magnitude of this economic improvement is currently a subject of debate tempered by political perspectives.

Throughout this period of economic fluctuation, post-9/11–era Veterans had higher unemployment rates than their non-Veteran counterparts.[85] A RAND report on this disparity found that, even after controlling for differences in sociodemographic factors such as gender and race, the employment disparity between younger Veterans and non-Veterans during the Great Recession persisted. This appeared to be a period effect because, with increased age, the level of Veteran unemployment decreased and the Veteran-based disparity disappeared. Most of the disparity was a function of new Veterans transitioning out of the military and taking time to locate employment.[86] Another study finds that female Veterans and Veterans with lower levels of education were particularly disadvantaged with regard to employment, while Black Veterans do not show such a disadvantage.[87] Unemployment levels reported in the most recent Bureau of Labor Statistics study show that, in the years following these studies, the unadjusted, Veteran-based disparity decreased as the overall unemployment rate went down.[88]

It is unclear how these employment dynamics affect homelessness on a population level. Insofar as education level stands in for socioeconomic status, Veteran status among people in poverty may be an additional disadvantage in finding employment and thereby could increase the risk for homelessness. Similarly, employment difficulties may increase vulnerability to homelessness among poor female Veterans but mitigate it some among poor Black Veterans. More direct links than this, however, are currently lacking. Taken together, unemployment and lower earnings disproportionately affect adults of younger age and younger Veterans in particular. This is consistent with individual accounts of Veterans, for whom the inability to find work is a major factor in the pathway to homelessness.[45,62,89] However, on a population level, there is as yet no clear indication that higher unemployment mediates higher homelessness risk among post-9/11–era Veterans compared with their non-Veteran peers.

Housing is another key dynamic linking the overall economy to homelessness. The United States has been experiencing an affordable housing crisis,[90,91] with housing affordability continuing to deteriorate and disproportionately affecting the low end of the housing and rental markets.[92] While housing affordability has become more critical overall, there is no evidence that this is a particular problem for Veterans. The only recent report to specifically focus on housing and Veterans concluded that:

> while overall, veteran households were less likely to experience a housing cost burden than non-veteran households, there were significant disparities among veteran households. In particular, veterans who are racial minorities, who are women, who have disabilities, and who served after September 11, 2001, have the greatest need for affordable housing.[93 (p. 1)]

This elevated housing need among post-9/11–era Veterans appears to be more a function of factors that they share with their non-Veteran peers, such as family formation and being less established vocationally, than it does with anything related to their military service.

## BEHAVIORAL HEALTH

Behavioral health issues, focusing on mental health and substance use disorders, are consistently among the most salient individual factors related to homelessness outcomes among both Veterans and non-Veterans. This appears to be the case for the post-9/11–era Veteran cohort as well.[25] A more general overview of behavioral health issues among homeless Veterans is the topic of Chapter 3. Beyond that, three specific behavioral health conditions have received additional scrutiny for their disproportionate effects on this cohort: PTSD (discussed earlier), suicide, and opioid misuse.

Considerable public concern has focused on rising suicide rates among military personnel and Veterans. With findings that suicide risk was 22% higher among Veterans than among non-Veterans,[94] the Trump Administration has made suicide prevention a top priority for VA policy. Among post-9/11 Veterans, suicide has been cast in the media as an epidemic.[95,96] While this appears hyperbolic, the rate of suicide for post-9/11 Veterans (regardless of deployment) is higher than that of the comparable non-Veteran population.[97] The media often casts Veteran suicide as an outcome of having experienced substantial wartime trauma, but research has offered inconsistent support for such a link among post-9/11 Veterans.[98,99] Similarly, while a link between Veteran suicide and homelessness has not been widely recognized in the research literature, one recent review[100] argues for such a connection based on evidence from several studies.[101–105] Given the priority that the VA has given to both issues,[15,106] more research on this topic is likely to emerge and add to a fuller understanding of how suicide and homelessness interact among Veterans from all eras.

Opioid abuse and overdoses, by prescription and illicit means, have also been cast as being at epidemic levels, with post-9/11–era Veterans being at particular risk.[107,108] In contrast, the most systematic assessment of opioid use among OEF/OIF/OND Veterans found "relatively modest" use and at a much lower level than suggested by the media and other research studies.[109] Among the post-9/11–era Veterans who do abuse opioids, the most common trajectory is one that starts through pain management for service-connected injuries and then diffuses to misuse for recreational purposes or to cope with (and ultimately exacerbate) transition-related issues.[110] Taken together, there are two perspectives here. On an individual level, Veterans who misuse opioids have an elevated risk for homelessness, particularly when combined with poverty and lack of family support. On a population level, however, there is no evidence to date that suggests anything about post-9/11 Veterans that renders them more vulnerable to opioid misuse or more likely to become homeless as a result of such misuse.

PTSD, suicide, and opioid abuse all carry stigma that have more generally colored military service during the post-9/11 era, particularly in conjunction with the Iraq and Afghanistan wars. The media documents a reluctance among employers to hire post-9/11 Veterans because of concerns related to PTSD and mental instability.[111,112] A commonly cited statistic of 22 Veterans per day committing suicide carries presumptions that most of these deaths are war related, when the majority of such suicides occur among older Veterans.[113] And the stigma of prescription opioid abuse now extends beyond Veterans to where the VA has received criticism for overprescribing opioids.[114] In a more systematic and nuanced view, Kleykamp and Hipes present evidence that print media coverage of Iraq and Afghanistan Veterans has indeed framed this cohort as damaged by their service but as nonetheless deserving of government benefits and assistance by virtue of their having suffered as a result of their military service.[115] This may help to marshal resources on behalf of post-9/11 Veterans but also risks casting these Veterans as damaged goods.

Smith and True associate, and differentiate, mental disorders such as these (and PTSD in particular) and the psychological distress more generally rooted in the identity conflicts inherent to transitioning back to a civilian milieu.[38] Central to this psychological distress is a sense of alienation from a civilian population that is increasingly detached from military culture.[116] This framing emphasizes the social dimension of psychological distress, as opposed to casting it in a clinical domain, and thereby lends itself better to explaining a Veteran-specific vulnerability to homelessness. Casting homelessness in more psychosocial terms avoids the inherent medicalization found in the more direct associations between behavioral health disorders and homelessness[117,118] and invites scrutiny on how social aspects of disorders such as PTSD, suicidal ideation, or opioid dependence (rather than the clinical aspects of the diagnoses) drive Veterans to homelessness.

## INTERACTIONS WITH THE VA: HEALTH CARE, BENEFITS, AND HOMELESSNESS ASSISTANCE

Veterans enjoy an "integrated web of institutional supports" that contrast with the "fragmented, conditional nature of the civilian welfare state."[119] The VA is by far the largest provider of such support services and provides eligible Veterans[f] with an extended safety net that includes health care, income supports, housing and homeless services, and education benefits. All OEF/OIF/OND Veterans with other-than-dishonorable discharge receive automatic eligibility for VA health care for five years following their service, and all post-9/11 Veterans who were discharged honorably can receive tuition and a living stipend in conjunction with enrollment in a post-secondary education program. Routine VA health care services and income assistance benefits have doubtlessly prevented homelessness for an uncountable number of Veterans of all eras. VA homeless services have provided more targeted emergency assistance and facilitated rehousing for hundreds of thousands of Veterans. Ending Veteran homelessness was a VA policy priority during the Obama Administration and continues to be a rallying cry backed by bipartisan support and a significant commitment of federal resources.[2]

There is no evidence that the post-9/11 cohort is making disproportionate use of VA homeless services. Conversely, beyond making efforts to better accommodate women and children, the VA has not substantially modified its homeless services to specifically target post-9/11 Veterans. One exception to this was a pilot program called the Veterans Homelessness Prevention Demonstration (VHPD) program. This joint effort between the VA, Department of Housing and Urban Development, and Department of Labor served almost 2,000 Veteran households (the majority serving during the post-9/11 era) in five locations (San Diego, CA; Tampa, FL; Killeen, TX; Tacoma, WA; and Watertown, NY)

[f] Eligibility is based primarily on nature of military service (i.e., active duty or service in a combat theater), discharge status (conditions other than dishonorable), presence of a service-connected medical or psychiatric condition, and income.

that were either literally homeless or at imminent risk for homelessness. These households received short-term housing and financial assistance, case management, and employment services in an effort to both stabilize their immediate housing situation and gain long-term self-sufficiency. Veterans, as noted in the program evaluation, presented needs that were very similar to those of non-Veterans, although the investigators found that Veterans, especially post-9/11–era Veterans, respond better to services that are competent in military culture and that engage Veterans in settings that are not specific to providing housing assistance (e.g., community-based locations or other types of service locations).[120] Although the VHPD showed positive outcomes in facilitating housing, employment and income gains among the Veteran households that were served, the program was not continued after this demonstration.

Post-9/11 Veterans have shown an ambivalence toward the VA. In a series of in-depth interviews, Veterans acknowledged and appreciated the health and mental health care services they received through the VA, as well as additional housing and homeless services that are not available to non-Veterans. However, like many Veterans generally, they often expressed frustration with the accessibility of VA health care services and the lengthy process required to gain VA disability benefits. One of the services from non-VA provider agencies that the respondents found most valuable was assistance in navigating a byzantine VA bureaucracy.[45]

## Looking Ahead

In this chapter, we have examined associations in the popular media and in the advocacy literature between the unique circumstances facing post-9/11–era Veterans and their vulnerabilities to homelessness. We have found that more systematic examinations of these associations often produce a more mixed and nuanced picture and that there are numerous and substantial gaps in research that hamper making clear conclusions about the nature of these associations. For all the attention and concern that homelessness among post-9/11–era Veterans has generated, it remains a poorly understood phenomenon.

Judging from the available evidence, homelessness among post-9/11 Veterans occurs on a magnitude comparable to other Veteran cohorts, and popular notions of why these Veterans become homeless, while often overstated, should not be discarded. For example, PTSD does not appear to be a primary driver of homelessness among this cohort as is widely believed, but homelessness is more difficult and prolonged for many post-9/11 Veterans because of PTSD and other combat sequelae.[44,45] In another example, onset of homelessness among most post-9/11 Veterans who experience homelessness appears to occur after transitioning back to civilian life, but the precursors to this homelessness likely emerge much sooner after separating from military service.

The advocacy group IAVA lists addressing homelessness as one of their 11 top policy priorities. Many of their specific recommendations apply more generally to homelessness among all Veterans.[27] Likewise, many of the elements we identified as key to the post-9/11 Veteran homelessness narrative, such as gender, psychological distress and disorder, and money management, extend beyond this cohort and are covered in their own right in other chapters in this book. Conversely, the Veteran-specific housing and homeless services initiatives that were launched and expanded in the previous decade have likely mitigated the rise in homelessness among this cohort because they have contributed to the dramatic decline in overall Veteran homelessness. As we turn to outstanding concerns related more specifically to this cohort, this broader accomplishment should not be overlooked.

One cohort-specific concern, also mentioned in IAVA's policy agenda, are for services that better accommodate the needs of Veterans who are homeless with children. Most Veteran families who experience homelessness are headed by single women of childbearing age, virtually guaranteeing that they will have served in the post-9/11 era. Providing homeless services to Veteran families represents unfamiliar terrain for the VA and other Veteran service providers because homeless Veterans in previous cohorts have been almost exclusively single men. In a broader context, it also challenges the VA in its more general efforts to provide a more gender-inclusive environment. In the absence of this, Veteran-headed families will be more likely to seek services through non-Veteran providers, a process that will deprive Veteran families of Veteran-specific assistance and can foster an alienation associated with their Veteran identities.

Another concern involves OTH discharges. OTH discharges and corresponding VA ineligibility occur disproportionately among post-9/11–era Veterans and are associated with high risk for becoming homeless.[37,76] Ironically, many of these Veterans are in particular need of the services that are unavailable to them. As the overall homeless Veteran population decreases, Veterans with OTH discharges will likely be more overrepresented among those who remain homeless. Some policy gains have been made recently toward giving Veterans with OTH discharges increased opportunities to upgrade discharges and access services, especially when the OTH discharge co-occurs with service-connected medical or mental health issues.[27,121] Further steps toward normalizing the Veteran status of this group likely also would reduce the homelessness risk among more than 125,000 post-9/11 Veterans with such discharges.

A third area concern involves transition. Currently and for the foreseeable future, all transitioning Veterans join the post-9/11 cohort on separation from the military, and only this cohort receives new ranks. While the onset of homelessness appears to most often occur well after transitioning out of the

military, the trajectory to homelessness, including issues such as financial stability, family support, and behavioral health issues, often appears in the transition period.[84] Focusing on such issues in a more prevention-oriented approach,
rather than focusing directly on imminent homelessness, may thus more effectively ward off homelessness over the long term. Furthermore, the fixed
number of new Veterans and the distinct process by which they leave the military makes initiating prevention initiatives more feasible. Here, separating
military personnel could receive assessments and briefings related to housing,
with DoD and VA administrative records, along with recent advances in predictive modeling techniques, providing a promising foundation for identifying
vulnerable Veterans. At-risk Veterans can then receive ongoing, largely passive
monitoring, with service interventions occurring at a point before housing instability becomes outright homelessness. Such a model, in better identifying
and addressing immediate transition-related issues, could thereby head off both
imminent and more distal threats of homelessness.

Finally, we offer some prognostication on the future based on trends
identified in the past three decades of contemporary homelessness. Figure 9.1
shows changes in the age distribution of Veterans served by VA homelessness
services over time. It shows a distinct cohort effect among the homeless Veteran
population, with the largest numbers of homeless Veterans belonging to the
post-Vietnam-era cohort[41] and experiencing similar socioeconomic dislocations
to their non-Veteran counterparts in this birth cohort.[122] While this figure
indicates that Veteran homelessness still primarily affects older Veterans, the

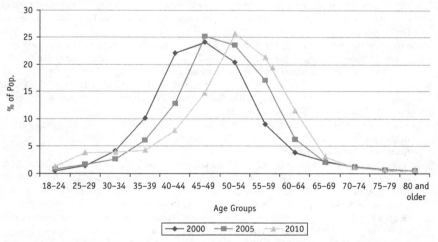

*Figure 9.1* Progressive age distribution for homeless Veterans served by U.S.
Department of Veterans Affairs programs.  Source: Unduplicated count of all Veterans
who completed Form X (an intake form for those receiving services from the VA's Health
Care for Homeless Veterans Program) in each year from 2000 to 2010.

2010 curve shows a small bump that represents the post-9/11 Veteran cohort. Were this bump to grow, it would form the kernel of a next generation of Veteran homelessness. It also underscores how Veterans from past eras have become homeless throughout their life course, and unless circumstances surrounding Veteran homelessness change, the trajectory of homelessness among post-9/11 Veterans is poised to increase along the lines seen in previous cohorts.

As such, this chapter, like the post-9/11 cohort itself, remains open-ended. In two years, the Afghanistan war will have spanned the entire lifetime of the military's youngest recruits, and right now some children are likely already serving in the same wars in which their parents served. As this cohort continues to grow and mortality continues to shrink an increasingly aging Veteran population, the post-9/11–era Veterans will simultaneously become more monolithic and variegated. Those who served in the earlier years of the era, who represent the bulk of those who are currently homeless in this cohort, will have very different experiences than the Veterans who will continue to join this cohort for the indefinite future. This will further enhance the challenges related to accurately portraying homelessness of Veterans from this era and to providing an evidentiary basis for efficient and effective responses to the problem into the future.

# References

1. Scotti M. Back from Iraq war, and alone. *CNN.com*. March 10, 2010. http://www.cnn.com/2010/OPINION/03/10/scotti.war.veterans/index.html. Accessed December 27, 2017.
2. US Interagency Council on Homelessness. *Opening doors: Federal strategic plan to prevent and end homelessness*. http://dev2.usich.gov/opening-doors. Published June 2015. Accessed December 27, 2017.
3. Disabled American Veterans. *Proceedings of Disabled American Veterans 2016 Convention*. https://www.dav.org/wp-content/uploads/2016_Convention_Proceedings.pdf. Published October 13, 2016. Accessed December 27, 2017.
4. Pew Research Center. *The military-civilian gap: War and sacrifice in the post-9/11 era*. http://www.pewsocialtrends.org/2011/10/05/war-and-sacrifice-in-the-post-911-era/. Published October 5, 2011. Accessed December 27, 2017.
5. Samet E. War, guilt and "thank you for your service." *Washington Monthly*. August 2, 2011. http://washingtonmonthly.com/2011/08/02/war-guilt-and-thank-you-for-your-service/ Accessed December 27, 2017.
6. Eckholm E. Surge seen in number of homeless veterans. *New York Times*. November 8, 2007. www.nytimes.com/2007/11/08/us/08vets.html. Accessed December 27, 2017.
7. Fairweather A. *Risk and protective factors for homelessness among OEF/OIF veterans*. San Francisco, CA: Swords to Plowshares Iraq Veteran Project; 2006.
8. Williamson V, Mulhall E. *Coming home: The housing crisis and homelessness threaten new veterans*. Iraq and Afghanistan Veterans of America. https://issuu.com/iava/docs/coming_home_2009. Published January 2009. Accessed December 27, 2017.
9. Zoroya G. Up to 48,000 Afghan, Iraq vets at risk for homelessness. *USA Today*. January 16, 2014. https://www.usatoday.com/story/news/nation/2014/01/16/veterans-homeless-afghanistan-iraq-wars/4526343/. Accessed December 27, 2017.

10. Schuetz A. The homecomer. *Am J Sociol.*1945;50(5):369–376. doi: 10.1086/219654.

11. Ahern J, Worthen M, Masters J, Lippman SA, Ozer EJ, Moos R. The challenges of Afghanistan and Iraq veterans' transition from military to civilian life and approaches to reconnection. *Plos ONE.* 2015;10(7):e0128599. doi:10.1371/journal.pone.0128599

12. Balshem H, Christensen V, Tuepker A, Kansagara D. *A critical review of the literature regarding homelessness among veterans.* VA-ESP Project #05-225. https://www.hsrd.research.va.gov/publications/esp/homelessness.cfm. Published April, 2011. Accessed December 27, 2017.

13. McGuire J. Closing a front door to homelessness among veterans. *J Prim Prev.* 2007;28:389–400. doi:10.1007/s10935-007-0091-y

14. Montgomery AE, Cutuli JJ, Evans-Chase M, Treglia D, Culhane DP. Relationship among adverse childhood experiences, history of active military service, and adult outcomes: Homelessness, mental health, and physical health. *Am J Public Health.* 2013;103(S2):S262–S268.

15. Perl L. *Veterans and homelessness.* Congressional Research Service. https://fas.org/sgp/crs/misc/RL34024.pdf. Published November 6, 2015. Accessed December 27, 2017.

16. Tsai J, Rosenheck RA. Risk factors for Homelessness Among US Veterans. *Epidemiol Rev.* 2015;37:177–195. doi:10.1093/epirev/mxu004.

17. FAQ About Homeless Veterans. National Coalition for Homeless Veterans website. http://nchv.org/index.php/news/media/background_and_statistics/. Accessed December 27, 2017.

18. D'Angelis T. More PTSD among homeless vets. *Monitor Psychol.* 2013;44(3):22. http://www.apa.org/monitor/2013/03/ptsd-vets.aspx. Accessed December 27, 2017.

19. Lee SJ. Speech in support of "Homes for Heroes Act." *Congressional Record,* Extension of Remarks. May 16, 2013. E675. https://www.congress.gov/crec/2013/05/16/CREC-2013-05-16-pt1-PgE675-4.pdf. Accessed December 27, 2017.

20. US Department of Housing and Urban Development, Office of Community Planning and Development and US Department of Veterans Affairs, National Center for Homelessness Among Veterans. *Veteran homelessness: A supplemental report to the 2010 Annual Homeless Assessment Report to Congress.* Washington DC: Authors; 2011. Available at: https://www.va.gov/HOMELESS/docs/2010AHARVeteransReport.pdf. Accessed December 27, 2017.

21. Culhane DP, Dejowski EF, Ibanez J, Needham E, Macchia I. Public shelter admission rates in Philadelphia and New York City: The implications of turnover for sheltered population counts. *Hous Policy Debate.* 1994;5(2):107–140. doi:10.1080/10511482.1994.9521155.

22. Culhane D, Metraux S. One-year rates of public shelter utilization by race/ethnicity, age, sex and poverty status for New York City (1990 and 1995) and Philadelphia (1995). *Popul Res Policy Rev.* 1999;18(3):219–236. doi: 10.1023/A:1006187611323.

23. Solari CD, Morris S, Shivji A, de Souza T. *The 2015 Annual Homeless Assessment Report (AHAR) to Congress.* The US Department of Housing and Urban Development, Office of Community Planning and Development. https://www.hudexchange.info/onecpd/assets/File/2015-AHAR-Part-2.pdf. Published October 2016. Accessed December 27, 2017.

24. US Department of Veterans Affairs, Office of Public Health. *VA health care utilization by recent veterans.* http://www.publichealth.va.gov/epidemiology/reports/oefoifond/health-care-utilization/index.asp. Published January 2017. Accessed December 27, 2017.

25. Metraux S, Clegg LX, Daigh JD, Culhane DP, Kane V. Risk factors for becoming homeless among a cohort of veterans who served in the era of the Iraq and Afghanistan conflicts. *Am J Public Health.* 2013;103(S2):S255–S261. doi: 10.2105/AJPH.2013.301432.

26. Henry M, Watt R, Rosenthal L, Shivji A. *The 2017 Annual Homeless Assessment Report (AHAR) to Congress.* The US Department of Housing and Urban Development, Office of Community Planning and Development. https://www.hudexchange.info/resources/documents/2017-AHAR-Part-1.pdf. Published December 2017. Accessed December 27, 2017.

27. Iraq and Afghanistan Veterans of America. *Policy agenda: Fulfill the promise.* https://iava.org/wp-content/uploads/2017/03/IAVA_Policy_2017_v8_125bleed.pdf. Published March 21, 2017. Accessed on December 27, 2017.

28. Vogel S. Donovan, Shinseki hit D.C. streets for national homeless count. *Washington Post*. February 1, 2013. https://www.washingtonpost.com/politics/donovan-shinseki-hit-dc-streets-for-national-homeless-count/2013/02/01/4c28c6e4-6c8f-11e2-bd36-c0fe61a205f6_story.html. Accessed December 27, 2017.

29. US Department of Veterans Affairs Office of the Inspector General. *Incidence of Homelessness among Veterans and Risk Factors for Becoming Homeless in Veterans*. https://www.va.gov/oig/pubs/VAOIG-11-03428-173.pdf. Published May 4, 2012. Accessed December 27, 2017.

30. Edens EL, Kasprow W, Tsai J, Rosenheck RA. Association of substance use and VA service-connected disability benefits with risk of homelessness among veterans: Substance use, VA disability and homelessness risk. *Am J Addict*. 2011;20(5):412–419. doi:10.1111/j.1521-0391.2011.00166.x.

31. Tsai J, Link B, Rosenheck RA, Pietrzak RH. Homelessness among a nationally representative sample of US veterans: Prevalence, service utilization, and correlates. *Soc Psychiatry Psychiatr Epidemiol*. 2016;51(6):907–916. doi:10.1007/s00127-016-1210-y.

32. Pietrzak RH, Cook JM. Psychological resilience in older US Veterans: Results from the National Health and Resilience in Veterans study. *Depress Anxiety*. 2013;30(5):432–443. doi:10.1002/da.22083.

33. Elbogen EB, Sullivan CP, Wolfe J, Wagner HR, Beckham JC. Homelessness and money mismanagement in Iraq and Afghanistan veterans. *Am J Public Health*. 2013;103(S2):S248–S254. doi: 10.2105/AJPH.2013.301335.

34. Blackstock OJ, Haskell SG, Brandt CA, Desai RA. Gender and the use of Veterans Health Administration homeless services programs among Iraq/Afghanistan veterans. *Med Care*. 2012;50(4):347–352. doi: 10.1097/MLR.0b013e318245a738.

35. Brignone E, Fargo JD, Blais RK, Carter ME, Samore MH, Gundlapalli AV. Non-routine discharge from military service: Mental illness, substance use disorders, and suicidality. *Am J Prev Med*. 2017;52(5):557–565. doi:10.1016/j.amepre.2016.11.015.

36. Fargo JD, Brignone E, Metraux S, et al. Homelessness following disability-related discharges from active duty military service in Afghanistan and Iraq. *Disabil Health J*. 2017;10(4):592–599. doi: 10.1016/j.dhjo.2017.03.003.

37. Gundlapalli AV, Fargo JD, Metraux S, et al. Military misconduct and Homelessness Among US Veterans separated from active duty, 2001–2012. *JAMA*. 2015;314(8):832–834. doi: 10.1001/jama.2015.8207.

38. Smith RT, True G. Warring identities: Identity conflict and the mental distress of American veterans of the wars in Iraq and Afghanistan. *Soc Ment Health*. 2014;4(2):147–161. doi:10.1177/2156869313512212.

39. Sundin J, Fear NT, Iversen A, Rona RJ, Wessely S. PTSD after deployment to Iraq: Conflicting rates, conflicting claims. *Psychol Med*. 2010;40(03):367. doi:10.1017/S0033291709990791.

40. Rosenheck RA, Leda C, Frisman LK, Lam J, Chung A. Homeless veterans. In: Baumohl J, ed. *Homelessness in America: A reference book* (pp. 97–108). Phoenix, AZ: Oryx Press; 1996.

41. Rosenheck RA, Fontana A. A model of homelessness among male veterans of the Vietnam War generation. *Am J Psychiatr*. 1994;151(3):421–427. doi:10.1176/ajp.151.3.421.

42. Tanelian T, Jaycox LH, eds. *Invisible wounds of war: Psychological and cognitive injuries, their consequences, and services to assist recovery*. Santa Monica, CA: Rand Corporation; 2008.

43. Murdoch M, Sayer NA, Spoont MR, et al. Long-term outcomes of disability benefits in US veterans with posttraumatic stress disorder. *Arch Gen Psychiatr*. 2011;68(10):1072–1080. doi:10.1001/archgenpsychiatry.2011.105.

44. Tsai J, Pietrzak RH, Rosenheck RA. Homeless veterans who served in Iraq and Afghanistan: Gender differences, combat exposure, and comparisons with previous cohorts of homeless veterans. *Adm Policy Ment Health*. 2013;40(5):400–405. doi:10.1007/s10488-012-0431-y.

45. Metraux S, Cusack M, Byrne TH, Hunt-Johnson N, True G. Pathways into homelessness among post-9/11-era veterans. *Psychol Serv*. 2017;14(2):229–237. doi:10.1037/ser0000136.

46. Barnes SM, Russell LM, Hostetter TA, Forster JE, Devore MD, Brenner LA. Characteristics of traumatic brain injuries sustained among veterans seeking homeless services. *J Health Care Poor U*. 2015;26(1):92–105. doi:10.1353/hpu.2015.0010.

47. Russell LM, Devore MD, Barnes SM, et al. Challenges associated with screening for traumatic brain injury among US veterans seeking homeless services. *Am J Public Health*. 2013;103(S2):S211:212. doi: 10.2105/AJPH.2013.301485

48. Brown PL. Honor betrayed: Trauma sets female veterans adrift back home. *New York Times*. February 28, 2013. http://www.nytimes.com/2013/02/28/us/female-veterans-face-limbo-in-lives-on-the-street.html. Accessed December 27, 2017.

49. Casura L. Homeless women veterans are veterans with an important difference. *Huffington Post*. May 16, 2017. https://www.huffingtonpost.com/entry/homeless-women-veterans-are-veterans-with-an-important_us_591a8d3ae4b03e1c81b00880. Accessed December 27, 2017.

50. Byrne T, Montgomery AE, Dichter ME. Homelessness among female veterans: A systematic review of the literature. *Women Health*. 2013;53(6):572–596. doi:10.1080/03630242.2013.817504.

51. Fargo J, Metraux S, Byrne T, et al. Prevalence and risk of Homelessness Among US Veterans. *Prev Chronic Dis*. 2012;9(1):110–112. doi:10.5888/pcd9.110112.

52. US Department of Veterans Affairs, National Center for Veterans Analysis and Statistics. *Profile of women veterans: 2014*. https://www.va.gov/vetdata/docs/SpecialReports/Women_Veterans_2014.pdf. Published March 2016. Accessed December 27, 2017.

53. Pavao J, Turchik JA, Hyun JK, et al. Military sexual trauma among homeless veterans. *J Gen Intern Med*. 2013;28(S2):536–541. doi:10.1007/s11606-013-2341-4.

54. Rosenheck RA. Risk factors for homelessness: VA patients and those who served in OIF/OEF. Paper presented at SAMHSA's Expert Panel on Homeless Veterans of Operations Enduring Freedom, Iraqi Freedom, and New Dawn. August 18, 2011. Washington DC. https://www.usich.gov/resources/uploads/asset_library/RPT_SAMHSA_Veterans_Expert_Panel_report_04_13_FINAL.pdf. Accessed December 27, 2017.

55. US Government Accountability Office. *Homeless women veterans: Actions needed to ensure safe and appropriate housing* (GAO-12-182). https://www.gao.gov/products/GAO-12-182. Published December 23, 2011. Accessed December 27, 2017.

56. Tsai J, Rosenheck RA, Kasprow WJ, Kane V. Characteristics and use of services among literally homeless and unstably housed US veterans with custody of minor children. *Psychiatr Serv*. 2015;66(10):1083–1090. doi:10.1176/appi.ps.201400300.

57. Wilson LC. The prevalence of military sexual trauma: A meta-analysis. *Trauma Violence Abuse*. December 2016:152483801668345. doi:10.1177/1524838016683459.

58. Benda BB. Survival analysis of social support and trauma among homeless male and female veterans who abuse substances. *Am J Orthopsychiatr* 2006;76(1):70–79. doi: 10.1037/0002-9432.76.1.70

59. Brignone E, Gundlapalli AV, Blais RK, et al. Differential risk for homelessness among US male and female veterans with a positive screen for military sexual trauma. *JAMA Psychiatr*. 2016;73(6):582. doi:10.1001/jamapsychiatry.2016.0101.

60. Hamilton AB, Poza I, Washington DL. "Homelessness and trauma go hand-in-hand": Pathways to homelessness among women veterans. *Womens Health Issues*. 2011;21(4):S203–S209. doi:10.1016/j.whi.2011.04.005.

61. Washington DL, Yano EM, McGuire J, Hines V, Lee M, Gelberg L. Risk factors for homelessness among women veterans. *J Health Care Poor U*. 2010;21(1):82–91. doi: 10.1353/hpu.0.0237.

62. Spitzer KA. Alone at home: Post-9/11 *Military Veterans and American Housing and Homelessness Policy*. (PhD dissertation). Massachusetts Institute of Technology; 2016. http://hdl.handle.net/1721.1/107083. Accessed December 27, 2017.

63. Street AE, Vogt D, Dutra L. A new generation of women veterans: Stressors faced by women deployed to Iraq and Afghanistan. *Clin Psychol Rev*. 2009;29(8):685–694. doi:10.1016/j.cpr.2009.08.007.

64. Rosenheck R, Frisman L, Chung AM. The proportion of veterans among homeless men. *Am J Public Health*. 1994;84(3):466–469. doi: 10.2105/AJPH.84.3.466.

65. Korb LJ, Duggan SE. An all-volunteer army? Recruitment and its problems. *Polit Sci Politics*. 2007;40(3):467–471. doi: 10.1017/S1049096507070953.

66. Kurtz A. Getting into the military is getting tougher. *CNN Money*. May 15, 2013. http://money.cnn.com/2013/05/15/news/economy/military-recruiting/. Accessed December 27, 2017.

67. Kane T. *Who are the recruits? The demographic characteristics of US military enlistment, 2003–2005*. Heritage Foundation. http://www.heritage.org/defense/report/who-are-the-recruits-the-demographic-characteristics-us-military-enlistment-2003. Published October 27, 2006. Accessed December 27, 2017.

68. Gallaway MS, Bell MR, Lagana-Riordan C, Fink DS, Meyer CE, Millikan AM. The association between US Army enlistment waivers and subsequent behavioral and social health outcomes and attrition from service. *Mil Med*. 2013;178(3):261–266. doi:10.7205/MILMED-D-12-00316.

69. Horton JL, Phillips CJ, White MR, LeardMann CA, Crum-Cianflone NF. Trends in new US Marine Corps accessions during the recent conflicts in Iraq and Afghanistan. *Mil Med*. 2014;179(1):62–70. doi:10.7205/MILMED-D-13-00329.

70. Institute of Medicine. *Returning home from Iraq and Afghanistan: Preliminary assessment of readjustment needs of veterans, service members, and their families*. http://nationalacademies.org/hmd/Reports/2013/Returning-Home-from-Iraq-and-Afghanistan.aspx. Published March 26, 2013. Accessed December 27, 2017.

71. Sayer NA, Carlson KF, Frazier PA. Reintegration challenges in US service members and veterans following combat deployment. *Soc Iss Policy Rev*. 2014;8:33–73. doi:10.1111/sipr.12001

72. Phillips D. Other than honorable. *The Gazette*. May 20, 2013. http://cdn.csgazette.biz/soldiers/. Accessed December 27, 2017.

73. Veterans Legal Clinic. *Underserved: How the VA wrongfully excludes veterans with bad paper*. https://www.swords-to-plowshares.org/2016/03/30/underserved/. Published March 10.1177/1536504213487702. 30, 2016. Accessed December 27, 2017.

74. US Government Accountability Office. *DOD health: Actions needed to ensure post-traumatic stress disorder and traumatic brain injury are considered in misconduct separations* (GAO-17-260). https://www.gao.gov/products/GAO-17-260. Published May 16, 2017. Accessed December 27, 2017.

75. Brooks-Holliday S, Pedersen ER. The association between discharge status, mental health, and substance misuse among young adult veterans. *Psychiatr Res*. 2017;256:428–434. doi:10.1016/j.psychres.2017.07.011.

76. Seamone ER, McGuire J, Sreenivasan S, Clark S, Smee D, Dow D. Moving upstream: Why rehabilitative justice in military discharge proceedings serves a public health interest. *Am J Public Health*. 2014;104(10):1805–1811. doi: 10.2105/AJPH.2014.302117.

77. Ismay J. "Bad paper" discharge can lead to homelessness, hopelessness. *WBEZ*. March 24, 2016. https://www.wbez.org/shows/american-homefront/bad-paper-discharge-can-lead-to-homelessness-hopelessness/a3670c26-15a1-4cce-bd15-56ae1815d3e5. Accessed December 18, 2017.

78. Wilder Research. *Homelessness in Minnesota: Findings from the 2015 Minnesota Homeless Study*. St. Paul MN: Wilder Foundation; 2016.

79. Sussman A. Iraq and Afghanistan war veterans join the homeless. *San Francisco Chronicle*. November 11, 2008. http://www.sfgate.com/opinion/article/Iraq-and-Afghanistan-war-veterans-join-the-3185473.php. Accessed December 27, 2017.

80. Robertson MJ. Homeless veterans: An emerging problem? In: *The homeless in contemporary society* (pp. 64–81). Newberry Park CA: Sage; 1987.

81. Fallows J. The tragedy of the American military. *Atlantic Monthly*. January 2015. https://www.theatlantic.com/magazine/archive/2015/01/the-tragedy-of-the-american-military/383516/. Accessed December 27, 2017.

82. Gomez D. The other side of the millennials in the military debate. *Task Purpose.* February 22, 2016. http://taskandpurpose.com/the-other-side-of-the-millennials-in-the-military-debate/. Accessed December 27, 2017.

83. Schafer A. The warrior caste. *Slate.* August 2, 2017. http://www.slate.com/articles/news_and_politics/politics/2017/08/the_warrior_caste_of_military_families_that_fight_america_s_wars.html. Accessed December 27, 2017.

84. Sherman MD, Larsen J, Borden LM. Broadening the focus in supporting reintegrating Iraq and Afghanistan veterans: Six key domains of functioning. *Prof Psychol-Res Pr.* 2015;46(5):355–365. doi:10.1037/pro0000043.

85. Bureau of Labor Statistics. *Employment Situation of Veterans—2013.* https://www.bls.gov/news.release/archives/vet_03202014.pdf. Published March 20, 2014. Accessed December 27, 2017.

86. Loughran DS. *Why is veteran unemployment so high?* https://www.rand.org/pubs/research_reports/RR284.html. Published June 25, 2014. Accessed December 27, 2017.

87. Kleykamp M. Unemployment, earnings and enrollment among post 9/11 veterans. *Soc Sci Res.* 2013;42(3):836–851. doi: 10.1016/j.ssresearch.2012.12.017.

88. Bureau of Labor Statistics. Employment situation of veterans—2016. https://www.bls.gov/news.release/pdf/vet.pdf. Published March 22, 2017. Accessed December 27, 2017.

89. Kintzle S, Keeling M, Xintarianos E, Taylor-Diggs K, Munch C, Hassan AM, Castro CA. Exploring the economic and employment challenges facing US Veterans: A qualitative study of volunteers of America service providers and veteran clients. https://www.voa.org/vets-study. Published May 2015. Accessed December 27, 2017.

90. Aurand A, Emmanuel D, Yentel D, Errico E, Pang M. *Out of reach: The high cost of housing. 2017.* Washington DC: National Low Income Housing Coalition; 2017. http://nlihc.org/sites/default/files/oor/OOR_2017.pdf. Released June 8, 2017. Accessed December 27, 2017.

91. Galvez M, Brennan M, Meixell B, Pendall R. *Housing as a safety net: Ensuring housing security for the most vulnerable. 2017.* Washington DC: Urban Institute. https://www.urban.org/sites/default/files/publication/93611/housing-as-a-safety-net_1.pdf. Accessed December 27, 2017.

92. Guddell S. *The US housing affordability crisis: How a rent and low-income problem is becoming everyone's problem.* Seattle, WA: Zillow Inc; 2016. https://www.zillow.com/research/housing-affordability-q4-2015-12111/. Accessed December 27, 2017.

93. Arnold A, Bolton M, Crowley S. *Housing instability among our nation's veterans.* Washington DC: National Low Income Housing Coalition; 2013. http://nlihc.org/sites/default/files/NLIHC-Veteran-Report-2013.pdf. Released November 12, 2013. Accessed December 27, 2017.

94. US Department of Veterans Affairs, Office of Suicide Prevention. *Suicide among veterans and other Americans: 2001–2014.* https://www.mentalhealth.va.gov/docs/2016suicidedatareport.pdf. Released August 3, 2016. Accessed December 27, 2017.

95. Keteyian A. (2007). The veteran suicide "epidemic." *CBS News.* November 13, 2007. https://www.cbsnews.com/news/the-veteran-suicide-epidemic/. Accessed December 27, 2017.

96. Pilkington E. US military struggling to stop suicide epidemic among war veterans. *The Guardian.* February 1, 2013. https://www.theguardian.com/world/2013/feb/01/us-military-suicide-epidemic-veteran. Accessed December 27, 2017.

97. Kang HK, Bullman TA, Smolenski DJ, Skopp NA, Gahm GA, Reger MA. Suicide risk among 1.3 million veterans who were on active duty during the Iraq and Afghanistan wars. *Ann Epidemiol.* 2015;25(2):96–100. doi:10.1016/j.annepidem.2014.11.020

98. Bullman T, Schneiderman A, Bossarte R. Suicide risk by unit component among veterans who served in Iraq or Afghanistan. *Arch Suicide Res.* March 2017:1–10. doi:10.1080/13811118.2017.1304308.

99. Elbogen EB, Wagner HR, Kimbrel NA, et al. Risk factors for concurrent suicidal ideation and violent impulses in military veterans. *Psychol Assess.* 2018;30(4):425–435. doi:10.1037/pas0000490.

100. Logan J, Bohnert A, Spies E, Jannausch M. Suicidal ideation among young Afghanistan/Iraq War Veterans and civilians: Individual, social, and environmental risk factors and perception of unmet mental healthcare needs, United States, 2013. *Psychiatr Res.* 2016;245:398–405. doi:10.1016/j.psychres.2016.08.054.

101. Hoffberg AS, Spitzer E, Mackelprang JL, Farro SA, Brenner LA. Suicidal self-directed violence among homeless US veterans: A systematic review. *Suicide Life-Threat.* July 2017. doi:10.1111/sltb.12369.

102. McCarthy JF, Bossarte RM, Katz IR, Thompson C, Kemp J, Hannemann CM, Nielson C, Schoenbaum M. Predictive modeling and concentration of the risk of suicide: Implications for preventive interventions in the US Department of Veterans Affairs. *Am J Public Health.* 2015 Sep;105(9):1935–1942. doi: 10.2105/AJPH.2015.302737.

103. Montgomery AE, Dichter ME, Thomasson AM, Roberts CB, Byrne T. Disparities in housing status among veterans with general medical, cognitive, and behavioral health conditions. *Psychiatr Serv.* 2015;66(3):317–320. doi: 10.1176/appi.ps.201400014.

104. Schinka JA, Schinka KC, Casey RJ, Kasprow W, Bossarte RM. Suicidal behavior in a national sample of older homeless veterans. *Am J Public Health.* 2012;102(S1):147–S153. doi: 10.2105/AJPH.2011.300436.

105. Tsai, J., Trevisan, L., Huang, M., & Pietrzak, R. H. (in press). Addressing veteran homelessness to prevent veteran suicides. *Psychiatric Services.* https://doi.org/10.1176/appi.ps.201700482

106. Bagalman E. *Health Care for Veterans: Suicide Prevention.* Congressional Research Service. https://fas.org/sgp/crs/misc/R42340.pdf. Published February 23, 2016. Accessed December 27, 2017.

107. Childress S. Veterans face greater risks amid opioid crisis. *PBS.* March 28, 2016. https://www.pbs.org/wgbh/frontline/article/veterans-face-greater-risks-amid-opioid-crisis. Accessed December 27, 2017.

108. Goldberg B. Opioid abuse crisis takes heavy toll on US veterans. *Reuters.* November 10, 2017. https://www.reuters.com/article/us-usa-veterans-opioids/opioid-abuse-crisis-takes-heavy-toll-on-u-s-veterans-idUSKBN1DA1B2. Accessed December 27, 2017.

109. Hudson TJ, Painter JT, Martin BC, et al. Pharmacoepidemiologic analyses of opioid use among OEF/OIF/OND veterans. *Pain.* 2017;158(6):1039–1045. doi:10.1097/j.pain.0000000000000874.

110. Bennett AS, Elliott L, Golub A. Opioid and other substance misuse, overdose risk, and the potential for prevention among a sample of OEF/OIF veterans in New York City. *Subst Use Misuse.* 2013;48(10):894–907. doi:10.3109/10826084.2013.796991.

111. Dillon PA. Memo to employers: Veterans aren't PTSD basketcases; they're disciplined and committed. *Forbes.* September 29, 2014. https://www.forbes.com/sites/realspin/2014/09/29/memo-to-employers-veterans-arent-ptsd-basketcases-theyre-disciplined-and-committed/#77171bd07f60. Accessed December 27, 2017.

112. Zoroya G. Recent war vets face hiring obstacle: PTSD bias. *USA Today.* April 9, 2013. https://www.usatoday.com/story/news/nation/2013/04/06/recent-war-vets-face-hiring-obstacle-ptsd-bias/2057857/. Accessed December 27, 2017.

113. Lee MYH. The missing context behind the widely cited statistic that there are 22 veteran suicides a day. *Washington Post.* February 4, 2015. https://www.washingtonpost.com/news/fact-checker/wp/2015/02/04/the-missing-context-behind-a-widely-cited-statistic-that-there-are-22-veteran-suicides-a-day/. Accessed December 27, 2017.

114. Levine A. How the VA fueled the national opioid crisis and is killing thousands of veterans. *Newsweek.* October 12, 2017. http://www.newsweek.com/2017/10/20/va-fueled-opioid-crisis-killing-veterans-681552.html. Accessed December 27, 2017.

115. Kleykamp M, Hipes C. Coverage of veterans of the wars in Iraq and Afghanistan in the US media. *Sociol Forum.* 2015;30(2):348–368. doi:10.1111/socf.12166.

116. Stein JY. The veteran's loneliness: Emergence, facets and implications for intervention. In: Lázár R, ed. *Psychology of loneliness: New research.* (pp. 1–36). Hauppauge NY: Nova Science Publishers, 2017.

117. Estroff S. Medicalizing the margins: On being disgraced, disordered, and deserving. *Psychosoc Rehabil J.* 1985;8(4):34–38. doi:10.1037/h0099662.

118. Snow DA, Baker SG, Anderson L, Martin M. The myth of pervasive mental illness among the homeless. *Soc Probl.* 1986;33(5):407–423. doi: 10.2307/800659

119. Kleykamp M, Hipes C. Social programs for soldiers and veterans. Oxford Handbooks. In Béland D, Morgan KJ, Howard C. *Oxford handbook of US social policy* (pp. 565–584). New York, NY: Oxford University Press; 2014.

120. Cunningham M, Biess J, Emam D, Burt MR. *Veterans homelessness prevention demonstration evaluation: Final report.* https://www.huduser.gov/portal/publications/homeless/veterans-homelessness-prevention-report.html. Published December 10, 2015. Accessed December 27, 2017.

121. Wentling N. Pentagon expands policy to upgrade vets' bad paper discharges. *Stars Stripes.* August 29, 2017. https://www.stripes.com/news/pentagon-expands-policy-to-upgrade-vets-bad-paper-discharges-1.485038. Accessed December 27, 2017.

122. Culhane DP, Metraux S, Byrne T, Stino M, Bainbridge J. Aging trends in homeless populations. *Contexts.* 2013;12(2):66–68. doi: 10.1177/1536504213487702.

# 10

# Aging and Mortality in Homeless Veterans

JOHN A. SCHINKA AND THOMAS H. BYRNE

Time is but the stream I go a-fishing in. I drink at it; but while
I drink I see the sandy bottom and detect how shallow it is. Its
thin current slides away, but eternity remains.
—Henry David Thoreau, *Walden*

## Homelessness in Veterans

Homelessness has long been a public health issue in the U.S. Veteran population. Perl's[1] review of community surveys of Veteran homelessness showed that
Veterans have been overrepresented in homeless populations since the 1980s.
In the 2016 national survey of homelessness,[2] Veterans represented 9.2% of
all homeless adults compared with only 6.9% of the total U.S. population. The
survey's point-in-time calculations provided an estimate of the number of homeless Veterans at 39,471, with 26,404 in sheltered (temporary emergency or transitional housing) sites and 13,067 in unsheltered locations. Detailed estimates
revealed that homeless Veterans are predominantly male (91.1%) and that the
small majority are non-Hispanic Whites (52%). African American Veterans are
especially overrepresented (32.9%). Notably, older Veterans (51 years and older)
make up the majority of the homeless Veteran population. Chapter 2 discusses
these and other issues related to the epidemiology of homelessness among
Veterans in more detail.

A substantial literature documents that the causes and consequences of
homelessness are varied and complex. A valuable perspective on homelessness
was provided by Koegel,[3] who proposed that causes and consequences could
best be understood by considering both structural factors and individual limitations. From a structural standpoint, it is clear that reductions in the stock
of affordable housing, a mental health movement that released seriously mentally ill from institutional care into local communities, limited employment for

unskilled workers, and national economic crises over the past three decades have produced an environment that has contributed to homelessness. These factors continue to create the potential for homelessness; however, who becomes homeless is not determined randomly. Koegel noted that a vulnerability to homelessness based on individual limitations is an equally critical factor in determining those who actually become homeless. The key concept in summarizing these individual limitations is vulnerability, which is produced by a long list of distal factors, including childhood homelessness and trauma, poverty, marginal work history, low educational achievement, health conditions, psychiatric disorders, and substance abuse. Based on their collective and interactive status on these factors, individuals will vary in their degree of vulnerability to homelessness. At any given level of structural risk, those with greater vulnerability will be more likely to become, and stay, homeless when faced with a proximal cause such as divorce or a health crisis.

A cardinal element in understanding health outcomes for homeless Veterans is that vulnerability factors for homelessness are also potent factors for accelerated biological aging and early mortality. Chronological age is the primary risk factor for chronic diseases, including cardiovascular, malignant, and neurodegenerative conditions. Vulnerability factors associated with homelessness can accelerate the impact of chronological aging on age of onset, progression, and comorbidity for chronic diseases and may contribute to accelerated biological aging. Biological aging reflects a reduction in the reparative and regenerative potential in tissues and organs. The mechanisms underlying accelerated biological aging are complex,[4] but the critical message is that individuals of the same chronological age can exhibit differential trajectories of biological age-related decline and mortality risk based on cumulative vulnerability.

To date, no known study has attempted to incorporate both perspectives on homelessness identified by Koegel, either in the general U.S. homeless population or in homeless Veterans. However, research addressing the individual vulnerability perspective has examined the influence of potential risk factors on homelessness, particularly in the Veteran population. The most informative study was conducted by Rosenheck and Fontana,[5] who examined vulnerability to homelessness among Vietnam-era Veterans. They analyzed data from the Vietnam Veterans Readjustment Study, examining risk factors in various domains (e.g., race, age, history of psychiatric treatment). Structural equation modeling analyses revealed that psychiatric disorder as an adult, substance abuse, and social isolation had significant direct effects on risk for homelessness. Indirect and smaller effects were found for other variables (e.g., childhood conduct disorder on subsequent substance abuse, combat exposure on psychiatric disorder). Subsequent studies have reported additional evidence that social isolation, adverse childhood experiences, and past incarceration may elevate homelessness risk.[6,7] These studies shed some light on the prevalence of vulnerability risk factors that impact risk for homelessness and have been shown to be related to biological aging.

In the following sections, we examine characteristics of the aging homeless Veteran population and the impact of age and other vulnerability factors on the ultimate measure of biological aging—early mortality.

## Prevalence and Risk for Homelessness Among Older Veterans

In this section, we focus on providing context about aging in the Veteran homeless population. This context is necessary for informing policy and programmatic decisions, specifically with respect to the scope and type of services needed. On the largest scale, this requires understanding basic epidemiological questions about the prevalence and risk for homelessness among older Veterans. It also requires examining how aging trends in the Veteran homeless population might result in changes to the future size and composition of Veterans in need of homeless assistance. Thus, we begin by addressing these questions. We then shift to questions that are focused at a more micro level, specifically with regard to the characteristics and service needs of older Veterans experiencing homelessness. This is important from the perspective of tailoring existing interventions (and possibly designing and implementing new ones) for which older Veterans are most likely to benefit.

How many older Veterans experience homelessness? How common is homelessness among Veterans? Are older Veterans at an increased risk for homelessness relative to their non-Veteran counterparts? Answers to these fundamental epidemiological questions about the scope, prevalence, and risk for homelessness among older Veterans are essential for understanding the nature of the problem and ultimately for informing policy and programmatic responses. Yet, answers to what seem like straightforward questions are complicated by what is considered to be an "older" Veteran.

If in keeping with the traditional retirement age, one uses a threshold of age 65 years, then older Veterans appear to constitute only a minority of the population of homeless Veterans. The Annual Homeless Assessment Report (AHAR) to Congress provides information about the number of Veterans nationwide who use a residential homeless assistance program at some point over the course of a year, stratified by discrete age groups. In this report, the oldest age group is composed of Veterans aged 62 years, which is a reasonable proxy for retirement age, given that it is the youngest age at which individuals can claim Social Security retirements benefits. According to the most recent available AHAR data, Veterans 62 years[8] and older accounted for 14.5% (or roughly

19,000 Veterans) of all Veterans who used an emergency shelter or transitional housing program at some point during 2015. By contrast, Veterans 62 years and older accounted for 54.8% of the overall Veteran population in the United States in 2015, suggesting that Veterans in this age bracket are grossly underrepresented among the population of homeless Veterans. Combining the AHAR estimates with estimates of the size and age distribution of the Veteran population from the 2015 American Community Survey results in an estimated annual prevalence rate of shelter or transitional housing use of 0.18% (one in 550 Veterans) among Veterans 62 years and older. Importantly, prior research suggests that the prevalence rate of homelessness among the oldest segment of Veterans varies as a function of sex and race, with the highest rates of homelessness among Veterans 65 years and older found among African American males.[7] Research on whether older Veterans face an increased risk for homelessness relative to the non-Veteran population offers findings that are similarly mixed based on race and sex: males Veterans (both African Americans and non–African Americans) 65 years and older do not appear to face an elevated risk for homelessness compared with their non-Veteran counterparts, although both non–African American and especially African American female Veterans in this age bracket do face an elevated risk for homelessness compared with non-Veterans.[8]

In light of evidence that persons 50 years and older experiencing homelessness experience geriatric conditions at rates that are on par with persons in the general population who are 20 years older,[9,10] it is arguably more appropriate to apply a threshold of 50 or 55 years for identifying "older" Veterans experiencing homelessness. Indeed, persons 50 years and older experiencing homelessness tend to self-identify as "old," and the broader body of research on older homeless adults tends to define "older" in this manner. Using such a lower age cutoff results in a somewhat different understanding of the scope of homelessness among older Veterans: according to the AHAR, Veterans 51 years and older accounted for 58% of all Veterans who used emergency shelter in 2015 (roughly 77,000 Veterans). Moreover, Veterans in the 51- to 61-year-old bracket appear to be highly overrepresented in the homeless Veteran population; they accounted for 43% of Veterans who used shelter in 2015 (roughly 57,500 Veterans) but only 18% of the overall U.S. Veteran population. Combining these AHAR estimates again with estimates of the overall Veteran population from the American Community Survey results in an estimated prevalence of sheltered homelessness among Veterans 51 years and older of 0.55% (or roughly one in 180 Veterans). Evidence also points to a higher risk for homelessness among Veterans in this approximate age range. Fargo and colleagues found that Veterans in the 55- to 64-year-old bracket all faced an elevated risk for homelessness relative to their non-Veteran counterparts, regardless of sex or race.

Regardless of whether one uses a relatively higher or lower age threshold to define "older," one important fact to emerge from national data is that the homeless Veteran population is aging. Indeed, as Figure 10.1 shows, older Veterans appear to represent an increasing share of homeless Veterans: in 2009, those 51 years and older made up about 47% of all Veterans who used emergency shelter over the course of a year, and Veterans 62 years and older made up about 8.7% of this total. However, by 2015 Veterans 51 years and older represented nearly three out of every five Veterans (57.8%) using emergency shelters, and those 62 years and older alone accounted for 14.5% of the total.

This trend means that while the overall number of Veterans experiencing homelessness appears to have gone down substantially since 2009, the number of older Veterans experiencing homelessness has actually increased. Indeed, applying the estimated proportion of Veterans 62 years and older to the annual AHAR estimates, it appears that the number of Veterans 62 years and older using shelter on an annual basis increased by 47% from roughly 13,000 to roughly 19,000. Importantly, this aging trend in the Veteran homeless population is distinct from that seen in the overall Veteran population. Specifically, data from the American Community Survey indicate that the number of Veterans 62 years and older in the general population declined by about 5% from 10.9 million to

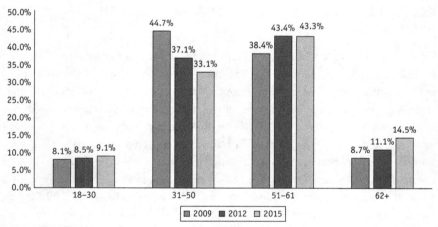

*Figure 10.1* Age distribution of the national population of Veterans using emergency shelter on an annual basis in 2009, 2012, and 2015. Source: 2012 Annual Homeless Assessment Report to Congress, Volume II and the 2015 Annual Homeless Assessment Report to Congress, Part 2. US Department of Housing and Urban Development. (2013). *The 2012 Annual Homeless Assessment Report (AHAR) to Congress: Volume II: Estimates of Homelessness in the United States.* https://www. hudexchange.info/resources/documents/2012-AHAR-Volume-2.pdf. US Department of Housing and Urban Development. (2016). *The 2015 Annual Homeless Assessment Report (AHAR) to Congress: Part 2: Estimates of Homelessness in the United States.* Retrieved from Washington, DC. https://www.hudexchange.info/onecpd/assets/File/ 2015-AHAR-Part-2.pdf

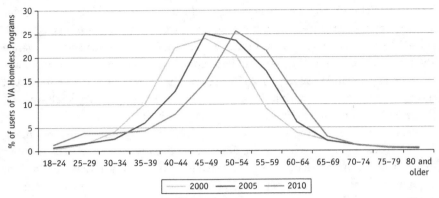

*Figure 10.2* Age distribution of users of VA specialized homeless programs, 2000–2010. Data sources: Author Tabulations of Health Care for Homeless Veterans Program Intake Assessments obtained from VA Form X in years 2000, 2005, and 2010.

10.4 million between 2009 and 2015. In the next section of this chapter, we expand on this trend, its origins, and its implications.

## AGE COHORT EFFECTS IN THE HOMELESS VETERAN POPULATION

The aging trend in the homeless Veteran population and the pattern of risk for homelessness among Veterans by age need to be understood in the context of evidence of a cohort effect in the population of Veterans experiencing homelessness, wherein those who served in the immediate post-Vietnam era (in the period after the implementation of the All-Volunteer Force in 1973) have consistently been at the greatest risk for homelessness. This cohort effect was first identified in data that are now more than 30 years old when Veterans in this age cohort (who were between the ages of 20 and 34 years at the time) were found to be at the highest risk for homelessness.[11] A study conducted in 1996 found the same age cohort (then 35–44 years) to be at the greatest risk for homelessness relative to non-Veterans,[12] and this cohort was again at the greatest risk for homelessness in a study using data from 2008 when they were in the 45- to 54-year-old bracket.[8]

It is this cohort effect that is responsible for the aging trend illustrated in Figure 10.1; persons in this cohort are now roughly aged 55 to 64 years and are thus shifting the age distribution of the shelter homeless population to the right. Figure 10.2 presents the age distribution of the population of Veterans using U.S. Department of Veterans Affairs (VA) homeless services between 2000 and 2010 to illustrate the progression of this trend before 2009. The hypothesized explanation for the persistently elevated risk for homelessness among persons is that this cohort lies in the introduction of the All-Volunteer Force, which is thought to have resulted in the enlistment of less-qualified recruits and those with fewer options beyond military service. A similar cohort effect with slightly different origins has been observed in the more general population of single homeless adults.[13] This cohort effect has affected persons born in the latter half of the Baby Boom generation (roughly between 1955 and 1965) who, while slightly younger than the Veteran age cohort that has been overrepresented in the Veteran homeless population for several decades, are nonetheless roughly comparable in age. The standard explanation offered for the cohort effect observed in the broader single adult homeless population is that those in the latter half of the Baby Boom generation faced extremely tight labor and housing markets because of the flooding of those markets by early Baby Boomers.[13] This fact, coupled with economic recessions that occurred in the late 1970s and early 1980s when this group was entering adulthood, as well as cuts in social safety net spending and the emergence of crack cocaine during the same time period, meant that the most disadvantaged members of this age cohort never gained a solid foothold in the labor and housing markets, placing them at increased risk for homelessness over the ensuing decades.[13] Although this explanation differs from the hypothesized origin of the cohort effect in the Veteran homeless population, it is likely that some of these same dynamics affected the Veterans in this age group as well and thus contributed to the cohort effect driving the aging of the homeless Veteran population.

The persistence of this cohort effect means that, even as the number of Veterans experiencing homelessness continues on a downward trend, the number of older Veterans experiencing homelessness is likely to continue to grow in the near term, thus potentially presenting new challenges to the serv - ice systems (and the VA health care system in particular) that have previously served relatively small numbers of older homeless Veterans. However, with the average life expectancy among homeless adults of roughly 64 years for males and 69 years for females,[14] the number of older homeless Veterans may ultimately level off (and subsequently decline) over the longer term as persons in this cohort attrite from homelessness because of mortality, receipt of additional income through Social Security, or eligibility for nursing home or senior housing programs. Thus, understanding the likely short-term and long-term trajectories of homelessness among older adults (and the likely impact on the VA health care system as a whole) is of obvious importance, and the next section describes the results of an attempt to project the changing size of the population of older homeless adults and discuss its potential impact on health care systems.

## PROJECTED TRAJECTORY OF HOMELESSNESS AMONG OLDER ADULTS AND IMPACT ON HEALTH CARE SYSTEM

Projections of the number of Veterans 60 years and older experiencing home-lessness over the course of the year were generated for the period from 2010 to 2025 using data from three sources: the 2010 AHAR, administrative data from the VA Health Care for Homeless Veterans (HCHV) program from the period from 2000 to 2010, and the VA Office of the Actuary's 2007 Veteran Population Projection Models (VetPop2007),[15] which forecast the size of the overall Veteran population 40 years into the future, stratified by age and sex and thus ac-counting for anticipated demographic changes in this population. The latter two data sources were combined to generate age-group stratified projections of the number of Veterans expected to use HCHV services in 2015, 2020, and 2025 using demographic methods that were similar to those applied elsewhere to proj-ect changes in the single adult homeless population.[16] However, users of HCHV services do not represent the extent of the population of Veterans experiencing homelessness by the definition used in the most official numbers available through the AHAR. Thus, we used the HCHV projections and AHAR data to impute estimates of the total number of Veterans accessing emergency shelters over the course of the year (as per the AHAR definition) in 2015, 2020, and 2025. The basic approach was to use the 2010 AHAR estimate[a] of the number of Veterans using emergency shelters as a baseline estimate and to allocate these Veterans to more fine-grained age groups than are available in the AHAR by as-suming that the age distribution of this population matched that of Veterans identified as HCHV users in 2010. We then multiplied the 2010 estimates by the estimated percentage change in each age group in 2015, 2020, and 2025 (relative to 2010) from the HCHV projections. This resulted in extrapolated age-stratified projections of the number of Veterans expected to use emergency shelter in future years, assuming that 2010 conditions prevailed.

Figure 10.3 shows the results of the projections. The figure suggests a roughly linear increase between 2010 and 2020 in the number of Veterans 60 years and older experiencing homelessness, with the number of older Veterans experiencing homelessness expected to increase by 14% overall— from 24,100 to 27,524—between 2010 and 2020. However, the projections suggest a sharp decline between 2020 and 2025 in the number of Veterans 60 years and older who are expected to use an emergency shelter at some point over the course of a year. This sharp decline is likely due to members of the age cohort described previously, who have been overrepresented in the Veteran homeless population for several decades, increasing exiting homelessness

---

[a] These projections were originally developed in 2013 and we thus used 2010 as the baseline year.

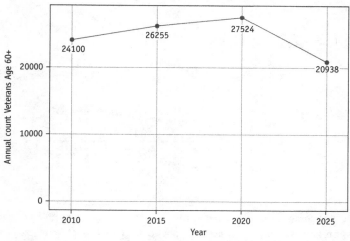

*Figure 10.3* Estimates of the national number of Veterans using emergency shelter on an annual basis, 2010–2025.  Data sources: Author forecasts based on Homeless Veterans Program Intake Assessments obtained from VA Form X, and overall Veteran population forecasts obtained from the US Department of Veterans Affairs, National Center for Veterans Analysis and Statistics, Veteran Population Projection Model 2007 (https://d3gqux9sl0z33u.cloudfront.net/AA/AT/gambillingonjustice-com/downloads/206143/VetPop07-ES-final.pdf)

through mortality, entering nursing homes, aging into eligibility for Social Security retirement other programs that allow them to access more stable housing, or other means.

Although the projections suggest that Veterans 60 years and older experiencing homelessness will continue to comprise a nontrivial share of the homeless Veteran population in 2025 and beyond, it appears that the greatest challenge in addressing the needs of an aging homeless Veteran population will unfold over the next decade or so. As this population continues to grow and approaches its life expectancy over the next several years, their health care needs and associated costs would be expected to increase. Indeed, Figure 10.4, which is based on data from VA specialized homeless programs and VA medical records, shows the estimated annual health care costs among users of VA homeless programs by age group. The figure clearly shows that health care costs and, in particular, inpatient costs increase with age among homeless Veterans. Among Veterans 60 years and older who use VA homeless programs, the figure shows that annual health care costs average roughly $17,000 per person. This far exceeds the cost of their younger counterparts and, in light of evidence of the high health care costs incurred by persons experiencing homelessness, likely exceeds that of their same-aged housed counterparts as well. In short, the overall aging trend in the Veteran homeless population in the coming years is

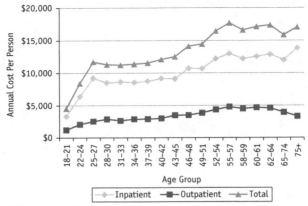

*Figure 10.4* Average annual per person VA health care costs among users of VA homeless programs. Data sources: Author population based on VA homeless program data obtained from the VA Homeless Operations and Management Evaluation System (HOMES) and Decision Support System (DSS) data obtained from the VA Corporate Data Warehouse. Figure represents average cost of VA health services use (from DSS) among all Veterans with a HOMES record during 2011.

likely to have a nontrivial impact on health care systems and on the VA health care system in particular.

## CHARACTERISTICS AND NEEDS OF OLDER VETERANS EXPERIENCING HOMELESSNESS

Older and younger Veterans experiencing homelessness are alike in that both groups constitute vulnerable segments of the Veteran population. By definition, younger and older Veterans experiencing homelessness universally have needs related to housing stability, and many in both groups will have other needs related to their overall well-being and long-term housing stability, including medical and behavioral health care, income, and social support. As such, interventions for Veterans experiencing homelessness, regardless of their age, need to consider all of these domains. However, older Veterans experiencing homelessness have unique needs that should be taken into consideration for modifying the implementation of existing interventions or for designing new ones that may be tailored specifically to older Veterans. Evidence points to three key issues in particular that need to be considered. First, older Veterans experiencing homelessness have different needs than their younger counterparts. Second, the population of older homeless adults is not homogeneous; there is meaningful heterogeneity with respect to their characteristics and housing and health care needs. Finally, the impact and suitability of housing interventions intended for Veterans may vary by age. We expand on each of these briefly next.

First, prior research conducted among the broader single homeless adult population underscores the complex and overlapping medical, behavioral health, and social challenges that many older Veterans experiencing homelessness are likely to face that distinguish them from their younger counterparts. One recent study conducted using a population-based sample of homeless adults 50 years and older found that rates of geriatric conditions (e.g., difficulties in completing activities of daily living, mobility impairments, experiencing falls, cognitive impairments, urinary incontinence) among the study sample exceeded those in a general population cohort who were, on average, 20 years older and also exceeded those observed in a cohort of persons in poverty who were 15 years older.[10] In the same study, an array of chronic medical conditions (e.g., hypertension, diabetes, arthritis) were highly prevalent, and more than 70% of participants reported having a lifetime history of mental health problems. These findings square with prior research comparing the medical and mental health needs of older and younger homeless Veterans.[17-19] Indeed, as might be expected, chronic medical conditions such as hypertension, cardiovascular problems, diabetes, and liver disease all appear to be much more common among older Veterans experiencing homelessness than their younger counterparts, although there are fewer differences with respect to mental health problems.[17] Similar age-based comparisons conducted among the more general homeless population have yielded comparable results with respect to the increased odds of chronic medical conditions among older homeless adults.[18] The story with respect to substance use disorders appears to be somewhat more complicated. While some evidence points to lower rates of substance abuse among older homeless adults,[19] one study found older homeless adults to be more likely to use heroin than their younger counterparts.[18] Regardless of whether older Veterans are more likely than their younger counterparts to have substance use disorders, rates of substance use among older adults experiencing homelessness are high—more than 50% reported illicit drug use in the population-based study described previously. And, when taken in conjunction with the complex and overlapping geriatric and chronic medical conditions that disproportionately affect older homeless adults, older Veterans experiencing homelessness are likely to have medical and behavioral health needs that are quite distinct (and more complicated) than their younger counterparts.

Second, there is meaningful heterogeneity within the population of older adults experiencing homelessness with respect to their demographic characteristics, medical and behavioral health diagnoses, and use of medical and behavioral health services. One study based on VA health care and homeless program data used latent class analysis (LCA) to identify distinct subgroups among Veterans 55 years and older who used VA homeless programs in 2014, using demographic and VA health services use variables as the manifest variables for identifying different subgroups.[20] That study identified five distinct profiles of older homeless adults. The first and largest profile group represented 42% of the entire study co-hort and comprised mainly middle-aged (55–59 years) African American males. Persons in this group had very low rates of VA health are use (only about one in 10 had an outpatient visit during the one-year observation period). The second group constituted 21.2% of all older Veterans using VA homeless programs and was markedly older (all were >60 years old with nearly one-third 70 years or older). Interestingly, this group did not have identified chronic medical or be-havioral health conditions and made very limited use of VA health care services. About one in five Veterans was in a third group, and nearly all of these Veterans were between the ages of 55 and 59 years. This group was characterized by low rates of chronic medical and behavioral health conditions and limited use of VA health care services. The fourth group comprised about 8% of all older Veterans using VA homeless programs. The defining characteristic of this group was its high rate of chronic medical conditions, which for about 10% of the sample were accompanied by a serious mental illness. The fifth and final group also accounted for 8% of the study sample and was defined primarily by its high rate of identified behavioral health conditions (38% overall, including 34% with a serious mental illness either alone or in combination with a substance abuse dis-order) and chronic medical conditions (72% with an identified chronic medical condition). This group also made heavy use of VA inpatient services, with nearly one in five having at least one inpatient stay during the one-year observation pe-riod. These Veterans also made much greater use of outpatient services than any other group. The documented heterogeneity in the population of older Veterans experiencing homelessness underscores that one-size-fits-all interventions are not likely to be sufficient for this group and that housing and related support should be tailored to their unique needs. Indeed, the analysis points to fairly sizeable segments of the older homeless Veteran population who may not have complex medical and behavioral health needs and for whom a less intensive in-tervention focused on providing them with a housing subsidy or other economic support may suffice.

Finally, there is some evidence that the impact of housing interventions for persons experiencing homelessness varies as a function of age. For example, one study found that while there were no significant differences between younger and older homeless adults in a Housing First program with respect to improved housing stability, older homeless adults experienced greater improvements in mental health and self-reported quality of life relative to their younger counterparts in the program.[21] On the other hand, a study conducted of the VA's Grant and Per Diem (GPD) transitional housing program found that older Veterans had longer stays in the program than their younger counterparts but were less likely to complete the program.[17] These two findings are not meant to necessarily suggest that Housing First is a better intervention for older Veterans than transitional housing but rather to underscore the point that the impact of housing interventions for persons experiencing homelessness may be moderated by age and that this fact needs to be considered in program planning decisions and in future research.

## Mortality in Homeless Veterans

Despite the size and older age of the homeless Veteran population, only a few studies have examined mortality in homeless Veterans. Kasprow and Rosenheck[22] retrospectively examined mortality in homeless and nonhomeless Veterans who had been treated in the VA specialized mental health programs. Mortality rates were compared with the reported rates for the general U.S. population. Standardized mortality rates for both Veteran groups were significantly higher than for the general population, and the rate for the homeless Veteran group was significantly higher than that for the nonhomeless group. Not surprisingly, increase in risk for homeless Veterans was greatest in the oldest age groups. In another retrospective analysis, Birgenheir, Lai, and Kilbourne[23] examined trends in mortality from 2000 through 2009 among Veterans categorized by severe mental illness (SMI) status and the use of VA homeless services. Homeless Veterans died younger than nonhomeless Veterans; years of potential life lost ranged from 18.9 to 24.3 over the study period. Serious mental illness was found to increase the years of life lost in both homeless categories; however, homelessness was a contributor to the years lost above and beyond serious mental illness. LePage, Bradshaw, Cipher, Crawford, and Hoosyhar[24] examined health care service use and mortality for 102,034 Veterans receiving care from the VA North Texas Health Care System in 2010. Homeless Veterans represented 2.1% of the cohort. Medical care and outcomes were analyzed in the following fiscal year. Homeless Veterans were found to have a 32.3% increase in all-cause mortality relative to nonhomeless Veterans. Higher all-cause mortality was found even after controlling for age, race, gender, SMI, substance abuse, and medical disease comorbidity (adjusted risk ratio = 1.23).

In summary, the few studies of Veterans who were homeless were consistent in suggesting that homelessness is associated with early mortality, even after adjustments were made for the presence of other variables known to contribute to early death. These estimates are questionably representative, however, given that the study samples were not selected from the population of homeless Veterans but were identified in records of medical care or were enrolled in general medical or psychiatric treatment programs. By definition, these samples were characterized by factors known to affect mortality, and results might therefore inflate mortality rates. As noted in the previous section, age is a potent factor for study among Veterans who are homeless, given the disproportionate number of older Veterans in the homeless Veteran population. More than 20% of Veterans who enter VA homelessness programs are 55 years or older.[25] Older homeless Veterans have substantial health problems[17] and report high rates of nonfatal suicidal behavior.[25] The vulnerability of Veterans who are homeless may be especially enhanced with increasing age.

To address methodological issues in extant studies of mortality in homeless Veterans, a study team lead by one of us (JAS) recently conducted three retrospective cohort studies[26–28] with the primary aim of describing mortality patterns in large samples of homeless Veterans identified solely by their entry into national VA homeless programs. Specifically, these studies examined differences between homeless and nonhomeless Veterans in all-cause and specific-cause mortality, including death by suicide. In the first study,[26] analyses focused on Veterans who were younger or middle-aged (30–54 years) at the time of entry into the homeless program. The second and third studies focused on the impact of age on mortality, examining mortality risk in Veterans who were 55 years or older at the time of entry into a homeless program. Additionally, risk factors associated with mortality in older homeless Veteran groups were explored. These studies are summarized next.

## MORTALITY IN YOUNGER AND MIDDLE-AGED HOMELESS VETERANS

In this research, data were merged from several sources to estimate mortality risk and explore factors contributing to risk. These sources included the VA Northeast Program Evaluation Center (NEPEC), the VA Corporate Data Warehouse (CDW), and the Epidemiology Program of the VA Office of Public Health. NEPEC provided administrative data for the registry of all Veterans aged 18 to 54 years who were admitted into VA homeless programs from 2000 to 2003. Veterans in these programs qualify for VA health care, but a significant percentage use community resources for some or all of their health care. The CDW provided administrative records containing age, date of birth, and sex for Veterans who received medical care from the VA from 2000 to 2003. These records were culled to select Veterans who were aged 18 to 54 years at the point of their first contact for medical care in the 2000 to 2003 time period. Veterans with a subsequent history of intervention in VA homeless programs as indicated in NEPEC data for 2000 to 2011 were dropped from consideration and constituted a pool of nonhomeless Veterans for the purposes of study analyses. Examination of the age distributions of the two samples revealed relatively few subjects in the homeless sample in younger ages (2.1% in the 18- to 29-year-old range). To match more closely the age distributions of the homeless and control samples on a group basis, the age range for the study samples was reduced to 30 to 54 years. The final homeless sample consisted of 23,898 Veterans; the final nonhomeless sample consisted of 65,198 Veterans. Because of limited data on the use of VA health care services by the homeless sample and of both samples for community-based care, no other variables were used in matching the groups.

The Epidemiology Program provided mortality data from the National Death Index maintained by the Centers for Disease Control and Prevention for the years 2000 to 2011. Homeless and nonhomeless records were matched against the National Death Index file to determine survival status, date of death, and cause of death. For mortality analyses, time to death was calculated as the date of death minus the entry date into the VA homeless program for home-less Veterans and the date of first contact for medical care service in the period 2000 to 2003 for nonhomeless Veterans. The follow-up period therefore ranged from 8 to 11 years, depending on the date of entry or first contact; mean follow-up was approximately 10 years. The World Health Organization *International Statistical Classification of Diseases and Related Health Problems,* 10th revision (ICD-10) codes provided in the National Death Index file were used to deter-mine categories of cause of death (e.g., cardiovascular diseases). Specific cause of death was also determined for death by suicide and homicide and for other external causes of death. Death by suicide was captured by examining the fol-lowing ICD-10 codes: Intentional self-harm, X60–X84 and Late effects of in-tentional self-harm, Y87.0. Death by homicide was determined by examining ICD-10 codes X92–Y09. Limited data on the use of VA health care services by the homeless sample and of both samples for community-based care precluded analyses adjusted for covariates other than sex and age.

Survival analyses revealed substantial differences in mortality between the homeless and nonhomeless groups. During the follow-up period, 16.3% of homeless Veterans died from all causes; a significantly and notably smaller proportion of the nonhomeless Veterans died from all causes (6.4%). The covariate-adjusted Cox regression analysis showed that increased risk for death for Veterans in the homeless sample was associated with a hazard ratio of 2.93. Homeless Veterans were slightly but significantly younger at time of death (52.3 years of age) than nonhomeless Veterans (53.2 years of age). Additionally, homeless Veterans survived significantly fewer months in the follow-up period (108.4) than did nonhomeless Veterans (115.7). Figure 10.5 presents the group survival functions, demonstrating substantive decline in survival for the home-less Veterans. These differences in survival were highly significant.

We found that only five ICD-10 categories represented the specific cause for the large majority of deaths: 76% in the homeless sample and 83% in the nonhomeless sample. For both groups, the most frequent categories of cause of death were cardiovascular diseases (homeless, 25%; nonhomeless, 29%), neoplasms (homeless, 16%; nonhomeless, 27%), external causes (home-less, 23%; nonhomeless, 13%), infection and parasitic disease (homeless, 7%; nonhomeless, 5%), and disorders of the digestive system (homeless, 9%;

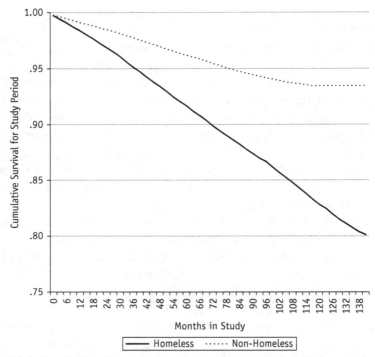

*Figure 10.5*  Survival functions for homeless and non-homeless Veterans, ages 30–54.  Data sources: US Department of Veterans Affairs (VA) Northeast Program Evaluation Center, the VA Corporate Data Warehouse, and the Epidemiology Program of the VA Office of Public Health. Study cohort identified in 2000–2003 and followed through 2011.

nonhomeless, 8%). A higher proportion was found in the homeless sample for deaths due to external causes (24% vs. 13%). The frequency of death due to neoplasms was higher in the nonhomeless sample (27% vs. 16%). There were no other substantive differences in specific cause of death categories between the samples. When we examined subcategories of external causes of death, we found that the majority (homeless, 91%; nonhomeless, 90%) were due to death by one of five specific causes: suicide, homicide, exposure to prescribed or illegal drugs (overdose), vehicle accidents, and nonvehicle accidents. Death by suicide was rare but occurred in 129 homeless and 148 nonhomeless cases during the follow-up period. The difference in proportions (0.54% for homeless sample vs. 0.22% for nonhomeless sample) was significant. Death by homicide was also rare, occurring in 75 (0.31%) of the homeless sample and 32 (0.04%) of the nonhomeless sample. In examining causes of death for those Veterans who did die, however, there was no difference between samples in the proportion of cases of death by suicide, with 4.15% of homeless deaths and 3.17% of nonhomeless deaths attributable to this cause. Among those who died, there was a significant difference between samples in the proportion of cases dying by homicide, with 1.92% of homeless deaths and 0.77% of nonhomeless deaths dying by this cause.

Not surprisingly, death due to exposure to drugs was significantly more frequent in the homeless sample (6%) than the nonhomeless sample (2%). This specific cause was responsible for 26% of the homeless Veteran external-cause deaths and 13% of the nonhomeless Veteran external-cause deaths. This difference was also significant. Deaths due to vehicle accidents did not differ between homeless and nonhomeless cases (3% for each); however, among those who died of external causes, there was a significant difference, with 13% of homeless deaths and 22% of nonhomeless deaths by this specific cause. In the homeless sample as a whole, 7% died in nonvehicle accidents such as falls, drowning, and electrical shock. This was significantly greater than the percentage (3%) for the sample of nonhomeless Veterans. These types of accidents were a significantly larger proportion of external-cause deaths in the homeless sample (30%) than in the nonhomeless sample (23%).

## Summary of Mortality in Younger Homeless Veterans Study

Our study of younger homeless Veterans found evidence of substantially increased mortality in Veterans identified exclusively by housing status. Frequency of all-cause death in the 10-year follow-up period was found to be more than twice as high for homeless than for nonhomeless Veterans. In contrast, national mortality statistics estimate that 6.8% of men in the age range of 25 to 54 years die over a time period equivalent to that used in this study's follow-up. We concluded that mortality in the homeless sample, therefore, not only was greater than that of nonhomeless Veterans but also appears to be approximately twice than expected on the basis of national mortality estimates. A notable finding from the study was that only a single category of cause of death, death due to external causes, was associated with a significant and meaningful proportional increase in homeless Veteran mortality compared with nonhomeless mortality. Almost one-fourth of homeless deaths were due to external causes that included drug overdose, suicide, homicide, and both vehicle and nonvehicle (e.g., falls, drowning, errors in operating machinery) accidents. While the large majority of these deaths were due to drug overdose, suicide, and homicide, a notable proportion were attributable to vehicle and especially nonvehicle accidents. One possible explanation for this specific increased mortality rate may be the documented high rate of alcohol and drug use in homeless Veterans and the fact that episodes of intoxication are associated with death by external causes due to accident.[29,30]

## MORTALITY IN OLDER HOMELESS VETERANS

In the second and third studies,[27,28] we conducted an expanded set of analyses on a cohort of Veterans aged 55 years and older. In addition to examining mortality risk and cause of death in an older group of Veterans, the research also examined the contribution of several potential factors, in addition to age, in increasing risk. The data for this study were obtained from the same sources as for their study of younger homeless Veterans: NEPEC, the Epidemiology Program of the VA Office of Public Health, and CDW. NEPEC provided administrative data for all Veterans 55 years and older who were admitted into VA homelessness programs in 2000 to 2003 and had program entry data as recorded on an administrative intake interview (Form X). This sample included 4,475 Veterans. A control group was created by using administrative records from the CDW containing age, date of birth, and sex for Veterans 55 years and older who received medical care from the VA from 2000 to 2003. Those with a subsequent history of intervention in VA homeless programs as indicated in NEPEC data for 2000 to 2011 were dropped from the analyses. The final control sample consisted of 20,071 Veterans. The age distributions of the two groups were matched by proportional sampling across three-year age intervals (e.g., 55–57, 58–60 years).

Again, homeless and control sample records were matched against the Centers for Disease Control and Prevention National Death Index file for the years 2000 to 2011 to determine survival status, date of death, and cause of death. ICD-10 codes provided in the National Death Index file were used to determine category (e.g., infectious disease) and specific causes of death for suicide, intentional self-harm, late effects of intentional self-harm, poisoning of undetermined intent, and other events of undetermined intent.

Analyses of mortality risk factors were conducted only on the homeless sample. Risk predictors were taken from Form X. Fifteen Form X variables from six domains (demographics, health, psychiatric condition, alcohol and substance abuse, employment, and housing) were selected to represent constructs found to be potent in previous studies of risk for homelessness. These variables served as predictors of survival.

We found that, during the follow-up period, mortality was almost twice that for the homeless group compared with the nonhomeless group. In the homeless group, 35% (1,560 of the 4,475) of Veterans died from all causes compared with a significantly smaller proportion (3,649 of 20,071, 18%) of the control sample. Veterans in the homeless sample were significantly younger at time of death (65 years of age) compared with the control sample (66.9 years of age). To examine the impact of age on survival more specifically, we examined all-cause mortality in old (55–59 years) and older (≥60 years) groups. Mean survival times were longest for old Veterans in the control sample (132 months), followed by older Veterans in the control sample (126.6 months) and both homeless groups

(116.2 months for old Veterans and 106.1 months for older Veterans). Survival rates were highest among old Veterans in the control sample (11,128 of 13,139, 85%), followed by older Veterans in the control sample (5,294 of 6,932, 76%), old Veterans in the homeless sample (2,031 of 2,938, 69%), and older Veterans in the homeless sample (884 of 1,537, 58%).

Figure 10.6 presents the group survival functions, demonstrating substantive decline in survival on the basis of both age and homelessness. Overall comparison of differences in survival among the four groups and all pairwise comparisons of the group survival distributions were significant. As Figure 10.6 indicates, the largest pairwise difference was between the distributions of older Veterans in the homeless sample and old Veterans in the control sample. With old Veterans in the control sample as the reference group, risk ratios (RRs) for all-cause mortality were increasingly positive for older Veterans in the control sample (RR = 1.58), old Veterans in the homeless sample (RR = 2.46), and older Veterans in the homeless sample (RR = 3.64).

Eleven ICD-10 categories made up the specific causes of death for 95% (1,489 of 1,560) of the homeless sample and 94% (3,424 of 3,649) of the control sample who did not survive through the follow-up period. For both samples, the most frequent categories were cardiovascular diseases (homeless, 33%; nonhomeless,

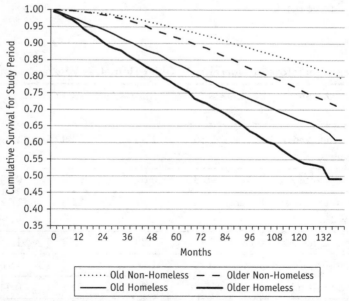

*Figure 10.6* Survival functions for homelessness and age. Data sources: US Department of Veterans Affairs (VA) Northeast Program Evaluation Center, the VA Corporate Data Warehouse, and the Epidemiology Program of the VA Office of Public Health. Study cohort identified in 2000–2003 and followed through 2011.

31%), neoplasms (homeless, 23%; nonhomeless, 30%), and respiratory diseases (homeless, 10%; nonhomeless, 11%). Compared with the nonhomeless sample, the homeless sample had higher proportions of deaths due to digestive diseases (7% vs. 5%), mental or behavioral disorders (5% vs. 2%), infectious or para-sitic diseases (4% vs. 2%), and accidents or self-harm (3% vs. 2%). Deaths due to neoplasms and to endocrine, nutritional, or metabolic diseases were more common in the nonhomeless sample than the homeless sample (30% vs. 23%, and 6% vs. 4%, respectively). The odds of dying by suicide were significantly higher among Veterans in the homeless (0.4%) than the nonhomeless (0.2%) samples (odds ratio = 1.93).

Examination of risk factors for mortality was explored in the homeless sample using Cox proportional hazards regression analysis to examine the rel-ative contribution of Form X variables. Table 10.1 presents the results of the analysis, showing the variable entering at each of eight sequential steps and the model statistics, including the adjusted hazard ratios (HRs). Five of the eight variables (presence of a serious health issue, history of hospitalization for al-cohol abuse, alcohol dependency, unemployment for three years or more, and age ≥60 years) were associated with increased risk for death, with HRs ranging from 1.13 to 1.32. Three variables (drug dependency, non-White, and dental problems) were associated with reduced risk, with HRs ranging from 0.62 to 0.84. Notably, variables related to homelessness (chronicity and frequency) were not found to be risk factors.

*Table 10.1*  **Predictors of Mortality in Older Homeless Veterans**

| Step | Variable Entering Equation | B | Hazard Ratio | 95% CI for Hazard Ratio | |
|------|---------------------------|------|--------------|-------------|------|
| 1 | Unemployed 3 years or more | 0.38 | 1.32 | 1.39 | 1.23 |
| 2 | Non-White | −0.32 | 0.62 | 0.78 | 0.44 |
| 3 | History of hospitalization for alcohol abuse | 0.31 | 1.27 | 1.35 | 1.17 |
| 4 | Serious medical problem | 0.35 | 1.30 | 1.38 | 1.21 |
| 5 | Age 60 years and older | 0.29 | 1.30 | 1.34 | 1.16 |
| 6 | Drug dependent | −0.28 | 0.67 | 0.87 | 0.44 |
| 7 | Dental problems | −0.15 | 0.84 | 0.96 | 0.70 |
| 8 | Alcohol dependent | 0.14 | 1.13 | 1.24 | 1.01 |

B = Unstandardized beta values.

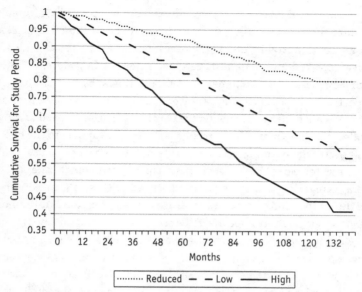

*Figure 10.7* Survival functions for three risk groups. Data sources: US Department of Veterans Affairs (VA) Northeast Program Evaluation Center, the VA Corporate Data Warehouse, and the Epidemiology Program of the VA Office of Public Health. Study cohort identified in 2000–2003 and followed through 2011.

To evaluate the efficacy of the group of predictor variables in predicting risk, a risk score was calculated. To compute the score, each of the eight variables in the regression model was unit weighted (+1 for variables with HRs >1 and –1 for variables with HRs <1), and a total risk score was calculated by summing the eight variable weights. The possible range of scores was –3 to +5. Based on the risk score, the full sample was classified into three risk groups: reduced risk (risk score less than 0, $N$ = 522), low risk (risk score of 0–2, $N$ = 2,466), and high risk (risk score greater than 2, $N$ = 632). Contingency table analysis showed a significant difference among the groups in the proportion of those dying (reduced-risk group, 17.8%; low-risk group, 34.4%; and high-risk group, 53.2%). Figure 10.7 presents the survival functions for the three groups. There was a significant difference in the survival functions of the three groups, and all pairwise comparisons of the functions of the groups revealed significant differences. There was also a significant difference in mean survival time in months for the three groups (reduced risk = 128.20, low risk = 113.31, and high risk = 94.90).

## Summary of Mortality in Older Homeless Veterans Studies

The unadjusted analyses of mortality among older Veterans identified exclusively by housing status and age revealed that the frequency of all-cause deaths in the 11-year follow-up period was approximately twice as high for the homeless sample (35%) compared with the control sample (18%). Notably, only 58% of homeless Veterans 60 years and older survived the study period. The RRs for all-cause mortality among homeless Veterans were comparable to those previously reported for a sample of Veterans who were homeless. [22,24] Mortality for both homeless and nonhomeless Veterans was substantially higher than that reported in the Schinka et al. study of younger Veterans (16% for homeless Veterans, 6% for nonhomeless Veterans) in the same time period and over the same follow-up time frame. These results lend further support to the hypothesis of excess mortality among Veterans who are homeless and provide estimates of mortality risk for older Veterans who have experienced homelessness.

Several categories of disease were associated with small and questionably meaningful proportional increases in deaths among Veterans in the homeless sample; no single category appeared to be critical in reducing survival time. Thus, older age did not appear to differentially affect vulnerability to specific disease categories. As was the case in the study of younger homeless Veterans, death by suicide was rare. However, again suicide was twice as common among the Veterans in the homeless sample compared with the control sample, a finding consistent with the relatively high frequency of reported suicidal behaviors among older Veterans who have been homeless.[25]

Results of regression analyses suggested that several variables contribute in both risk and protective directions to mortality. Five of these variables were associated with increased risk for death (presence of a serious health issue, history of hospitalization for alcohol abuse, alcohol dependency, unemployment for three years or more, and age ≥60 years). The most significant risk variable was unemployment for three years or more. There is a large literature on the study of unemployment and its association with health and mortality (e.g., Lundin, Lundberg, Hallsten, Ottosson, & Hemmingsson),[31] much of which has focused on untangling the coping (unemployment produces adverse changes in health) versus "health vulnerability" (preexisting health conditions and behaviors lead to unemployment) hypotheses. An informative study by Martikainen, Maki, and Jantti[32] found an HR for all-cause mortality of 1.30 following unemployment after adjustment for psychiatric diagnosis, education and income, drug and alcohol abuse, and socioeconomic factors, suggesting that unemployment does have an adverse effect on health beyond those explained by other vulnerability factors. Homelessness in Veterans is associated with a large number of associated conditions, such as mental illness and substance abuse, associated with unemployment. In our study, unemployment may have served as a proxy for the effect of several other measured and unmeasured factors. This finding is consistent with the report by Kasprow and Rosenheck[22] on reduced risk for mortality for homeless Veterans who were employed.

The findings for alcohol abuse and health issues are consistent with previous reports. The association of chronic alcohol abuse and mortality is well documented.[33] In a recent study,[34] at-risk drinking was shown to be associated with a modest estimated mortality HR of 1.20. Both of the alcohol use–related variables were found to have HRs of the same size. As anticipated, serious health issues and age contributed to the risk for death, consistent with regularly reported national mortality statistics.[35] Notably, three variables were associated with reduced risk for mortality: non-White status, drug dependence, and dental problems. We have suggested that non-White status and drug dependence may be protective because health services from both VA and non-VA sources are more readily available in the impoverished locales of large cities where most homeless and drug-dependent Veterans are found. In a previous study,[36] it was shown that homeless Veterans receiving dental care as part of homeless services had significantly improved employment and housing outcomes. This result was attributed to the direct effect of dental care (e.g., reduction in pain, improved nutrition, and enhanced appearance) and the indirect effect that Veterans remained in the program longer to receive dental care, thereby promoting greater exposure to other therapeutic and training modalities.

Of note, measures of homelessness severity (chronicity, frequency of homeless episodes) were not found to be risk factors for early mortality. In conjunction with the other findings, this suggests that the vulnerability factors for homelessness operate on mortality risk and not the condition of homelessness itself.

## Biological Aging and Mortality Risk in Homeless Veterans

The extant research and recent studies by Schinka et al.[26–28] provide substantive evidence that homelessness is associated with early mortality in both younger and old Veterans. As expected, chronological age is a major contributing factor because risk for early death is accelerated in older Veterans. With the exception of death due to external causes in younger homeless Veterans, the same diseases and disorders are the causes of death in both homeless and nonhomeless Veterans. Of note, chronicity of homelessness and frequency of homeless episodes were not found to be risk factors in older homeless Veterans. These findings suggest that (1) vulnerability factors common to homelessness and biological aging, and not homelessness per se, contribute to mortality risk; and (2) accelerated biological aging is the mechanism by which the same set of diseases and disorders produce earlier death in homeless Veterans, likely owing to diminished repair and regeneration in widespread organ systems. Support for this interpretation can be found in recent studies[10,37] of geriatric conditions (e.g., falls, cognitive impairment, frailty, sensory impairment, urinary incontinence) in homeless adults

50 years and older. The prevalence of these conditions was found to be higher than that seen in housed adults 20 years older and was associated with vulnerability factors common to homelessness and biological aging—limited education, medical comorbidities, and alcohol and drug use problems.

# Implications for Housing and Health Care Interventions

The increasing age of Veterans who have experienced homelessness and the evidence suggesting that these Veterans experience accelerated biological aging have important implications for housing and health care interventions for homeless Veterans who have reached or are approaching age 60 years. Permanent supportive housing, defined as subsidized housing with closely linked or onsite supportive services, may reduce acute care use among homeless adults.[38-40] Currently, many older homeless adults who have functional impairment and other geriatric conditions may be placed in nursing homes because of a lack of other appropriate options.[41] However, permanent supportive housing may be able to meet the needs of the aging homeless population, with modifications including personal care attendants and environmental adaptations. Further study is needed to determine whether such adapted housing programs could allow formerly homeless individuals to age in place, delaying or preventing the need for nursing home care.

In addition, modifications to training for staff of permanent supportive housing and other specialized homeless assistance programs will be an important part of adapting these models to better address the needs of older homeless Veterans. Staff in these programs, who may have previously focused primarily on ensuring housing stability and addressing behavioral health issues, may need to be trained so that they are better equipped to deal with issues related to chronic disease management and end-of-life care, which are likely to be increasingly common among Veterans they work with and which they report feeling unable to address in an adequate manner.[42] Likewise, evidence of high rates of mortality among formerly chronically homeless adults in permanent supportive housing has led some to suggest that it may be important to have additional grief support in place for staff to help them cope with client deaths.[43]

Older Veterans also need a professional health care workforce that coordinates medical management on a routine basis. While the VA Homeless Patient-Aligned Care Team (HPACT) program is a very positive step in promoting access to health care for homeless Veterans, the focus of the HPACT approach is generalist ambulatory care. For older Veterans, a facilitated path to assessment by a geriatrician or referral to a geriatric evolution unit would enhance care and help to avoid more intense levels of treatment.

Relatedly, geriatric specialty care providers may also need to adapt service models and practices to address the unique needs of Veterans experiencing homelessness, who face additional barriers to care than their housed counterparts accessing the same services. One study involving a survey of end-of-life programs in the VA health care system found that such programs reported lack of appropriate housing as the most critical challenge they faced in providing care to their Veteran patients.[44] Greater coordination between VA homeless assistance and housing programs and geriatric specialty care providers could prove highly valuable. Moreover, VA homeless assistance programs should collaborate with community-based providers of homeless assistance to identify and engage older Veterans experiencing homelessness who access the mainstream homeless assistance system but do not use VA homeless services for which they may be eligible and which may be a crucial resource for ending their homelessness.

Older Veterans have less social support, more significant health care needs, and perhaps more motivation to change.[45] Given their frequently brittle health care status, it appears that access to homeless programs and geriatric-informed health care for older Veterans could be enhanced by using media outlets that promote the connection between homeless programs and VA clinics/hospitals that treat geriatric health care needs. Enlisting older Veterans to conduct peer outreach in homeless shelters touting the benefits of VA homelessness programs is an unexplored but potentially valuable tool.

That the older homeless Veteran population is growing has only recently been recognized. There is a need to provide more comprehensive education to homeless program staff on important geriatric issues in housing placement and support as well as health care assessment, treatment, and referral.

# References

1. Perl L. *Veterans and homelessness*. Washington, DC: Congressional Research Service; 2014.
2. US Department of Housing and Urban Development. *The 2016 Annual Homeless Assessment Report to Congress: Part 1—Point in Time Estimates of Homelessness in the U.S.* Washington, DC; 2016. Retrieved from https://www.hudexchange.info/ resources/documents/ 2016-AHAR-Part-1.pdf.
3. Koegel P, Burnam MA, Baumohl J. The causes of homelessness. In J. Baumohl, ed. *Homelessness in America*. Phoenix: Oryx Press; 1996.
4. Khan SS, Singer BD, Vaughan DE. Molecular and physiological manifestations and measurement of aging in humans. *Aging Cell*. 2017;16(4):624–633.
5. Rosenheck RA, Fontana AF. Race and outcome of treatment for veterans suffering from PTSD. *J Trauma Stress*. 1996;9:343–351.
6. Tsai K, Rosenheck RA. Risk factors for Homelessness Among US Veterans. *Epidemiol Rev*. 2015;37:177–195.

7. US Department of Housing and Urban Development. *The 2015 Annual Homeless Assesment Report to Congress: Part 2—Estimates of Homelessness in the U.S.* Washington, DC; 2016.
8. Fargo J, Metraux S, Byrne T, et al. Prevalence and risk of Homelessness Among US Veterans. *Prev Chronic Dis.* 2012;9:E45.
9. Brown RT, Kiely DK, Bharel M, Mitchell SL. Geriatric syndromes in older homeless adults. *J Gen Intern Med.* 2012;27(1):16–22.
10. Brown RT, Hemati K, Riley ED, et al. Geriatric conditions in a population-based sample of older homeless adults. *Gerontologist.* 2017;57(4):757–766.
11. Rosenheck R, Frisman L, Chung A. The proportion of veterans among homeless men. *Am J Public Health.* 1994;84(3):466–469.
12. Gamache G, Rosenheck R, Tessler R. The proportion of veterans among homeless men: A decade later. *Soc Psychiatry Psychiatr Epidemiol.* 2001;36(10):481–485.
13. Culhane DP, Metraux S, Byrne T, Stino M, Bainbridge J. The age structure of contemporary homelessness: Evidence and implications for public policy. *Anal Soc Issues Public Policy.* 2013;13(1):228–244.
14. Metraux S, Eng N, Bainbridge J, Culhane DP. The impact of shelter use and housing placement on mortality hazard for unaccompanied adults and adults in family households entering New York City shelters: 1990–2002. *J Urban Heal.* 2011;88(6):1091–1104.
15. US Department of Veterans Affairs Office of the Actuary. Veteran Population Projection Model—VetPop2014. http://www.va.gov/vetdata/Veteran_population.asp. Accessed March 6, 2016.
16. Sharygin E, Smith HL, Miranda V, Byrne T, Culhane D. How can we guess how many will be living in shelters in the next U.S. Census? University of Pennsylvania Population Studies Center, no date.
17. Brown LM, Barnett SD, Frahm KA, Schinka JA, Schonfeld L, Casey RJ. Health risk factors and differences in outcomes between younger and older veterans using VA transitional housing. *Psychiatr Serv.* 2015;66(1):33–40.
18. Garibaldi B, Conde-Martel A, O'Toole TP. Self-reported comorbidities, perceived needs, and sources for usual care for older and younger homeless adults. *J Gen Intern Med.* 2005;20(8):726–730.
19. Hecht L, Coyle B. Elderly homeless: A comparison of older and younger adult emergency shelter seekers in Bakersfield, California. *Am Behav Sci.* 2001;45(1):66–79.
20. Byrne T, Montgomery AE, Fargo, JD. Unsheltered homelessness among veterans: Correlates and profiles. Paper presented at the 2016 National Coalition for Homeless Veterans; June, 2016; Washington, DC.
21. Chung TE, Gozdzik A, Palma Lazgare LI, et al. Housing First for older homeless adults with mental illness: A subgroup analysis of the At Home/Chez Soi randomized controlled trial. *Int J Geriatr Psychiatry.* 2018;33(1):85–95.
22. Kasprow WJ, Rosenheck R. Mortality among homeless and nonhomeless mentally ill veterans. *J Nerv Ment Dis* 2000;188:141–147.
23. Birgenheir DG, Lai Z, Kilbourne AM. Trends in mortality among homeless VA patients with severe mental illness. *Psychiatr Serv.* 2013;64:608.
24. LePage JP, Bradshaw LD, Cipher DJ, et al. The effects of homelessness on veterans' health care service use: An evaluation of independence from comorbidities. *Pub Health.* 2014;128:985–992.
25. Schinka JA, Schinka KC, Casey RJ, et al. Suicidal behavior in a national sample of older homeless veterans. *Am J Publ Health.* 2012;102:S147–S153.
26. Schinka JA, Leventhal KC, Casey RJ. Mortality risk and early death in homeless veterans. Paper presented at the 2016 National Coalition for Homeless Veterans; June, 2016; Washington, DC.
27. Schinka JA, Bossarte RM, Curtiss G, Lapcevic WA, Casey RJ. Increased mortality among older veterans admitted to VA homelessness programs. *Psychiatr Serv.* 2016;67:465–468.
28. Schinka JA, Curtiss G, Leventhal K, Bossarte RM, Lapcevic W, Casey R. Predictors of mortality in older homeless veterans. *J Gerontol B Psychol Sci Soc Sci.* 2017;72(6):1103–1109.

29. Miller TR, Spicer RS. Hospital-admitted injury attributable to alcohol. *Alc Clin Exp Res.* 2012;36:104–112.

30. Smith GS, Branas CC, Miller TR. Fatal nontraffic injuries involving alcohol: A meta-analysis. *Ann Emerg Med.* 1999; 33:659–668.

31. Lundin A, Lundberg I, Hallsten L, Ottosson J, Hemmingsson T. (2010). Unemployment and mortality: A longitudinal prospective study on selection and causation in 49321 Swedish middle-aged men. *J Epidemiol Community Health.* 2010;64:22–28.

32. Martikainen P, Mäki N, Jäntti M. The effects of unemployment on mortality following workplace downsizing and workplace closure: A register-based follow-up study of Finnish men and women during economic boom and recession. *Am J Epidemiol.* 2007;165:1070–1075.

33. Rehm J, Dawson D, Frick U, et al. Burden of disease associated with alcohol use disorders in the United States. *Alc Clin Exp Res.* 2014;38:1068–1077.

34. Moore AA, Giuli L, Gould R, et al. Alcohol use, comorbidity, and mortality. *J Am Geriatr Soc.* 2006;54:757–762.

35. Kochanek KD, Murphy SL, Xu J, Arias E. Mortality in the United States, 2013. *NCHS Data Brief.* 2014;178:1–8.

36. Nunez E, Gibson G, Jones JA, Schinka JA. Evaluating the impact of dental care on housing intervention program outcomes among homeless veterans. *Am J Publ Health.* 2013;103(suppl 2):S368–S373.

37. Brown RT, Kiely DK, Bharel M, Mitchell SL. Factors associated with geriatric syndromes in older homeless adults. *J Health Care Poor Underserved.* 2013;24:456–468.

38. Sadowski LS, Kee RA, VanderWeele TJ, Buchanan D. Effect of a housing and case management program on emergency department visits and hospitalizations among chronically ill homeless adults: a randomized trial. *JAMA.* 2009;301:1771–1778.

39. Stergiopoulos V, Herrmann N. Old and homeless: A review and survey of older adults who use shelters in an urban setting. *Can J Psychiatry.* 2003;48:374–380.

40. Stergiopoulos V, Gozdzik A, Misir V, et al. Effectiveness of Housing First with intensive case management in an ethnically diverse sample of homeless adults with mental illness: A randomized controlled trial. *PLoS One.* 2015;10:1–21.

41. Bamberger JD, Dobbins SK. A research note: Long-term cost effectiveness of placing homeless seniors in permanent supportive housing. *Cityscape.* 2014;17(2):269–277.

42. Henwood BF, Katz ML, Gilmer TP. Aging in place within permanent supportive housing. *Int J Geriatr Psychiatry.* 2015;30(1):80–87.

43. Henwood BF, Byrne T, Scriber B. Examining mortality among formerly homeless adults enrolled in Housing First: An observational study. *BMC Public Health.* 2015;15(1):1209.

44. Hutt E, Whitfield E, Min S-J, et al. Challenges of providing end-of-life care for homeless veterans. *Am J Hosp Palliat Med.* 2016;33(4):381–389.

45. Molinari VA, Brown LM, Frahm KA, Schinka JA, Casey R. Perceptions of homelessness in older homeless veterans, VA homeless program staff liaisons, and housing intervention providers. *J Health Care Poor Underserved.* 2013;24:487–498.

## 11

# Homeless Veterans and Use of Information Technology

### D. KEITH MCINNES AND SARAH L. CUTRONA

*I've been able to feel my way through [the PHR] with the help of what you people showed me, and I order my medicines through it now. Before I used to have to [use] the phone system. This way I can go over the computer line and it's a lot quicker. It's less hassle. I can keep track of it very easy.*
—Unstably housed Veteran, Massachusetts[1] (pp. S64–S65)

## Introduction

Not long ago, it was assumed that homeless Veterans had minimal access to technologies. Lack of income and the high costs of computers, cell phones, and cell phone service plans were seen as prohibitive. Early, small-scale studies of homeless men and women from the general population changed this perception, finding surprisingly high rates of access to cell phones. In addition, these studies noted that many homeless persons used computers and the Internet, with a 2011 study indicating that 47% had used a computer in the past 30 days,[2] and a 2010 study of homeless adolescents reporting that 84% used the Internet at least weekly.[3] Several mechanisms offer likely explanations for these findings. Public libraries, community centers, and some homeless shelters offered free computer access.[4,5] At the same time, government support provided free or reduced-price phones to the indigent.[6,7] Prices of technology have dropped; what was once a luxury has become a relatively inexpensive necessity for many Americans. Social factors also play a role. Homeless men and women are increasingly likely to have peers who have and use technology. Internet access and use of social media can maintain or extend valuable social connections, providing social support, social capital, and access to other needed resources.

## Overview

Available information on use of technology by homeless Veterans is limited. To place our discussion in context, we begin with a brief review of statistics on use of technology in the general U.S. population and then among the separate subgroups represented in the population of homeless Veterans, that is, homeless persons and U.S. Veterans. We then describe a conceptual model, the Technology Adoption Model (TAM), for understanding factors that influence uptake and use of technology by homeless Veterans. TAM's strengths are in explaining individual behaviors, placing less emphasis on social factors influencing technology use. For this reason we have augmented TAM by considering the social milieu occupied by the homeless Veteran because both the social influence of peers and considerations of social capital may influence uptake and use.

Following this discussion, we shift to focus on our main topic, a discussion of available literature on technology use in homeless Veterans. We include a discussion of use of technology among special Veteran populations, including ones that, while not homeless, may be at higher risk for housing instability compared with other Veteran groups. We include in this group those with stigmatized conditions including mental health disorders, HIV, or hepatitis C. We discuss technology use broadly, including available information on cell phone and smart phone use, texting, Internet access, telehealth (devices connecting to a landline for transmission of health-related information), and electronic personal health records (PHRs). We provide information on technology use for health-related purposes where available.

At the conclusion of this review, we provide recommendations for how the U.S. Department of Veterans Affairs (VA) and other organizations can improve homeless Veterans' access to and meaningful use of these technologies. We offer suggestions for future research, related to understanding variation in access among homeless Veterans (e.g., by age, sex), the types of uses of these technologies, and ways that the VA could use technology to help homeless Veterans manage chronic conditions and achieve better health. Expanding on current patterns of use and enabling access for those who previously had none can offer benefits to homeless Veterans and to the greater society. A note about terminology: in this chapter the terms "cell phone" and "mobile phone" are inclusive of smartphones and feature phones (the latter are typically not Internet connected and do not have the ability to use apps), unless otherwise specified.

# Use of Information Technology in the U.S. Population and in Relevant Subgroups

## U.S. POPULATION AND INFORMATION TECHNOLOGY USE

The United States has seen rapid proliferation of mobile phone ownership over the past 10 years. Cell phone ownership among U.S. adults, reaching just over half of the population (65%) in 2004, increased to 91% by the end of 2013.[8] Smartphone ownership rose from 35% in 2011 to 77% at the end of 2016,[9] and Internet use was reported by 87% of U.S. adults in 2016, up from 52% in 2000.[9,10]

## U.S. HOMELESS POPULATION AND INFORMATION TECHNOLOGY USE

Available statistics on use of information technology (IT) among the general homeless population have significant limitations. In many cases, samples may not be representative of their target population.[11] Studies demonstrate frequent reliance on convenience sampling over relatively short time periods and have small sample sizes. A 2013 systematic review[11] focused on use of IT among the homeless, defining IT broadly to encompass computers, the Internet, mobile phones, iPods, and applications (apps). The authors used an encompassing definition of what it means to be homeless, ranging from living on the streets to staying in homeless shelters, living in transitional housing, or doubling up (i.e., "couch surfing") with a friend or a relative.

The 16 articles that authors retrieved[12–27] (reflecting 12 studies) had a combined sample size of 1,082 homeless persons; six articles described homeless adults[15,16,18–21] and six articles described homeless adolescents.[22–27] All articles described populations within the United States. Available data on access to and use of IT (e.g., Internet, mobile phones, texting) was gathered using structured surveys with sample sizes ranging from 39 to 265 individuals. Studies were conducted in limited geographic areas, usually in a single city (and all the reports related to homeless adolescents came from Los Angeles). Highlights from this systematic review include:

- *Mobile phone ownership*: mobile phone ownership ranged from 44% to 62% (including direct ownership, long-term borrowing and renting).
- *Texting*: Among mobile phone users, 61% had texted at least once and 20% had accessed the Internet at least once on their phones.
- *Computer access*: Computer access and use ranged from 47% to 55%.
- *Locations used to access computers and the Internet*: Common locations from which individuals accessed a computer included public libraries (most

common), followed by social service agencies, university libraries, coffee shops, churches, friends' homes, work, and hotel lobbies.

- *Rates of Internet use*: Internet use ranged from 19% to 84%. The 19% represents use in the past 30 days and comes from a study of 265 homeless drug users; while the 84% represents those accessing the Internet at least weekly, among 201 homeless adolescents from Hollywood, California.
- *Health-related uses*: Uses included connecting with health care providers, looking online for general health information, and looking online for information about infectious disease testing.

## U.S. VETERAN POPULATION AND INFORMATION TECHNOLOGY USE

Existing studies suggest that IT use among U.S. Veterans is similar to the use among the U.S. non-Veteran population. A 2013 joint VA and Pew random-digit dialed survey examined this comparison.[28] There were 353 Veteran respondents in the sample and 2,637 non-Veterans; Internet use was similar between Veterans and non-Veterans (67% and 69%, respectively). On both general Internet use and a wide variety of health-related uses, ranging from managing chronic pain to medical test results and environmental health, there were no differences between Veterans and non-Veterans. Additional similarities included rates of cell phone ownership (84% vs. 83%), watching online health-related videos, and tracking weight, exercise, or other health indicators.

These findings align with an earlier population-based study that found no statistically significant difference between Veterans and non-Veterans in access to the Internet or in use of the Internet for health.[29] In the study's 12,878 randomly selected adults there were 3,408 Veterans. The survey, conducted in 2002, found that 54% of Veterans and 53% of non-Veterans were using the Internet. Among those who used the Internet, 29% of Veterans and 33% of non-Veterans used the Internet to look for health information.

## MODEL FOR UNDERSTANDING FACTORS INFLUENCING USE OF TECHNOLOGY AMONG HOMELESS VETERANS

We propose the TAM[30,31] as a guide for gaining a deeper understanding of factors influencing use of technology among homeless Veterans (Figure 11.1).

Central to the TAM are perceived usefulness and perceived ease of use. Perceived usefulness is the degree to which a person believes that using a particular system would enhance his or her personal objectives, while perceived ease of use is the degree to which a person believes that using a particular

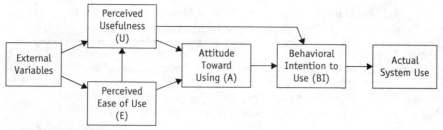

*Figure 11.1* A model of technology acceptance among homeless Veterans. (Davis, Bagozzi & Warshaw 1989, p985)

system requires little effort or specialized skills.[30] External variables influence both perceived ease of use and perceived usefulness; these perceptions in turn influence attitudes toward use, behavioral intention, and ultimately, actual use. Homeless Veterans are influenced by a variety of unique external variables, suggesting that perceptions of technology's usefulness and ease of use may likewise have characteristics unique to this population. In Table 11.1, we describe factors (e.g. external variables) relevant to homeless Veterans' use of technology. As external variables we consider five issues that are commonly associated with IT use, especially among populations with fewer resources: (1) material and logistical issues; (2) safety, security, health, and privacy; (3) educational level, general literacy, and English language literacy; (4) technological literacy; and (5) social influences and the role of social capital.

As alluded to earlier and as shown in the last row of Table 11.1, the social environment in which a homeless Veteran moves is important when considering technology uptake. Social factors can act at multiple points within the TAM model, and we will discuss later the role of social influences on the potential technology user, including concepts from social capital theory. IT offers a means of enhancing social capital. Social capital has been defined as the value of social relationships and networks that an individual must cultivate and from which an individual gains benefits, such as friendship, instrumental or informational social support, and job and housing opportunities.[32,33] For persons experiencing indigency and homelessness, there may, generally speaking, be limited opportunities for diverse kinds of social interaction. The use of IT, however, may represent significant and growing opportunities for expanding social capital in this population.

Social capital has been divided into three types—bridging, bonding, and maintained. The first two forms of social capital (bridging and bonding) were popularized in Putnam's 2001 book, *Bowling Alone*.[33] *Bridging social capital*, he tells us, is created by connecting with people who are different from oneself, for example, of another social class or income level or different racial or ethnic

**Table 11.1** External Variables Relevant to Homeless Veterans that Influence Uptake and Use of Information Technology (IT)

| External Variables | Influence of External Variables on Perceived Usefulness | Influence of External Variables on Perceived Ease of Use |
|---|---|---|
| **Material and logistical issues** | **IT provides access to:**<br>• Information on resources (housing, employment, benefits, food, and temporary shelter)<br>• Health care (phone and Internet-based communication with physician and other health care providers, pharmacies); ability to identify nearby clinics | **How easy is access to:**<br>• IT device ownership (considerations include cost of individually owned device, portability)<br>• Ongoing service (cost, locations where person spends time)<br>• Free or low-cost IT access, including use of computers and Wi-Fi at libraries and other locations; considerations include limited hours and homeless persons feeling unwelcome |
| **Safety, security, health, and privacy** | **IT provides ability to:**<br>• Quickly access assistance in a medical emergency or when threatened with bodily harm<br>• Directly access information without confiding in others<br>• Access to health care providers and helping professionals for routine care | **How concerned is person about:**<br>• Ease or difficulty of securing information and maintaining privacy of data, such as through the use of a password or biometrics |
| **Educational level, general literacy, and English language literacy** | **IT tools can inform and educate:**<br>• IT tools (e.g., Wikipedia, Google, dictionary, videos on medication or device use) can assist with defining words and concepts; may be especially helpful for medical terms and jargon. | **Does the person's educational level and literacy enable them to locate, read (or watch/listen to), and understand:**<br>• General information<br>• Technology-based communications<br>• Health-related communication<br>• Information in English and other available languages |

(continued)

*Table 11.1* **Continued**

| External Variables | Influence of External Variables on Perceived Usefulness | Influence of External Variables on Perceived Ease of Use |
|---|---|---|
| **Technological literacy issues** | **Use of IT builds skills:**<br>• IT provides opportunities to learn, practice, and perfect technology-related skills | **To engage with technology effectively, does the person have:**<br>• Ability to navigate parts of device<br>• Ability to explore Internet and software programs/apps<br>• Ability to navigate secure pathways (remember, retrieve, and use passwords)<br>• Ability to download and store for future use (information, new apps)<br>• Prior experience with technology (i.e., growing digitization of equipment and systems in the military) |
| **Social influences and role of social capital** | **Benefits of virtual social networks:**<br>• IT offers a platform for communication with social networks<br>• Can enhance social capital by building connections and supporting others<br>• May address feelings of isolation<br>• Access to members of unique populations (Veterans, homeless, persons with a particular medical condition) | **Does person perceive peers as engaged with similar technology (social norms), such as:**<br>• Observing peers using technology or receiving support/training from others, which may help to increase perceived ease of use<br>• Ease/complexity of social media tools (e.g., texting, Facebook, Twitter, LinkedIn) |

group. This kind of bridging may bring people access to resources (e.g., finances, employment, information) that they might not have been able to access if their interactions were limited to persons similar to themselves. Alternatively, *bonding social capital* is formed when interacting with persons who are similar (e.g., of the same socio-economic class) or who are going through similar life experiences. Finally, *maintained social capital* refers to keeping in touch with communities that one has had for some time and possibly has moved away from, such as family, hometown friends, or Veterans who served in the same military unit.[34]

As an example of IT contributing to social capital for persons experiencing homelessness, when a person has a cell phone number or email address, this can create the semblance of permanence, concealing the lack of a permanent home. This appearance of stability may facilitate creation of bridging social capital if a person feels that disclosing his or her lack of permanent housing would create a rift between oneself and persons who have never experienced homelessness. Thus, a homeless Veteran can cultivate ties with employers (current or potential) and colleagues, including those in different life circumstances and of higher socio-economic position. Outside of the work environment, IT can allow homeless Veterans to keep in touch with similar others (bonding social capital—e.g., other persons who are homeless, other Veterans) and can enable new connections through online searches and use of social media to find shelters and transitional housing supportive of Veterans or through support groups that are especially welcoming to Veterans (e.g., Veteran coffee meetings or 12-step groups known to be frequented by Veterans).

## Use of Information Technology Among Homeless Veterans

In this section we review existing literature on IT use among homeless Veterans. We continue to draw on TAM, and we also consider the role of IT in enhancing social influence and social capital. A limited number of studies address IT use among homeless Veterans. The studies are both qualitative and quantitative in nature, most with relatively small sample sizes. They address homeless Veterans' access to IT and provide insight into attitudes toward IT, including perceptions of usefulness, ease of use, and barriers to IT use. Where available, we include information on the role of social factors. The section ends with a case example in which a new telehealth intervention was implemented with homeless Veterans who had been placed in voucher-based long-term housing in greater Los Angeles.

## INFORMATION TECHNOLOGY ACCESS AND USE AMONG HOMELESS VETERANS RESIDING IN SHELTERS AND TRANSITIONAL HOUSING

In a cross-sectional survey[35] conducted between January 2012 and February 2013, researchers recruited a convenience sample of 106 Veterans drawn from a variety of homeless programs within Massachusetts. The study's goal was to document access to IT and attitudes toward use of technology for needed health services among this population. The survey was administered by interviewers at the sites where Veterans resided. It included sociodemographic characteristics as well as information on access to and use of mobile phones, Internet, text messaging, and email. In addition, questions sought to identify purposes for use of these technologies, explored participant willingness to be contacted by mobile phone call or text message for appointment reminders or scheduling, and assessed barriers to mobile phone use.

The vast majority (89%) of the 106 surveyed Veterans in this study had a mobile phone (one-third were smartphones), and 76% used the Internet. Of mobile phone users, 71% used text messages. These technologies were perceived as useful and were employed in a diverse range of functions, including information acquisition and communication related to health, housing, and jobs. For mobile phones, Veterans reported that their top three categories for use were connecting with friends and family, health purposes, and VA benefits. For the Internet, the top three uses included connecting with friends and family, entertainment, and health. Nearly all respondents were interested in receiving mobile phone health care appointment reminders (93%) or receiving outreach to schedule a needed health care appointment (88%). In the 30 days preceding the survey, barriers to easy use included phones being out of power (35% of 94 respondents with mobile phones), running out of minutes (16%), or reaching text limits (6%). In this study, social factors (e.g., desire to connect with friends and family) were found to play a prominent role as one of the top three motivating factors for use of both mobile phones and the Internet.

## PERCEPTIONS OF INFORMATION TECHNOLOGY AMONG HOMELESS VETERANS

In a substudy of the work described previously, researchers conducted semi-structured qualitative interviews with 30 homeless Veterans (drawn from the sample of 106) to understand what types of health-related technology use would be of interest.[36] Their sample, drawn from Massachusetts, included nine Veterans from a community emergency shelter and nine from a domiciliary (a VA-run program providing three to four months of housing and group sessions for homeless Veterans with substance use disorders, located on a VA medical campus); additionally, six Veterans were participating in a transitional housing program run by a nonprofit on a VA medical campus, and six were participants in a Grant Per Diem program (apartment units run by a community organization, with VA funding). There were 26 men and four women, with a mean age of 54 years. Veterans voiced interest in learning to use computers, the Internet, and texting.

Use of cell phones was a special focus of this study. Using cell phones to provide text message reminders was perceived as useful, and a number of Veterans reported that they currently received automated phone call reminders about appointments:

> A lot of us Vets our memories aren't that great and to receive something on a cell phone like a text message letting me know two days from now I have an appointment, that way I wouldn't forget about it. Yeah, that would be helpful.[36] (p. 9)

Respondents liked the fact that text messages provide a written record that can be easily reviewed multiple times (e.g., with the date and time of an appointment). One respondent noted that someone not comfortable with English can show a text to a friend for translation.

Some Veterans perceived text reminders as useful, while others voiced concerns and identified barriers. Concerns addressed the quality of message content, costs incurred, and frequency of message receipt. Text messages could be confusing if they did not indicate which doctor's office they are coming from and which clinic to go to (VA uses safeguards with text messaging to protect confidential information so that no texts go out saying, e.g., "You have a 10 a.m. appointment at the HIV clinic"). Some worried about incurring additional costs of text messages; others cautioned that text messages sent too often would become annoying. Text message reminders for medication taking were generally seen positively if the number of text messages was limited, and reminder text messages for prescription refills were viewed more favorably than daily text reminders to take a medication. In this study, the idea of using text messages for social support was well received. Study participants liked the idea of "check-in" or "caring outreach" messages that ask a person how he or she is doing:

> [Text messages asking if you are doing ok] . . . would be a huge help, and then if you say "No" well, okay, then they transfer you and then either you're texting or phoning with somebody to try to help you get immediate help. Um, yeah that would be huge.[36] (p. 9)

## TEXT MESSAGING AS A MEANS OF CHANGING BEHAVIOR OF VETERANS EXPERIENCING HOMELESSNESS

One of the first tests of text messaging in VA health care was with home-less Veterans.[37] The VA has specialized clinics that focus on the health issues of homeless Veterans. These clinics, called Homeless Patient-Aligned Care Teams (HPACTs), face challenges with Veterans who do not keep scheduled appointments ("no-shows"). The pilot test, with 20 Veterans, was aimed at re-ducing HPACT clinic no-shows. Participating Veterans were sent text message reminders five days and two days before patients' appointments. These were one-way messages that simply contained the date, time, and name of the VA hospital where the appointment was taking place and a phone number to call to change or cancel the appointment. An example text was, "Remember on Friday, May 24 at 8:30 a.m. you have an appointment at [Name of VA Medical Center]. If you have questions or to cancel call xxx-xxx-xxxx. Thanks."

After an eight-week intervention period, the VA electronic medical record was examined to see whether use patterns were different in the eight-week period before the intervention compared with the eight-week intervention period. There were changes in all four measures of use: patient cancellations of appointments; no-shows to outpatient visits; emergency department (ED) visits, and hospitalizations. For the group of 20 participants combined, pa-tient appointment cancellations went from 53 to 37, no-shows dropped from 31 to 25, ED visits were reduced from 15 to 5, and hospitalizations went from 3 to 0. Only the reduction in ED visits, however, was statistically significant ($P = 0.01$).

The authors conducted a cost analysis based on preventing cancelled visits, preventing no-shows, and preventing ED visits, based on unit costs from VA reports.[38–42] There was wide variation due to confidence intervals surrounding point estimates, but the cost estimates ranged from a low of $2.3 million sav-ings to the VA annually up to a high of $115.7 million annual savings. This is solely health system cost and does not include any monetary valuation of the improved health that would likely also be an outcome of greater patient attend-ance at scheduled outpatient visits.

While the previous three studies yielded valuable information about attitudes toward IT and quantitative outcomes, such as appointment no-show rates and ED use, they lack the viewpoints of Veterans in the process of adopting (or trying to adopt) a new health IT. They also did not explore the issues related to implementing an IT intervention in a homeless Veteran population. In-depth examination, using qualitative methods, of persons adopting and using a tech-nology can improve our understanding of human interaction with technology that may not be possible with structured questionnaires or studies that examine outcomes only. In the next section we provide a case example of IT adoption and use among a sample of 14 homeless Veterans. We examine this study through the framework of TAM.

## Case Example: Home Telehealth for Formerly Homeless Veterans

We have chosen this case to provide details of a quality improvement health IT initiative for homeless Veterans served by the Los Angeles VA health care system. It illustrates the relative advantages that many homeless Veterans have (because of their access to VA health care services) compared with non-Veteran homeless persons. It also demonstrates how technologies, in this population, appear to be more acceptable when paired with face-to-face or phone interactions with human helpers. Gabrielian et al.[43] examined the use of home telehealth with homeless Veterans who had been placed in housing through the U.S. Department of Housing and Urban Development–VA Supportive Housing (HUD-VASH) program, which provides housing vouchers and wraparound services to Veterans. Despite the small sample, the ability to draw lessons from this study should not be underestimated. Thousands of homeless Veterans were provided HUD-VASH housing vouchers starting in 2008. While there are many benefits of this program (not least being long-term housing provided to thousands of Veterans), the program comes with risks such as social isolation because Veterans often have to adjust to housing in parts of town they may not be familiar with.[44] IT provides opportunities to lessen social isolation, which, if not addressed, can lead to psychological and physical deterioration that in turn may lead to loss of housing.

In this study Veterans were provided with a small device (telehealth hardware) that connected to a landline. Veterans were also provided health measurement tools, such as blood pressure cuffs, scales, and blood glucose monitors, as needed for their chronic medical conditions. The telehealth device sent questions to Veterans daily about their clinical status that day, to which the Veterans were expected to respond using a keypad on the device—entering readings from the measuring devices they had been provided (e.g., blood pressure cuff, scale). Veterans' answers sent by the keypad were reviewed daily by VA nurses. When a Veteran did not respond to the daily questions, the telehealth nurses would call the Veteran to gather the health measures over the phone and ask why the Veteran had not sent in his or her readings by the telehealth device. Each Veteran was also offered the assistance of a peer support specialist who could meet with the Veteran in person, have phone conversations, and provide emotional and social support. Peer specialists are used widely in VA health care system to assist

Veterans in recovery, including Veterans addressing mental health conditions, substance use disorders, housing instability, and homelessness.[45]

The goal of this study was to learn whether home telehealth could improve access to health care and provide supportive assistance to Veterans in HUD-VASH who were living on their own in community apartments. In this type of "scattered-site" housing (i.e., spread throughout the community in privately owned apartment buildings), there are concerns that recently homeless Veterans may feel disconnected from friends and support systems and feel isolated because of transportation barriers. Home telehealth may be able to reduce the sense of isolation, at least from one's clinical care team, and the clinical monitoring may help identify when chronic conditions are poorly managed, allowing outpatient follow-up before there is a serious exacerbation that requires an ED visit or hospitalization. The intervention addressed the social support concern by offering peer support specialists to participating Veterans.

Even at the study recruitment phase there were important findings about these Veterans' relationship with technology. The semi-structured qualitative interviews helped to uncover Veterans' attitudes and beliefs. Some of the Veterans who declined to participate had concerns that the VA had ulterior motives for providing Veterans with the in-home telehealth devices. Those concerns included the belief that the devices were monitoring other aspects of the Veterans' lives beyond just the few health-related biometrics. By necessity, homeless persons must be vigilant on streets and in crowded shelters—this may predispose them to suspicion when presented with the opportunity to try new technology devices. Additionally, there are relatively high rates of incarceration experience, other criminal justice system involvement, and mental illness among homeless persons,[46] which may increase their wariness of devices that appear to have monitoring functions.

There were 14 Veterans who agreed to use the home telehealth devices. Table 11.2 examines this intervention through the lens of TAM. Most who enrolled found the devices relatively easy to use. Veterans believed the program helped them to control their chronic conditions. They also appreciated the human aspects of this intervention. Nurse phone calls and the contacts with peer support specialists were seen as positive and may have helped to reduce social isolation.

There were downsides to having the intervention centered on a technology. The technology was not immediately attractive to potential participants, and many declined the offer to participate. Among those who enrolled in the intervention, some found the interaction with the device (e.g., answering questions with numbers on the keypad) to be impersonal, while others reported it was monotonous getting the same question day after day.

As Table 11.2 shows, while there were a number of aspects of the IT that suggested that users generally found it useful and easy to use, there were some

*Table 11.2*  **Home Telehealth with Veterans Who were Formerly Homeless, Viewed Through the Technology Acceptance Model (TAM)**

| Study Findings | Considerations for Homeless Veterans |
|---|---|
| **Perceived Usefulness: Positives** | |
| Most felt the home telehealth equipment combined with the nursing intervention helped control their illness. | The live interaction is valued by persons with limited social support |
| Veterans liked the health education messages (e.g., advice on controlling high blood sugar) and disease monitoring that was part of home telehealth. | Technology may be perceived as nonjudgmental when a participant does not meet a health target. |
| **Perceived Usefulness: Limitations** | |
| While there was appreciation of what telehealth messaging did, there was desire for personal contact to augment the home-telehealth technology component. The phone calls with live VA staff were helpful. | The live interaction is valued by persons with limited social support |
| Some found the messaging system impersonal, and it could be monotonous to receive the same message repeated over several days. | |
| **Perceived Ease of Use: Positives** | |
| Veterans generally found the home telehealth device easy to use. Most said the prompts on the message machine facilitated use. Some said the peers were also helpful in learning how to use the home telehealth device. | Technology skills may be more limited than for nonhomeless populations; conversely, Veterans' military experience may have provided opportunities to gain technological skills. |
| **Perceived Ease of Use: Limitations** | |
| One patient reported difficulty doing the blood pressure monitoring with the device; he attributed the difficulties to his own cognitive limitations. | There may be higher levels of cognitive impairment among formerly homeless because of harsh living conditions and, for many, histories of substance use. Additionally, among Veterans there is a higher prevalence of traumatic brain injury, which may affect cognition. |

*(continued)*

*Table 11.2* **Continued**

| Study Findings | Considerations for Homeless Veterans |
| --- | --- |
| **External Variables** | |
| Skepticism and wariness about the monitoring aspects of the telehealth device: During recruitment it was found that for many Veterans there was a lack of interest in enrolling in home telehealth. | Concern about more general monitoring of behavior, beyond just health. This may be related to mental health conditions, experiences in shelters, and incarceration. |
| Social isolation: Veterans brought up social isolation, depression, and loneliness. The peers seemed to lessen that isolation. | Social isolation is common among homeless and exacerbated when placed in new apartment housing situations. Technology alone may not address some needs. |

aspects that may have hampered the overall Veteran experience with this telehealth intervention. In this population with limited social ties, the technology is more likely to be successfully used when it is paired with personal connections from a nurse or peer support specialist. In these formerly homeless Veterans, the relatively limited social capital (few family ties, few friends or neighbors who can be called on for assistance with technology) suggests that interventions should include substantial social support.

In this study the social aspects of the intervention—phone calls with nurses and in-person interactions with peers—were seen as positive. These aspects may have been especially valuable for homeless Veterans who had recently been placed in an apartment (and who may have been experiencing feelings of isolation). Veterans voiced appreciation for the content of the chronic disease management messages. Because the technology delivered messages in a nonjudgmental way, this may have elicited more honest responses from the Veterans about their health behaviors. Homeless persons are often subjected to overt or unconscious reproach and experience general lack of respect when seeking services such as health care. The interaction with an unbiased and nonjudgmental telehealth device, in contrast, may be a welcome means of interacting with the health care system.

In the final section of this chapter we discuss Veteran populations that, while they may not be currently homeless, represent populations that may be at risk for homelessness or have health issues that are highly prevalent among homeless populations (and/or may contribute to homelessness).

# Use of Information Technology Among Special Populations (Veterans at Risk for Homelessness)

Use of technology has been assessed among other Veteran populations that, while not necessarily homeless at the time of the study, are at increased risk for homelessness or have important shared characteristics with homeless populations. Here we describe some of the literature on IT use in such populations.

## VETERANS SEEKING MENTAL HEALTH CARE

Miller et al. reported on findings from a survey of Veterans who were receiving mental health services.[47] We know that Veterans who are homeless or who have had periods of homelessness are overrepresented in populations who use VA mental health services.[48,49] A survey questionnaire was mailed to 300 Veterans using general mental health clinics in the VA health care system. There were 74 respondents.

The survey included questions about access to, use of, and interest in different types of IT that can be used for health-related purposes. Nearly all respondents (97%) had a cell phone, of which half (49%) were smartphones. Access to the Internet was very common, with 86% reporting such access through either a cell phone, computer, or tablet device. Interest in using computers and other IT for health-related purposes varied by task but generally was more than 50% among those who had a computer. Interest in using a computer for health-related tasks included interest in receiving laboratory results online (68%), interest in reporting symptoms to their providers (63%), and interest in communicating with their health care providers through secure email messages (61%). Areas where interest was lower included use of live video mental health sessions with providers (46%) and receipt of messages reminding the recipient to take medications (34%). When asked about using cell phones for these same health-related tasks, the results were similar, though with somewhat lower levels of interest. For example, 39% would want lab results by cell phone, 28% would want to report symptoms, 31% would want to exchange secure messages with providers about health, 15% were interested in live video mental health sessions, and 27% were interested in reminder messages to take medications.

Again, while this is not a homeless population, it is likely relevant to homeless Veterans, a large proportion of whom have mental illness.[48,50] These findings suggest greater interest in interacting with providers and the health care system by computer as opposed to cell phone; they also suggest that the level of interest in using IT is dependent on the type of task (e.g., getting lab results, communicating with provider). The larger screens and keyboards on computers may make some tasks easier compared with cell phones. With a homeless Veteran population (as opposed to this general Veteran mental health population), one might expect relatively less difference between computers and cell phones in the level of interest in using technology for health-related tasks because of the greater access to cell phones than to computers among this population.[35]

## VETERANS WITH HIV AND HEPATITIS C

In 2013, VA researchers and colleagues published findings from an intervention involving training in the use of the VA's electronic PHR use for Veterans with HIV or hepatitis C virus.[1] Of the 14 Veterans participating, six (43%) were unstably housed (defined as living in a homeless shelter, hospital, domiciliary, drug treatment facility, or with a friend or relative). The intervention was aimed at increasing skills in health-related Internet and PHR use for vulnerable populations with limited computer and Internet experience. Weekly, two-hour group training sessions were conducted over four weeks in hospital classrooms at two VHA medical centers in the northeastern United States. Sessions included discussion and hands-on training in the areas of computers, Internet and Internet searches, how to evaluate quality of health information on the Internet, use of VA's PHR (viewing of medication lists, medication refills, self-entering of data), and productive ways to engage care providers in a discussion about health information found online. Participants were included if they had low income, were infected with HIV or hepatitis C, used VA health care, and had limited computer experience (based on completion of a screening questionnaire). Pre-evaluation and post-evaluation assessments were performed using quantitative surveys, semi-structured interviews, focus groups, and ethnographic observation. Two follow-ups (one immediately at the end of training and one three months later) were performed. Cost evaluation was also performed.

Among study participants, at baseline, Internet use was 21% never; 36% weekly or less, and 43% more often than weekly. The intervention was associated with patient-reported increased frequency of use of the VA's PHR and of the Internet for health-related searches. There was also an increase in self-efficacy for technology use related to health, from a mean of 7.12 to a mean of 8.60 ($P = 0.009$), and a significant difference was maintained at second follow-up. Patient activation (measure of patient engagement and self-efficacy in managing one's health)[51] showed an increase at the second follow-up (but not the first follow-up), and improvement in disease knowledge was borderline significant. Average per-participant cost was $287 per four-session training. In qualitative interviews, participants indicated that online medication refills were very convenient, and many liked the PHR, with some finding it more personal than automated phone systems. Some less experienced computer users experienced challenges and anxiety related to the PHR login procedures.

> I just get nervous going into [the PHR], but that's me going, "Okay, is it gonna let me in?" And sometimes I make mistakes, and I have to re-login. And then there's times when it will tell me that I've tried too many times, and I won't be able to do it for 24 hours.[1 (p. S65)]

Participants reported that training increased their confidence in talking to health providers. Ethnographic observations indicated that during training sessions, more computer-savvy participants helped less-skilled participants. The authors suggest that future trainings of this type consider creating more formal roles for peer-to-peer support. It not only would contribute to learning but could help with self-esteem and self-efficacy for the peers assisting with the training. Because many people attribute their non-use of the Internet to lack of relevance, lack of skills, and poor usability,[52] interventions that demonstrate the relevance of the Internet and PHRs to patients' lives and address usability problems through hands-on instruction on difficult features may be beneficial.

### Personal Health Record Use and Medication Adherence Among Veterans with HIV

IT is increasingly being used to support patients' medication adherence. VA researchers conducted a study published in 2013 in which they examined the association between Veteran PHR use and adherence to antiretroviral medications.[53] Data were collected by survey and through access to the data warehouse for the VA's electronic medical record system. Authors studied 1,871 HIV-positive Veterans, of whom 18.7% (322) were either currently homeless or had previously been homeless. Of those with current or past history of homelessness, 34% had good adherence levels (at or above 90%, which is considered sufficient for controlling the HIV virus) compared with 44% of those without history of homelessness. Adherence was based on VA pharmacy refill data to estimate proportion of days without medication. In multivariable analyses, homeless status was not associated with PHR use (odds ratio = 0.90, 95% confidence interval = 0.64–1.26). In other words, stably housed Veterans and homeless Veterans were equally likely to use the My HealtheVet PHR in the past 12 months. Authors found that use of an electronic PHR in the overall Veteran sample (housed and homeless) was associated with higher levels of adherence, controlling for sociodemographic characteristics (including homelessness) and for other factors (e.g., self-reported health, geographic location of care).

# Conclusion and Future Directions

In this chapter we have demonstrated that homelessness is not an absolute bar-rier for those seeking to access and to use IT. IT provides homeless persons with the appearances and some of the attributes of having a home; this is signified by terminology used in IT such as email *address*, and mobile phone numbers increasingly replace home phones as a person's phone number of choice. For persons experiencing homelessness, transient living quarters generally make landline communication impractical or impossible. At the same time, a homeless man or women may have numerous high-stakes communication needs. These include identifying living quarters, seeking employment, and investigating available options for benefits, health care, food, and other necessities. For Veterans, there are valuable benefits to apply for (e.g., financial assistance, legal assistance, housing support, health care). Beyond helping to meet basic needs, the online world may provide homeless persons with a sense of equality and may help diminish self-consciousness and stigma associated with being home-less. Some authors have proposed that IT can help reduce social isolation and promote well-being by enhancing an individual's sense of "mattering." Here, mattering means a person's sense of importance and of being acknowledged and relied on by others.[54] More than many populations, persons experiencing home-lessness may have a particular need for validation and a need to feel that they matter. Veterans in particular, whose identities have been tied to membership in a highly interdependent military unit, may be especially prone to the need for validation.

The social aspects of IT are also growing in prominence. IT can help a person build and maintain social networks that may provide assistance, both in the short term and the longer term. By keeping in touch with other homeless or at-risk persons *(bonding social capital),* persons experiencing homelessness may learn of resources more quickly than otherwise, such as housing, food, and em-ployment. Veterans are a special group in that they share a similar training, military culture, and service to country—thus, there is likely to be consider-able social capital in Veteran networks. Nevertheless, those networks must be maintained, and IT is an efficient means of doing so and is within reach of per-sons who have very few resources.

To find opportunities to transition out of homelessness, *bridging social cap-ital* (connecting with persons different from oneself, with access to different re-sources) is valuable. IT can help connect with case managers, employers, and health care providers, many of whom are committed to seeking paths out of homelessness for their clients and/or employees. Veterans experiencing home-lessness, compared with non-Veterans who are homeless, again have some advantages. Many are eligible for VA health care and the wraparound resources provided at (or through) many VA medical centers such as supported employment, supported education, legal services, and housing vouchers. Access to and use of IT can facilitate the connections to VA providers and resources. The need is becoming increasingly important as more VA services provide online options (e.g., seeing one's medical record online); additional important uses include receiving cell phone text message reminders related to appointments, medication taking, and other health-related tasks.

## FUTURE ADVANCES IN IT RELEVANT TO VETERANS EXPERIENCING HOMELESSNESS

Other technologies, as their effectiveness increases and costs drop, may also become well suited for homeless persons. Rapid developments mean that some of these cutting-edge technologies may be appropriate for homeless Veterans in the near future. Some examples include voice-activated devices, wearables, and implantable devices. **Voice-activated devices and software** (e.g., dictation software) may become much easier to use than keypad-reliant technologies. They will increase the ease of use for emailing and text messaging, for example. Keypads and small screens can be challenging for people who may have less finger dexterity, poorer eyesight due to rough living conditions, and less access to and use of health care services. **Wearables** (e.g., wristbands, in clothing) track exercise, motion, vital signs, and sleep. They can remove some of the onus on homeless Veterans to connect to providers, report symptoms, and self-manage health. As their costs drop, these devices may also be equipped to wirelessly upload information to health system computers and thus help providers monitor patients' health. Devices can also assist with self-management, such as pill boxes that remind patients to take their medications (e.g., with sound or vibration) and also transmit information about openings (or the absence thereof) to clinical teams to help them detect poor adherence.

**Implantable devices** represent a more invasive use of technology, but their use could further reduce the effort to monitor and self-manage chronic health conditions. They can transmit metrics to health care providers such as vital signs, blood sugar, and blood pressure. Again, these may have special benefits for homeless populations for whom tracking health and communicating with providers can be quite challenging. All devices, especially wearables and implantables, come with a number of ethical considerations to prevent misuse of the information that they transmit. This is especially so with homeless, who, as this chapter has indicated, may be more sensitive to electronic monitoring than some populations. They are also, unfortunately, more susceptible to coercion because of the great financial needs they often have.

Despite the potential benefits of technologies and their growing use in homeless populations, we believe that a number of challenges remain for technology use in this population.

1. *Ownership of devices and payment for service:* Despite declining costs, they nevertheless represent substantial costs for many homeless persons. And after the device is obtained (e.g., cell phone, laptop), costs for ongoing service can remain a hindrance and can lead to interruptions in service and changing phone numbers. This makes it harder for health care providers to reach patients. Bulk purchases, for example by large systems such as the VA, can help lower costs.
2. *Theft and loss of devices:* Because of the vagaries of shelters and living on the street, theft and loss of belongings (including cell phones, tablets, etc.) are bigger barriers than for most people.
3. *Keeping devices charged:* There are fewer opportunities to charge devices than for persons with permanent housing, further leading to interruptions in service.
4. *Access to broadband:* This is a challenge for homeless persons who may have to go to libraries, cafes, and other public sites for Internet or Wi-Fi. In rural areas the difficulties are even greater given the lower penetration of Internet access.
5. *Training and learning opportunities are limited:* Even when opportunities to use IT exist for homeless Veterans, learning to use technology can create self-consciousness and anxiety. Here, the lessons from peer assistance may be valuable—such as in the study of home telehealth in Los Angeles and the study of technology training for Veterans with HIV and hepatitis C. Peer trainers who themselves have had homelessness experience may be able to present information and train others on use of technology in a way that limits embarrassment and increases ability to learn new skills.
6. *Social isolation:* Access to IT does not overcome some of the sense of isolation that is felt by persons who are homeless, whether they are living on the streets or in shelters or have recently been housed, such as through HUD-VASH programs. Health IT may diminish the isolation somewhat, as we have discussed, through social networks that are online. There is also the potential for unintended consequences, with technology replacing previous phone or face-to-face interactions, thereby exacerbating feelings of social isolation. Future interventions would do well to consider the pairing of technology with human interventions to achieve the greatest impact among Veterans who are currently homeless or were homeless in the recent past.

We conclude that there is significant potential for technology to enhance health and self-efficacy among Veterans who are homeless. To realize this potential, the VA will need to continue to explore and adopt innovative practices to ensure that Veterans who are homeless are given opportunities to use and receive support in technology use.

# References

1. McInnes DK, Solomon JL, Shimada SL, et al. Development and evaluation of an Internet and personal health record training program for low-income patients with HIV or hepatitis C. *Med Care.* 2013;51(3 suppl 1):S62–S66.
2. Eyrich-Garg KM. Sheltered in cyberspace? Computer use among the unsheltered "street" homeless. *Comput Human Behav.* 2011;27:296–303.
3. Rice E, Monro W, Barman-Adhikari A, Young SD. Internet use, social networking, and HIV/AIDS risk for homeless adolescents. *J Adolesc Health.* 2010;47(6):610–613.
4. Rainie L. Internet access at libraries. *Pew Research Center's Internet and American Life Project.* Dec 28, 2012.
5. Bertot JC, Sigler K, McDermott A, DeCoster E, Katz S, Langa LA, Grimes JM. 2010–2011 Public Library Funding and Technology Access Survey: Survey findings and results. *Information Policy and Access Center: University of Maryland.* 2011.
6. Lifeline Program for Low Income Consumers. https://www.fcc.gov/general/lifeline-program-low-income-consumers
7. Deschamps AE, De Geest S, Vandamme AM, Bobbaers H, Peetermans WE, Van Wijngaerden E. Diagnostic value of different adherence measures using electronic monitoring and virologic failure as reference standards. *AIDS Patient Care STDS.* 2008;22(9):735–743.
8. Cell phone ownership hits 91% of adults. *Pew Research Center's Internet and American Life Project.* June 6, 2013.
9. Mobile phone ownership. *Pew Internet and American Life Project.* January 11, 2017.
10. Anderson, M., Perrin, A., & Jiang, J. (2018). 11% of Americans don't use the internet. Who are they? Pew Research Center. Retrieved from http://www.pewresearch.org/fact-tank/2018/03/05/some-americans-dont-use-the-internet-who-are-they/.
11. McInnes DK, Li AE, Hogan TP. Opportunities for engaging low-income, vulnerable populations in health care: A systematic review of homeless persons' access to and use of information technologies. *Am J Public Health.* 2013;103(suppl 2):e11–e24.
12. Stennett CR, Weissenborn MR, Fisher GD, Cook RL. Identifying an effective way to communicate with homeless populations. *Public Health.* 2012;126(1):54–56.
13. Barman-Adhikari A, Rice E. Sexual health information seeking online among runaway and homeless youth. *J Soc Social Work Res.* 2011;2(2):88–103.
14. Bure C. Digital inclusion without social inclusion: The consumption of information and communication technologies (ICTs) within homeless subculture in Scotland. *J Commun Inform.* 2006;2(2):116–133.
15. Eyrich-Garg KM. Mobile phone technology: A new paradigm for the prevention, treatment, and research of the non-sheltered "street" homeless? *J Urban Health.* 2010;87(3):365–380.
16. Eyrich-Garg KM. Sheltered in cyberspace? Computer use among the unsheltered "street" homeless. *Comput Hum Behav.* 2011;27(1):296–303.
17. Hersberger J. Are the economically poor information poor? Does the digital divide affect the homeless and access to information? *Can J Inf Lib Sci.* **2003**;27(3):44–63.
18. Le Dantec CA, Edwards WK. Designs on dignity: Perceptions of technology among the homeless. *CHI '08: Proceedings of the SIGCHI Conference on Human Factors in Computing Systems.* New York, NY: Association for Computing Machinery; 2008:627–636.

19. Miller KS, Bunch-Harrison S, Brumbaugh B, Kutty RS, FitzGerald K. The meaning of computers to a group of men who are homeless. *Am J Occup Ther.* 2005;59(2):191–197.

20. Moser MA. Test "superpowers": A study of computers in homeless shelters. *Sci Technol Hum Values.* 2009;34(6):705–740.

21. Redpath DP, Reynolds GL, Jaffe A, Fisher DG, Edwards JW, Deaugustine N. Internet access and use among homeless and indigent drug users in Long Beach, California. *Cyberpsychol Behav.* 2006;9(5):548–551.

22. Rice E. The positive role of social networks and social networking technology in the condom-using behaviors of homeless young people. *Public Health Rep.* 2010;125(4):588–595.

23. Rice E, Kurzban S, Ray D. Homeless but connected: The role of heterogeneous social network ties and social networking technology in the mental health outcomes of street-living adolescents. *Community Ment Health J.* 2012;48(6):692–698.

24. Rice E, Lee A, Taitt S. Cell phone use among homeless youth: Potential for new health interventions and research. *J Urban Health.* 2011;88(6):1175–1182.

25. Rice E, Milburn NG, Monro W. Social networking technology, social network composition, and reductions in substance use among homeless adolescents. *Prev Sci.* 2011;12(1): 80–88.

26. Rice E, Monro W, Barman-Adhikari A, Young SD. Internet use, social networking, and HIV/AIDS risk for homeless adolescents. *J Adolesc Health.* 2010;47(6):610–613.

27. Young SD, Rice E. Online social networking technologies, HIV knowledge, and sexual risk and testing behaviors among homeless youth. *AIDS Behav.* 2011;15(2):253–260.

28. Houston TK, Volkman JE, Feng H, Nazi KM, Shimada SL, Fox S. Veteran internet use and engagement with health information online. *Mil Med.* 2013;178(4):394–400.

29. McInnes DK, Gifford AL, Kazis LE, Wagner TH. Disparities in health-related internet use by US Veterans: Results from a national survey. *Inform Prim Care.* 2010;18(1):59–68.

30. Davis FD, Bagozzi RP, Warshaw PR. User acceptance of computer technology: A comparison of two theoretical models. *Manage Sci.* 1989;35(8):982–1003.

31. Venkatesh V, Davis FD. A theoretical extension of the technology acceptance model: Four longitudinal field studies. *Manage Sci.* 2000;46(2):186–204.

32. Lin N. Building a network theory of social capital. *Connections.* 1999;22(1):28–51.

33. Putnam RD. *Bowling alone: The collapse and revival of American community.* New York: Simon and Schuster; 2001.

34. Ellison NB, Steinfield C, Lampe C. The benefits of Facebook "friends:" Social capital and college students' use of online social network sites. *J Comput-Mediat Commun.* 2007;12(4):1143–1168.

35. McInnes DK, Sawh L, Petrakis BA, et al. The potential for health-related uses of mobile phones and internet with homeless Veterans: Results from a multisite survey. *Telemed J E Health.* 2014;20(9):801–809.

36. McInnes DK, Fix GM, Solomon JL, Petrakis BA, Sawh L, Smelson DA. Preliminary needs assessment of mobile technology use for healthcare among homeless Veterans. *Peer J.* 2015;3:e1096.

37. McInnes DK, Petrakis BA, Gifford AL, et al. Retaining homeless Veterans in outpatient care: A pilot study of mobile phone text message appointment reminders. *Am J Public Health.* 2014;104(suppl 4):S588–S594.

38. Depart of Veterans Affairs Office of Inspector General. *Audit of Veterans Health Administration's efforts to reduce unused outpatient appointments.* Washington, DC: Author; 2008.

39. Drummond MF, O'Brien B, Stoddart GL, Torrance GW. *Methods for the economic evaluation of health care programmes.* New York, NY: Oxford University Press; 1999.

40. Vankirk KK, Horner MD, Turner TH, Dismuke CE, Muzzy W. Hospital service utilization is reduced following neuropsychological evaluation in a sample of U.S. Veterans. *Clin Neuropsychol.* 2013;27(5):750–761.

41. Koshy E, Car J, Majeed A. Effectiveness of mobile-phone short message service (SMS) reminders for ophthalmology outpatient appointments: Observational study. *BMC Ophthalmol.* 2008;8:9.

42. Franklin VL, Waller A, Pagliari C, Greene SA. A randomized controlled trial of Sweet Talk, a text-messaging system to support young people with diabetes. *Diabet Med.* 2006;23(12):1332–1338.

43. Gabrielian S, Yuan A, Andersen RM, et al. Chronic disease management for recently homeless Veterans: A clinical practice improvement program to apply home telehealth technology to a vulnerable population. *Med Care.* 2013;51(3 suppl 1):S44–S51.

44. Tsai J, Mares AS, Rosenheck RA. Does housing chronically homeless adults lead to social integration? *Psychiatr Serv.* 2012;63(5):427–434.

45. Chinman M, McInnes DK, Eisen S, et al. Establishing a research agenda for understanding the role and impact of mental health peer specialists. *Psychiatr Serv.* 2017;68(9):955–957.

46. Greenberg GA, Rosenheck RA. Jail incarceration, homelessness, and mental health: A national study. *Psychiatr Serv.* 2008;59(2):170–177.

47. Miller CJ, McInnes DK, Stolzmann K, Bauer MS. Interest in use of technology for healthcare among veterans receiving treatment for mental health. *Telemed J E Health.* 2016;22(10):847–854.

48. O'Toole TP, Conde-Martel A, Gibbon JL, Hanusa BH, Fine MJ. Health care of homeless Veterans. *J Gen Intern Med.* 2003;18(11):929–933.

49. McCarthy JF, Blow FC, Valenstein M, et al. Veterans Affairs Health System and mental health treatment retention among patients with serious mental illness: Evaluating accessibility and availability barriers. *Health Serv Res.* 2007;42(3p1):1042–1060.

50. Rosenheck R, Leda C, Gallup P. Combat stress, psychosocial adjustment, and service use among homeless Vietnam Veterans. *Psychiatr Serv.* 1992;43(2):145–149.

51. Greene J, Hibbard JH, Sacks R, Overton V, Parrotta CD. When patient activation levels change, health outcomes and costs change, too. *Health Affairs.* 2015;34(3):431–437.

52. Smith A. *Home broadband 2010.* Washington, DC: Pew Internet & American Life Project, Pew Research Center; 2010.

53. McInnes DK, Shimada SL, Rao SR, et al. Personal health record use and its association with antiretroviral adherence: Survey and medical record data from 1871 US Veterans infected with HIV. *AIDS Behav.* 2013;17(9):3091–3100.

54. Francis J, Rikard R, Cotten SR, Kadylak T. Does ICT use matter? How information and communication technology use affects perceived mattering among a predominantly female sample of older adults residing in retirement communities. *Inform Commun Soc.* 2017:1–14.

# Index